Managing
Client Care

Managing Client Care

Elizabeth F. Wywialowski, EdD, MS, BSN, CRRN, RN, C
Clinical Nurse Specialist
Veterans Administration Medical Center
Milwaukee, Wisconsin
Former ADN Curriculum Development Coordinator
Lakeshore Technical College
Cleveland, Wisconsin

With illustrations by
Bob Rich
New Haven, Connecticut

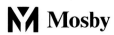 Mosby

St. Louis Baltimore Boston Chicago London Philadelphia Sydney Toronto

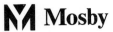

Dedicated to Publishing Excellence

Executive Editor: N. Darlene Como
Associate Developmental Editor: Brigitte Pocta
Project Manager: Carol Sullivan Wiseman
Senior Production Editor: David S. Brown
Designer: David Zielinski

FIRST EDITION

Printed in the United States of America

Mosby–Year Book, Inc.
11830 Westline Industrial Drive
St. Louis, Missouri 63146

Library of Congress Cataloging in Publication Data

Wywialowski, Elizabeth F.
    Managing client care / Elizabeth F. Wywialowski ; with
illustrations by Bob Rich.—1st ed.
            p.   cm.
    Includes bibliographical references and index.
    ISBN 0–8016–6529–9
    1. Nursing services—Administration.   I. Title.
    [DNLM: 1. Nursing—organization & administration.   2. Nursing
Care—organization & administration.   3. Patient Care Planning-
-organization & administration.   WY 105 W999m]
    RT42.W88   1993
    362.1'73'068—dc20
    DNLM/DLC
    for Library of Congress   92–48764
                                                                CIP

93 94 95 96 97   UG/D   9 8 7 6 5 4 3 2 1

**In Memory of
Barbara E. Doyle**

PREFACE

As a department chairperson, I repeatedly heard nurse employers express concern about the need for new graduates to learn more about managing client care. As a nurse educator instructing students in both the classroom and clinical agencies, I became aware of the lack of a textbook that addressed the management concepts and skills needed by entry-level staff nurses. Many of the current nursing management/leadership textbooks contain some of the needed information while omitting other major areas. Consequently, other nursing faculty and I continually searched for a textbook written specifically to help students develop skills required to manage the care needed by a group of clients for a specific time period; concurrently, faculty developed related instructional materials without one. The curriculum content and time allotted to the client care manager role were unintentionally minimized.

This textbook was written to fill the need of advanced nursing students to learn to manage client care in the capacity of a beginning staff nurse. It was the author's good fortune to have findings of three DACUM (developing a curriculum) charts that clearly delineated what management skills were expected of beginning staff nurses. The skills were described in staff nurse language and in the context that they are used.

This textbook is based on the belief that staff nurses and their immediate supervisors are best able to identify competencies required to succeed as an entry-level nurse. Using the DACUM method, the skills needed to manage client care described in this book were identified by exemplary nurses. They were recommended by their peers and believed that these skills were critical to their success. The DACUM method is a process designed to accurately and efficiently identify competencies required of a specific category of worker before developing competency-based or performance-based instructional programs.

Competency-based instructional programs differ from more traditional curricula. They are consistent with educational trends that emphasize research-based criteria and accountability to the learners. They focus on the desired behaviors that learners need to succeed in an occupational endeavor rather than emphasizing predetermined content or a specified number of instructional hours. They emphasize demonstrated performance of required skills and criteria inherent in safe, reliable practice. Competency-based instruction relies heavily on building more complex skills upon previously learned, less complex skills. Accordingly, the client care management skills described in this text build upon previously acquired competencies needed to provide client care and fulfill responsibilities as a member of the discipline of nursing. In addition, it is organized according to competencies needed to manage client care, rather than topics related to it. Each of the chapters describes a specific competency needed by beginning staff nurses to manage client care effectively and efficiently.

Consistent with principles of learning, each competency is described using language common to staff nurses, defining key concepts in the context in which they are applied. This knowledge is required before clinical application. Principles and processes are discussed to clarify their application in fulfilling nursing obligations and duties of entry-level staff nurses. Numerous examples are given.

Managing Client Care is organized in four units. Unit One includes competencies related to understanding the client care environment. Unit Two includes management competencies needed by the nurse to help the nursing work group provide care during a specific time period and coordinate efforts of the interdisciplinary team. Unit Three includes competencies needed to creatively enhance the effectiveness of individuals and the work group as a whole. Chapters 14 and 15 describe competencies needed to manage client care that build upon core competencies required of members of the discipline of nursing. The Epiloque addresses skills needed to manage one's career in a rapidly changing and demanding nursing practice environment.

This text was written to prepare student nurses to successfully make the transition from student to practitioner and effectively manage care of a group of clients in today's complex and rapidly changing health care settings. It is a client care management primer for nursing students about to enter the work force rather than an encyclopedia of "everything a staff nurse might need to know but did not remember to ask" about managing client care. It provides a foundation designed to help the staff nurse begin to manage client care effectively and efficiently while acknowledging that continuous effort will be required to remain competent throughout her or his career.

ACKNOWLEDGMENTS

Writing this book has taught me that an author needs many hours of solitude to allow for the needed concentration combined with a great deal of mental energy. Without the encouragement, help, and support of many people, I could not have written it. I acknowledge them here with sincere gratitude.

- My dear friend, Barb, who continuously encouraged me to "write, write, write." She persuaded me to make time rather than wait until I had the time to do so.
- Another dear friend, Roxanne Sieracki, who proofread and critiqued early drafts to ensure that the specific management competencies were addressed with clarity and who developed a very useful Instructor's Resource Manual to accompany the text.
- The executive editor, Darlene Como, and developmental editor, Brigitte Pocta, at Mosby-Year Book, Inc., whose persistent encouragement, guidance, and good humor nurtured the book's development and publication. They were also instrumental in enabling me to work with Bob Rich, who magically captured in his cartoons what I could only describe in words. Their attention to detail was almost surpassed by Dave Brown and the production editing staff. I truly believe that all of their efforts will be appreciated by readers.
- Those people who enabled me to do the library work before committing my thoughts to a word processor. They included Laura Adams at the UW-Oshkosh Polk Library in Oshkosh, Wisconsin, Dan Eckert at Holy Family Memorial Medical Center in Manitowoc, Wisconsin, and staff at the Educational Resource Center at Lakeshore Technical College in Cleveland, Wisconsin.
- My nursing colleagues and friends who listened carefully as I described my progress and enthusiastically endorsed the development of this text. They substantiated the information provided by the nurses who identified the competencies addressed in this book. Their input made writing the book possible.
- My family, who repeatedly recognized my need for time to complete the book. They revised many plans so that the time we could spend together inspired me to finish the book without delay.

Elizabeth F. Wywialowski

CONTENTS

UNDERSTANDING THE CLIENT CARE ENVIRONMENT

chapter one

INTRODUCTION TO CLIENT CARE MANAGEMENT

Completing this chapter should enable you to:

1. List components of client care management.
2. Describe the relationship of nursing roles and skills to the client care manager role.
3. Explain the differences between nursing management and nursing leadership.
4. Describe the primary purposes of organizations.
5. Describe three common types of organizational structures.
6. Explain the differences between formal and informal organizations.
7. Describe four common management theories of human motivation.

nursing role
core nursing roles
context
client care manager role
nursing management
nursing leadership
organization of a work group
bureaucracy
adhocracy
matrix organization

formal organization
informal organization
human motivations
Maslow's hierarchy of needs
Theory X
Theory Y
Theory A
Theory Z
Situational leadership

This book is about client care management. It was written primarily for nursing students preparing to become entry-level staff nurses employed in inpatient settings. Entry-level staff nurses manage care for a specified period of time, such as a shift, as contrasted to other nurses who manage care throughout a client's stay.

To succeed as a staff nurse, client care management skills are essential. Without these skills, entry-level staff nurses cannot effectively practice nursing in inpatient settings. In the past, most nurses developed client care management skills after graduation from their basic nursing programs. Often, these skills were learned through trial and error. Yet because client care management skills are essential, nursing students need to begin to develop them before they begin practicing. Entry-level staff nurses are likely to find that developing these skills is an ongoing process.

COMPETENCIES OF CLIENT CARE MANAGERS

What are the competencies (skills) expected of entry-level staff nurses as client care managers? They include using organizational resources and routines, providing direct client care, using time productively, collaborating with the interdisciplinary team, and using leadership characteristics to manage others on the nursing team. More specifically, to manage client care, entry-level nurses are expected to

1. Identify organizational resources and determine when they are needed.
2. Work within various nursing service delivery patterns.
3. Use position descriptions to establish the scope and limitations of their own and other nursing team member practices.
4. Manage time purposefully and productively.
5. Prioritize client needs and related care.
6. Exhibit flexibility in providing care within available time constraints.
7. Show initiative and creativity as leadership qualities.
8. Use decision-making skills.
9. Defend their own decisions.
10. Work with other health team members.
11. Resolve conflicts within the team.
12. Delegate appropriately.

RELATIONSHIP OF OTHER NURSING ROLES TO THE CLIENT CARE MANAGER ROLE

The practice of nursing is made up of several interrelated roles. A **nursing role** is a set of expectations of the nurse, including knowledge, attitudes, and behaviors. **Core nursing roles** are roles that are common to all practicing nurses. They include provider of care, member of the profession, and manager of client care. Other common roles include communicator, client teacher, and investigator. These common roles have been identified by nursing educators and administrators as a convenient way to organize components of nursing practice.

This book is based on information gathered from nurses practicing in inpatient settings and is focused on the management of client care. It covers skills expected of entry-level staff nurses employed in acute and long-term settings. The competencies discussed in this book were identified by entry-level staff nurses and their immediate supervisors, who indicated that these skills were essential for successful practice by beginning staff nurses. They arranged these skills and tasks in order of increasing complexity. This arrangement was used to organize the learning activities in this book to help nursing students learn less complex client care management skills before attempting more complex ones. This approach is based on the belief that client care management involves the use of agency resources to effectively and efficiently provide needed services.

In practice, the beginning staff nurse performs various aspects of each of the interrelated nursing roles identified earlier, depending on the client's needs and resources available to meet these needs. In addition, the nurse uses various skills adapted to the setting, or **context**. That is, the nurse behaves in ways that are appropriate in the specific nursing practice environment. Each nursing practice environment is affected by its organizational system, its primary purposes, routines, policies, and procedures. In the larger social context, the nurse is expected to adhere to various laws and codes of ethics. The nurse's practice environment significantly influences the nurses activities.

The process of learning to practice nursing is not universal, but there are common patterns. Learning to perform each nursing role usually proceeds from less complex to more complex activities.

Only those skills that are basic to client care management are addressed in this book. Basic nursing skills used to fulfill the roles of member of the profession and client care provider roles such as identifying one's limitations or performing specific nursing procedures are not addressed. However, basic nursing skills are necessary to develop client care management skills and to succeed as an entry-level staff nurse.

Typically, nursing students learn to use the nursing process before they learn to teach clients about the complexities of self-care. While learning to apply the nursing process, students develop communication skills, identify legal and ethical issues, and adhere to codes of conduct. Based on their individual strengths and limitations, students learn to accept responsibility for self-directed learning early in their careers and when they need assistance with client care. As they progress through their instructional activities, they learn about legal and ethical issues and various client needs and health problems throughout the life span. As they learn about ethical issues and legal constraints associated with various treatment options, they are expected to respond to client needs within the context of an agency's policies and procedures and state laws influencing nursing practice. The nursing student applies knowledge of legal and ethical issues to identify priorities for individual clients. Fulfilling role requirements as a member of the profession prepares the student for the client care manager role. The **client care manager role** requires the nursing student to address the priorities of an assigned group of clients for a specified time period.

Often, depending on the amount of time available, nursing students gain "management" experience immediately prior to graduation. Nursing procedures frequently used in practice are readily learned, depending upon the client's priority needs and the nature of the organizational setting. Some skills, such as CPR, are infrequently used, but are learned because a client's survival may depend on the nurse's immediate response.

When caring for any client or clients, nursing students are expected to demonstrate their skills as providers of care and members of the profession. When students advance beyond caring for more than one or two clients, they are asked to demonstrate skills needed to manage client care for a group of clients. This progression suggests that in most inpatient settings, client care management skills evolve from existing skills in less complex roles. In other words, some client care management skills are dependent on mastering less complex and interrelated nursing roles. Accordingly, learners tend to learn client management skills after they acquire other less complex nursing skills.

All nurses do not learn the many nursing skills in the same sequence. However, students who are striving to develop client care management skills will be presumed to have developed the ability to effectively carry out the following activities: using nursing process skills to provide bedside care; communicating with clients, peers, and other team members in face-to-face situations; identifying specific agency's resources; teaching clients and families about self-care; and adhering to the legal and ethical guidelines of nursing practice in various inpatient settings.

The client manager role is generally more complex than the provider-of-care and member-of-the-profession roles. This does not mean that the client care manager role is a combination of the other roles. Rather, the client care manager role is different, but requires skills needed to fulfill other nursing roles. Client care management skills entail applying knowledge and sensitivity to organizational variables in the health care environment, coordinating other health team members to meet client goals, and managing the efforts of others on the nursing team.

NURSING MANAGEMENT COMPARED TO NURSING LEADERSHIP

Sometimes the terms "nursing management" and "nursing leadership" are used as if they mean the same thing. They do not. Nor are these terms mutually exclusive. That is, many effective staff nurses are both managers and leaders.

Nursing management, refers to the judicious use of resources to achieve identified client goals. It implies responsibility for both directing and controlling. **Nursing leadership,** in comparison, refers to the ability to influence others to respond in desired ways, for example, to relate to others in ways that encourage them to voluntarily follow. Leadership implies providing direction that followers accept voluntarily, without organizational authority. Obviously, nursing management is less difficult if the nurse has leadership ability to influence others to respond in desired ways. However, nursing management implies more accountability to clients in terms of the use of resources within the organizational context. To be sure, all nurse leaders are not nurse managers, nor is every nurse manager a leader. However, nurse managers need leadership qualities to be effective and efficient.

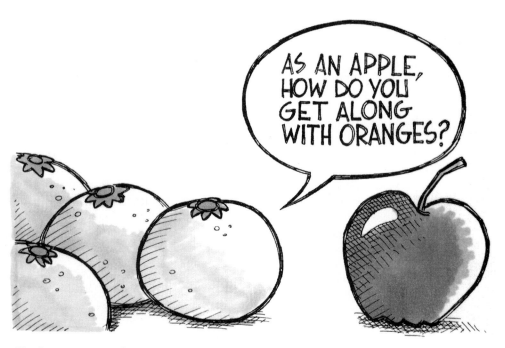

AS AN APPLE, HOW DO YOU GET ALONG WITH ORANGES?

Nursing management is not synonymous with nursing leadership.

ORGANIZATIONS

The organizations within which client care managers function in inpatient settings exist because the work to be done cannot be accomplished by one person. Groups of people are divided according to the type of work and how and when it needs to be done. The **organization of a work group** evolves to provide for the interdependencies of various subgroups or divisions of the work to be done. It helps these groups meet their overall common goals. The organizational structure divides the work and reflects how decisions are made within the structure. Since health care organizations evolve in response to client needs, the more complex the client care, the more complex the organizations designed to provide it are likely to be. Entry-level staff nurses need information about their organizational systems to direct available resources and communicate effectively with other health team members to address client needs (Martin, 1988, pp. 64I, 64J, 64M).

Common Types of Organizational Structures

Nurses usually practice within one or more of three common types of organizations. These are bureaucracy, adhocracy, and matrix organizations. Any type of organization is neither good or bad. Rather, the organization's effectiveness depends on the interaction of several variables. These variables are the needs of the organization's clientele; the needs of the workers attempting to meet client needs; the organization's need to respond to change; its size; the stability of the environment; and the use of technology (Dubrin, Ireland, and Williams, 1989, pp. 224–226).

In the past, most nurses were employed in bureaucratic organizational structures. This type of organizational structure divides the work along centralized departmental or functional lines. Figure 1-1 depicts the linkages or relationships of a **bureaucracy.** Most of the decision-making authority is vested in the upper levels of the organization. In bureaucratic organizations, many nurses experience difficulty responding to the diverse needs of clients because they lack the autonomy or authority to make the decisions required for quality nursing care.

As greater emphasis is placed on customer-oriented service, more attention has been given to an organizational structure known as a decentralized organization or an **adhocracy.** This type of organization provides for decentralized decision making and considerable employee participation. Figure 1-2 depicts the typical linkages or relationships of an adhocracy. Some nurses, practicing in environments characterized by frequent changes in technology, skilled personnel, and client needs often experience less frustration in adhocracies because they participate in decision-making processes.

As the complexity of health care continues to demand highly skilled workers in specialized work units, **matrix organizations** may be used to organize functional work groups. Matrix organizations allow a manager with special skills to guide workers who report directly to another manager. Figure 1-3 depicts a typical pattern of relationships within a matrix organization. A matrix organization allows the work group to solve special problems while retaining the original organizational structure. Nurses practicing in highly complex environments such as research centers might practice within a matrix organization.

Combinations of organizational structures are sometimes used. These combinations typically attempt to maximize the advantages and minimize the disadvantages of each type of structure to best meet the organization's purposes and goals.

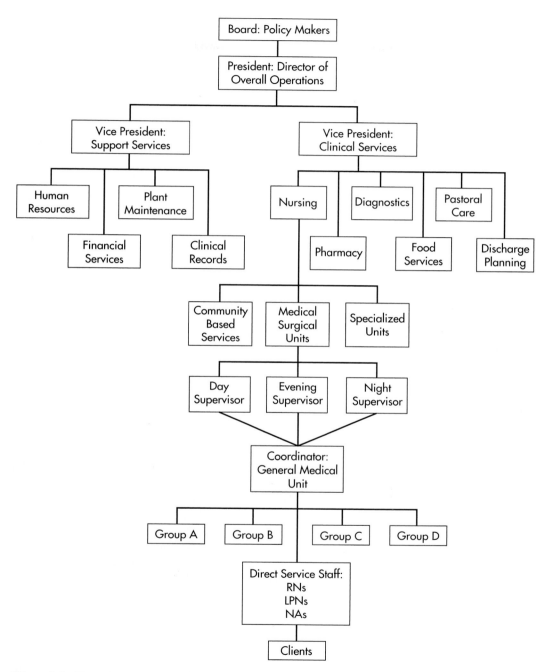

Figure 1-1   Bureaucratic (or centralized) organization.

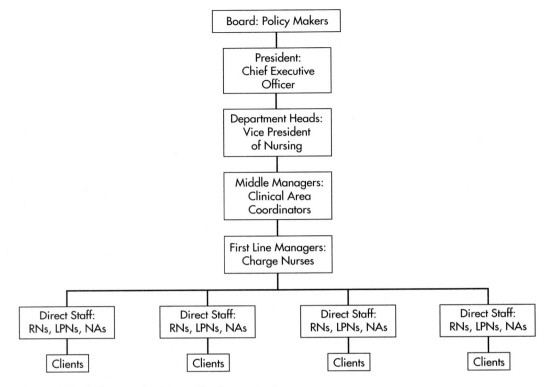

Figure 1-2   Adhocracy (or decentralized) organization.

Formal and Informal Organizations

The preceding discussion concerned **formal organizations.** These structures can be readily diagrammed to depict the work division and decision-making processes. An organization's formal structure is often presented in materials describing the governance and administrative processes in effect for the organization.

In contrast, **informal organizations** evolve from the many human variables within work groups. Informal organizational structures are not diagrammed or officially approved. They may evolve from informational sources, from positions based on knowledge but lacking formal organizational authority, or from spontaneous human responses to issues within or outside the organization. Often, informal organizations evolve around daily communications between members of work groups (Wurzbach, 1985, pp. 89–91). The "rumor mill" is typically a part of the informal organization. Though often described negatively, informal organizations help maintain meaningful communications among their members.

■■■ HUMAN MOTIVATIONS

Historically, early studies of work organizations involved manufacturing industries. These studies were designed to learn about the **human motivations** of workers or the reasons employees responded to work situations as they did. By using this information, managers tried to increase the effectiveness of their organizations. Consequently, many of the

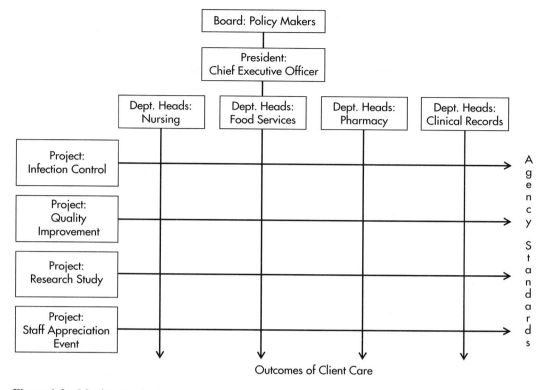

Figure 1-3   Matrix organization.

organizational and management theories adopted by service organizations were more suited to manufacturers than to health service providers.

Several theories contributed to the evolution of current management styles. Some of these theories are described to provide insight into the motivations of human behavior in work organizations.

Maslow's Hierarchy of Needs

A theory of human motivation that many nursing students learn is **Maslow's hierarchy of needs.** Basically, managers following Maslow's theory believe that workers have a hierarchy of needs that drive them to make choices in a predictable manner. According to this theory, physiological needs must be satisfied first for survival. Safety needs are the next level of need in the hierarchy; workers strive to meet safety needs once their physiological needs are satisfied. The safety level includes physical as well as psychological needs. Following the satisfaction of a worker's need to feel safe in the work environment is the need for love and belonging. Workers who gain a sense of love and belonging reach the next level and strive to gain a sense of self-esteem. When workers perceive that their contributions are valued, and feel positive about themselves, they are likely to seek self-actualization. In Maslow's hierarchy, self-actualization is the highest level need that workers experience in their quest for fulfillment.

Though Maslow's theory describes a positive approach to the motivations of workers, studies testing this theory revealed that satisfied needs are not motivators. Rather, unsatisfied needs, such as the need for self-actualization were more consistent motivators. Studies also found it difficult to demonstrate that everyone has the same need hierarchy (Miner, 1980, pp. 28–37).

Theories X and Y

Theory X has been quoted frequently as a set of assumptions about people that a manager might use to manage workers. Douglas McGregor, summarizing common management approaches in use at the time (1960), described the three major assumptions about employees that reflect **Theory X.** Managers assume

1. Employees avoid work because they dislike it.
2. That they must control, direct, coerce, and threaten employees to get them to strive toward organizational goals.
3. Employees lack ambition; therefore, they prefer to be directed, to avoid responsibility, and to seek security through work.

McGregor sought to stimulate more humanistic management practices, offering Theory Y as an alternative to Theory X. Assumptions underlying **Theory Y** reflect a more optimistic view of employees. Theory Y includes the following assumptions:

1. Employees do not dislike work, rather they view physical and mental work as a natural part of life.
2. Employees are self-motivated to achieve goals to which they are commited.
3. Employees remain committed to goals for which they are rewarded when achieved.
4. Employees seek and accept responsibility under favorable conditions.
5. Employees are innovative in solving job-related problems.
6. Human potential is underutilized in most job settings (Dubrin, Ireland, and Williams, 1989, p. 336).

McGregor succeeded in stimulating interest in developing participative management methods.

Theory A

Other popular human motivation theories that are increasingly advocated are Theory A and Theory Z. **Theory A** describes the traditional American management style for work organizations of "typical American firms," including

1. Short-term employment
2. Predominantly downward communication patterns
3. Individual decision making
4. Rapid evaluation and promotion
5. A segmented concern for employees (emphasizing hierarchical instead of functional work groups involved in mutual goal setting).

In the evolving global economy, many organizational analysts have advocated a change from use of Theory A to use of Theory Z to remain competitive.

Theory Z

Theory Z describes the beliefs underlying the Japanese style of managing. **Theory Z** emphasizes

1. Long-term employment
2. Open communication patterns
3. Harmonious work group or consensus decision making

4. Slow evaluation and promotion
5. Holistic concern for employees

Though there is considerable popular support for this style of management, there is reason to question whether this style of management is suitable for organizations that require significant amounts of individual flexibility and creativity (Dubrin, Ireland, and Williams, 1989, pp. 638–643). Indeed, these concerns may be difficult to resolve for people who are culturally rewarded for individual achievement, and when creativity and flexibility are critical employee characteristics. Health service organizations are highly dependent on creative and flexible employees.

Situational Leadership

Perhaps the most adaptable approach to human motivation that incorporates many of the variables important to client care managers is **situational leadership.** This theory of management incorporates the needs of the work group and their responses to the tasks to be done. The leader adopts a management style corresponding to the workers' response to the situation.

The goal of situational leadership, according to Hersey and Blanchard (1982, p. 312), is to "help people understand and share expectations in their environment so that they can gradually learn to supervise their own behavior and become responsible, self-motivated individuals." This theory incorporates the individual employee and work group needs, types of work tasks, and leadership styles. It advocates that managers attend to these variables in the work situation prior to identifying desired leadership behaviors to promote organizational effectiveness. This theory assumes that, just as there is no perfect organizational

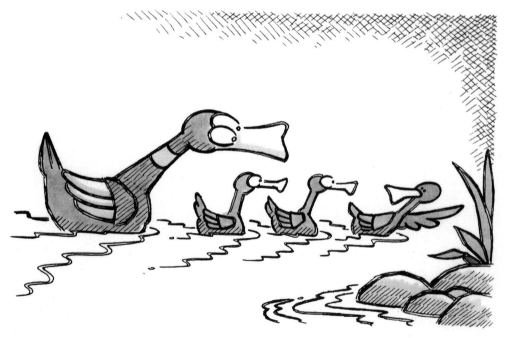

A situational leader adopts a management style corresponding to the workers' responses.

structure that fits every work group, there is no motivational theory that fits every employee.

Much has been learned through systematic study of managerial thought and human motivation. In the past, theories of human motivation often evolved from the study of industrial settings. As the industrial era is replaced by the information era, new theories of human motivation will be tested. As appropriate organizations evolve to support customer-oriented client care managers, more useful theories of human motivation will be developed (Albrecht, 1990, pp. 84–84). At present, management theories advocate sensitivity to human needs as well as close attention to environmental variables and contexts.

SUMMARY

The client care manager role is an essential component of the practice of entry-level staff nurses. Current elements of the client care manager role, as defined in this book, were delineated by entry-level staff nurses and supervisors of such nurses. These nurses were employed in inpatient settings.

Client care management skills depend upon the prior development of other interrelated nursing roles and skills. Client care management skills needed by entry-level staff nurses include the ability to use organizational routines and resources, provide direct client care, collaborate with the interdisciplinary team, manage time purposefully, and use leadership qualities to manage others on the nursing team.

Nursing management is not the same as nursing leadership. Nor are these terms mutually exclusive. Nursing management refers to the judicious use of resources to achieve client goals. Nursing leadership implies providing direction, without organizational authority, that followers accept voluntarily.

Three types of organizational structures within which nurses might work are bureaucracy, adhocracy, and matrix organizations. The different types of organizational structures have varied patterns of work division and decision making. Informal organizations coexist with formal organizational structures.

Managers' beliefs about the motivation of human behavior affect the people they manage. Maslow's hierarchy of needs theory has been popular, but it has been difficult to demonstrate that everyone in an organization has the same needs, as Maslow's theory stipulates. Theories X, Y, A, and Z have been used to help managers maximize the effectiveness of human resources, primarily in industrial settings. Situational leadership theory incorporates individual and work group needs, types of work tasks, and leadership styles. To date, there is no motivational theory that fits every employee. As service-oriented organizations evolve to support client care managers, suitable theories will evolve to help them respond in a sensitive manner to their fellow employees and clients.

APPLICATION EXERCISES

a. As you completed each nursing course, you developed nursing knowledge and skills to fulfill your core nursing roles. List the management skills you have already developed and those you will need to develop to be a successful staff nurse.

b. Compare characteristics of nurse managers and leaders that you prefer to those identified by your peers.

c. You have completed various client care assignments in a large medical center located in an urban area in the past. Now you are assigned to practice your "client care management" skills in a long-term care facility in a suburban community that has a capacity for 60 clients. Describe how the context of the long-term care facility will influence your nursing practice.

d. Review the organizational chart of your assigned agency. What type of formal organization is it?

e. In groups of two or more, debate the pros and cons of each of the management theories used to motivate employees. Which theory would you want your employer to use?

REFERENCES

Albrecht K: *Moving toward an internal service culture,* Northwood, Ill, 1990, Jones-Irwin.

DuBrin A, Ireland JRD, Williams JC: *Management & organization,* Cincinnati, Ohio, 1989, South Western Publishing Co.

Hersey P, Blanchard KH: *Management of organization behavior: utilizing human resources,* ed 4, Englewood Cliffs, NJ, 1982, Prentice-Hall.

Martin PA: Knowledge about your organizational system is power, *Nurs Manage* 19(4):64I 64J, 64M. (April, 1988).

Miner JB: *Theories of organizational behavior,* Hinsdale, Ill, 1980, The Dryden Press.

Wurzbach ME: Rumors. *Nurs* 85 (11):89–91. (November, 1985).

chapter two

UNDERSTANDING THE HEALTH CARE SYSTEM

OBJECTIVES

Completing this chapter should enable you to:

1. Describe trends of societal change that influence health care delivery systems.
2. Describe the agencies commonly involved in the health care continuum.
3. List agencies commonly used to make referrals to provide for continuity of client care.

KEY CONCEPTS

trends
information era
external support system
health care continuum
types of health care agencies
  public

private
proprietary
nonprofit
types of services
  institutionally based services
  community based services

TRENDS AFFECTING HEALTH CARE

Nursing practice, like any other activity, cannot be analyzed in isolation or out of context. The context of factors surrounding the practice of nursing includes demographic, economic, political, social, and technological needs. **Trends** (patterns of change) in these areas affect health care and influence nursing practice to evolve in certain directions. The nurse uses information on trends when discussing the desirability of various options with clients and when interacting with various health care agencies on the client's behalf. These trends also provide clues to future developments of the health care system. This chapter is designed to help entry-level staff nurses understand evolving health care trends. Some primary societal changes will be discussed. Examples of how these trends affect health care delivery will be provided.

Primary Societal Trends

Several futurists (predictors of future trends) have described primary trends in major societal changes. Alvin Toffler has written in detail about the transformation of the industrial era into the **information era.** This change, he explained, will entail an increased focus on contexts, relationships, and holism (Toffler, 1980, p. 301). Later findings support Toffler's predictions (Naisbitt and Aburdene, 1990).

Some important consequences of these trends include increased emphasis on self-help, individual choice, and representative participation in decisions affecting oneself (Toffler, 1980, pp. 265–288). Technology has enabled the mass media to provide a great variety of information in many diverse forms, not only in the workplace, but also at home for personal use. Individuals use various print and electronic media to obtain information to meet their personal needs and interests. Computers, as vehicles for processing and transmitting information, have altered work, the work place, and lifestyles. As the information era establishes itself, more people are using computers to manage and transmit information.

Evolving technology has increased individual choices. Adherence to a common schedule and perception of time is no longer emphasized. More individuals are taking an active role in decision making about the use of their time and resources. (For example, fewer people are working the same 9 to 5 work schedule as in the past.) In keeping with these trends, more clients expect to be included in decisions affecting their health care (Schwertel and Pitzer, 1990, pp. 37–39). In addition, they expect to make choices about health care options to suit their lifestyles.

The emerging roles of women in response to demands of the changing work place are altering the divisions of work within the family. The traditional nuclear family is being replaced by many diverse family structures and roles. Family care-giving patterns are changing as family structures and roles shift.

As the evolution of the information era continues, the pace of change is expected to increase, placing greater demands upon managers of organizational resources. Computerized information management systems and reference resources are examples of organizational resources associated with the information era. Staff nurses are expected to use organizational information in managing client care (Sinclair, 1990, pp. 60–65). In addition to including clients in decision making, the nurse will need to keep up-to-date on information that is constantly changing at an accelerating pace. This constant change is related to the dynamics of the community environment and other external health care and social agencies. Many client care managers perceive the constancy of change as a persistent stressor.

To effectively manage information, client care managers need to be computer literate. Computer literacy skills are used to gain access to information using technology increasingly available at the work site. For example, instead of relying on printed references, client care managers will rely increasingly on computer data bases to obtain information.

The nature of organizational structures is also changing to reflect increased emphasis on holism. Corporations, as business organizations, are coming to serve several purposes rather than a single primary function. For example, acute care health agencies frequently provide services to the sick and injured as inpatients, episodic outpatient care, and health promotion services designed to prevent and detect diseases. Corporations are being held legally accountable for the products and services they produce and for their positive and negative impact on the environment. Health agencies, as legal entities, are expected to use technology and human resources to improve the quality of the communities and environments in which they are located. The public expects these agencies to promote the well-being of the community while providing services to individual clients. For example, hospitals are expected to provide care for ill individuals and to promote the health of community residents. Consistent with the trend toward greater holism, health care agencies are involved locally, regionally, and nationally to promote positive images as providers of health services instead of illness-oriented care.

Closely related to public perception of corporate interconnectedness is the increased emphasis on preserving environmental integrity. The public is aware for example, of the growing difficulties in safely disposing of wastes. Wastes, including those that are very toxic to people and the environment, are increasing in volume. More people are changing their lifestyles to reduce wastes to preserve a safe environment. Environmental goals include safe water, air, and food chains for future generations. Many people are willing to pay more for food grown and preserved naturally without chemicals to maintain their health and that of the environment.

Emerging basic values held by increasing numbers of people are resulting in greater commitment to integrate nature in human activities, rather than striving to dominate it. Client care managers are expected to incorporate knowledge of these trends when managing wastes within the work environment and when assessing client needs and identifying options to meet them. They are expected, for example, to dispose of toxic, infectious, or otherwise dangerous wastes in a very carefully prescribed manner, and to assist their coworkers to do the same.

The environmental health movement is intricately involved with the increased interdependencies and complexities of multinational corporations. People involved with these multinational corporations are more mobile and culturally diverse than formerly. Widespread global migration will stimulate changes in ethnic and racial composition of American communities (Raymond, 1990, p. 1, A6). As a result, the lifestyles and health care needs of the evolving community populations will be increasingly culturally diverse. Client care managers need knowledge about diverse cultures to communicate with a wide variety of people.

Demographic Trends

Several demographic trends influence population needs for nursing services. The proportion of elderly persons living in the United States is increasing. This trend is related to many factors, including the types of health services available throughout the life span (U.S. National Center for Health Statistics, 1985, p. 2). As the U.S. population ages, long-term care may come to predominate the health care continuum (Estes, 1990, pp. 4–8).

The U.S. population continues to shift from rural to metropolitan areas. Concentrating populations in environments with increased pollution increases risks to health. These risks continue to stimulate political interest in reducing pollution and maintaining a safe environment. This population shift is likely to increase the need for nursing services to promote and maintain health and care for sick people.

Another major trend related to demographics is that many factors contributing to common health problems of the U.S. population reflect individual lifestyle choices and are preventable (U.S. National Center for Health Statistics, 1985, pp. 17–19). Personal choice will continue to influence individuals to reduce risk factors under their control. Nursing services will be needed to assess risk factors and help individuals change their lifestyles.

Economic Trends

Economic interests shape the evolution of technology and health care. Client care managers know that health care is often highly valued. However, the type of health care services delivered is limited by other factors, such as the cost constraints. These costs are produced by health care services that require highly skilled providers and very complex equipment and supplies. Clients and providers need to consider the costs, benefits, and financing of health care within the context of a global economy. Health services compete

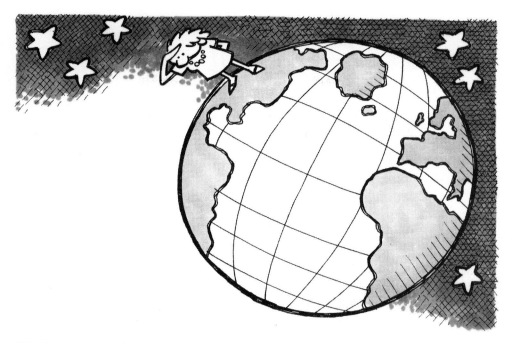

With the emergence of a global marketplace, economic forces have greater influence upon health care programs.

with other types of human needs and services, such as education, transportation, and public safety. Economic trends will probably continue to dominate the evolution of the health care system.

Economists speak about marketing goods and services in a global economy. Economic interests are interwined with political relationships. Increased public participation in decisions at various governmental levels is likely to result in greater interest in satisfying political and social human needs. People with vested interests are more likely to express their perceptions and needs in an attempt to influence political decisions affecting them. For example, despite the fact that health care is highly valued, the public has limits upon health care costs. As costs have increased, individuals must pay more of the actual cost of health care, rather than relying on government or private insurance programs. With the emergence of a global marketplace, economic forces have greater influence upon health care programs. Clearly, these trends are likely to continue. Health care financing trends will be described in more detail later in this section.

Technological Trends

The evolution of technology is driven by economic benefits. Consequently, much information is gathered and used to analyze aspects of a corporation's products or services to determine technological approaches to reducing costs. In accordance with these trends, it should not surprise client care managers to see cost-cutting technological innovations designed to be used in various health care settings.

Technology is used in health care to gather and transmit information in a timely manner to various providers, between health care agencies, and within various departments of

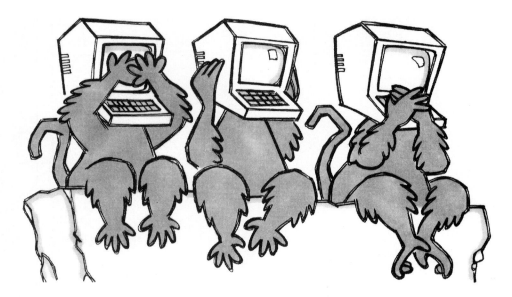

Information technology, such as computers, cannot perceive truth or error.

agencies. Nurses need to use computerized information systems to gather information and communicate with others. This information is integral to providing cost-effective nursing services. Considerable effort is needed to assure the accuracy of this information and to ensure that access is limited to approved users. Computerized information systems will be used increasingly to analyze patterns of care, with an emphasis on costs, benefits, and effectiveness.

Nurses need to remember that the technology used in health care increases the complexity of care. They need to use it properly and realize that it cannot and will not replace their professional skills and judgments. Information technology, such as computers, cannot perceive truth or errors. Technology provides additional tools to help nurses practice their profession. Nurses will need to rely on their own analysis of available data in the health care context to help them determine its relevance to a client's care.

Trends in Financing Health Care

As indicated earlier, the financing mechanisms for health care have changed. Individuals are required to assumed greater responsibility for paying for their health care. Most people must pay increasingly large deductibles before becoming eligible for insurance benefits. Health care financing mechanisms are closely tied to government regulations. Government agencies have assumed greater responsibility for the cost of health care for high-risk groups such as the very young or aged, the poor, or unemployed people. Consequently, government payment for health care increasingly uses prospective payment mechanisms, which pay a specified amount for specific categories of care (Diagnosis Related Groups) regardless of actual costs. Because government payments are now limited, health care agencies have attempted to control their costs by controlling the clients' length of stay. Unfortunately, in some cases, cost-effective quality care may be compromised. Many health care organizations have focused on shortening lengths of stay, while unintentionally deemphasizing individual client needs (Smeltzer, 1990, pp. 1–10). Government programs have generated increased regulations as the primary method of maintaining quality care. Public acceptance of care that is increasingly regulated by government has declined since individual clients have decreased opportunities to participate in decisions affecting their care. Thus, political support for further changes in the health care system is increasing.

As mentioned earlier, the number of elderly persons has been increasing, and this trend is expected to continue. Increasing government involvement in financing health care seems inevitable due to spiraling costs and the increase in the number of high-risk individuals such as the elderly.

Perhaps the most widely known methods of government financing of health care are the Medicare insurance programs, Parts A and B, which are administered through the Social Security Administration. Medicare is sometimes referred to as the Title XVIII program. It is a health insurance program for disabled or elderly persons and their dependents. Medicare Part A pays for some acute and convalescent care. Medicare Part B provides benefits to pay for physician and other treatment services, such as those provided in ambulatory care departments or medical clinics. Indeed, the financing mechanisms of Medicare have been very influential in increasing the number of health care clinics and treatments offered on an ambulatory basis. Printed materials about Medicare programs can be obtained from local post offices or local offices of the Social Security Administration.

As the population of eligible Medicare participants has increased, the costs of health care have increased, but the percentage of total health care costs paid by Medicare has decreased. Individual annual deductibles have also increased since 1967. The amount of payment for services varies and is determined by fiscal intermediates, which are large insurance companies that have contracted with the federal government to manage reimbursement. As a result of these changes in Medicare payments, many people obtain private supplementary insurance to help pay for the actual costs of their health care.

Closely associated with the Medicare insurance program is Medicaid, a health insurance program for financially needy people of all ages. Medicaid is sometimes referred to as the Title XIX program. Part of the Medicaid insurance program is state funded. To be eligible for Medicaid, a client must meet stringent financial requirements and typically must apply at authorized local welfare agencies. Given the high costs of health care, it is not uncommon for clients to become eligible for Medicaid after experiencing extensive injuries or catastrophic illnesses that require expensive treatment. Further information about eligibility requirements can usually be obtained from social service staff employed by various health agencies or local social welfare departments.

To receive payment from either Medicare or Medicaid, health care agencies are required to meet a wide variety of "Conditions of Participation" such as requirements for life safety, staffing, and types of services provided. These conditions are detailed in the *Federal Register,* a government publication of federal regulations. In addition, states have their own criteria for licensing health care agencies, so health care agencies are often required to meet two different standards of care due to differences in state and federal requirements. In such cases, they often attempt to meet the higher standards to obtain maximum reimbursement for services.

Professional Organization Trends

As previously described, recipients of health care expect to participate in decisions affecting them. The providers of health care also want to participate in the development of a system that addresses their needs.

As the complexities of health care increase, the variety of providers and care givers and the number of corresponding professional organizations is increasing. These organizations help socialize health care providers into their various professional roles (sets of expected behaviors for meeting societal needs).

Each profession has one or more representative organizations. For example, the American Nurses' Association (ANA) is the national professional organization for nurses. There are also numerous specialty nursing organizations. Each professional organization attempts to (1) guide the profession in meeting societal needs and (2) safeguard the interests of its members.

To guide their profession, members develop standards of care and codes of conduct, which are made available to the public. Though membership in a professional organization and adherence to standards of care and codes of conduct are voluntary, these criteria are often used as guidelines to evaluate safe practice.

To assure that their interests are addressed, care providers participate in shaping the health care system through the political activities of their organizations. Professional organizations function as advocates of health care providers and ultimately influence the evolution of the health care system. Professional organizations also influence health care legislation.

Political Trends

The cost of health care has increased faster than the cost of living, and as costs increase fewer people can afford it. Because there are many vested interests in the systems that provide quality health care and pay for it, political conflicts have arisen in many areas. Individuals and insurance companies have been required to use a larger proportion of their resources to pay for health care, for example. Many employers providing health insurance benefits to their employees have argued that these increasing costs of health care benefits have increased the costs of their products or services, and this has interfered with their ability to compete in the global economy.

As the pace of change in the information era accelerates and health care costs increase, financing health care is likely to remain a political issue. In the future, related issues such as living wills, assisted deaths, and personal responsibilities for maintaining health, will become common topics of political discussion (Nornhold, 1990, pp. 35–41). Individual expectations to participate in decisions affecting health care are also likely to persist.

As the American population increases in age and more people become entitled to health care financed by the government, health care will grow as a social concern. As demographic changes are integrated into the political system, legislation will be enacted to address issues in accordance with the basic social values of the public.

Client care managers need to be aware of the effects of current legislation on their nursing practice and on the quality of care afforded individuals throughout the health care continuum. As professionals and citizens, they are expected to communicate their concerns to their employers and elected political representatives.

In summary, the health care delivery system has been powerfully affected by the transformation of the industrial era to the information era. Change is constant. Concerns about individual choice, participation in decisions affecting oneself, and sensitivities to the contexts in which health care is provided are some primary social trends. The world has become a global market driven by changing technology and characterized by complex political interdependence. Clusters of various trends lead to societal changes that affect the

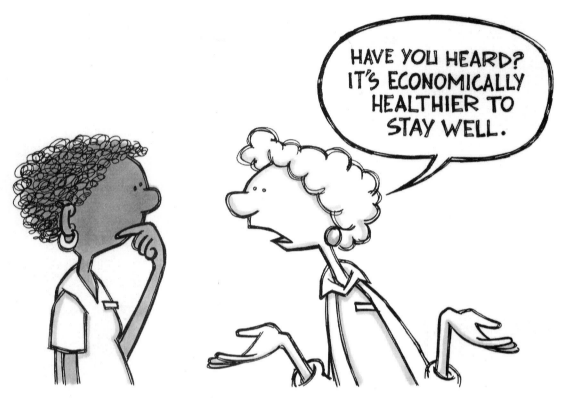

Health promotion and maintenance are preferable to the current focus on high-tech, costly illness care.

health care systems (see fig. 2-1). Given the nursing focus on the whole person over the individual's lifespan, health promotion and maintenance are preferrable to the current focus on high-tech, costly illness care.

EXTERNAL SUPPORT SYSTEMS

Nurses are expected to use knowledge of external support systems to help clients meet their health care needs. An **external support system** includes all the agencies that provide health services to clients separately or in cooperation with a specific inpatient health care agency. In the information era, external support systems have numerous and varied interrelationships, which depend on the agencies involved.

In the interest of the client, the nurse is expected to assess individual health needs and help the client select satisfactory options from the array of available services. Due to the rising costs of care, paid increasingly by individuals, clients need referrals to less costly services to meet their health needs. Though the mass media are very helpful to the public in providing general information about available community resources, the nurse is expected to make appropriate specific referrals for needed care.

Clients expect to be involved in decisions affecting their lives and health care. Many

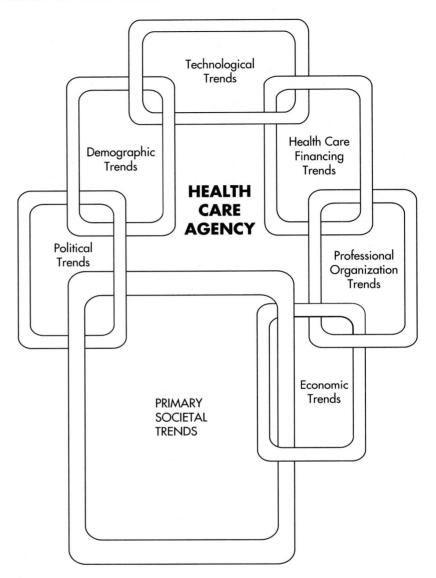

Figure 2-1   Health care trends.

clients know, for example, how long they will be hospitalized prior to their admission. However, they often do not know about the various options likely to best meet their health needs or about the consequences of selecting them. Nurses are expected to regularly evaluate individual client progress toward desired goals related to changing or discontinuing health services. Based upon feedback about their progress, clients expect to participate in their discharge planning. Either they or their families should assume responsibility for making arrangements for continued care with help from health care providers.

Nurses are expected to take initiative and be creative in helping clients address their health needs. Nurses use information from various sources to help clients select the options best suited to their health and insurance needs. Both client and nurse assume responsibility for satisfying health care needs within the limits of cost and available resources.

THE HEALTH CARE CONTINUUM

The characteristics of a health care system reflect (1) common strategies used to access publicly funded health care programs, (2) the many public and private agencies used throughout the health care continuum, and (3) clients' needs. Each health care agency is likely to have numerous printed, technological, and human resources available to help nurses maintain current sources of information about the evolving health care continuum.

The entry-level staff nurse uses knowledge of agencies involved in the health-care continuum to initiate referrals and make discharge plans. The type and purpose of an agency affects the eligibility or admission requirements clients must meet to receive the agency's services. The client's options for care are often affected by the increasing governmental financing of health care and by the availability of health insurance benefits. Though this is very controversial, for many agencies the financing mechanisms of health care dictate who receives which services.

The staff nurse is expected to use knowledge of various agencies and financing mechanisms to plan and evaluate client care. This information is used to determine the client's needs, plan priorities of care, and estimate the client's length of stay, based upon available community options. The staff nurse is expected to use available community options to provide cost-effective efficient client care.

The context or setting of a health care agency is very influential in shaping nursing practice (Lee, 1988, p. 13). The primary purpose of an agency is determined by the context and the types of clients it serves. The context affects not only what the nurse does, but how it is done, as influenced by available organizational resources. For example, hospitals are very different from nursing homes in terms of staffing, equipment, and supplies.

Another important variable related to the context of an agency is its relative location on the health care continuum. The **health care continuum** is the range of all health care services from those that promote and maintain health or optimum well-being to those that support services requisite for a peaceful death. Figure 2-2 depicts the health care continuum.

The next section focuses on the predominant functions of common types of agencies. There is, however, considerable overlap in the functions of various agencies. Since many health care organizations are multipurpose, an agency might declare that it both promotes and maintains health and treats illnesses of clients. However, each agency has one or two predominant functions that dictate their clients' eligibility requirements and the type of care delivered. Various methods of paying for services also affect the context of care.

Types of Agencies

Basically, there are two major **types of health care agencies:** public and private. First, various types of public agencies will be discussed.

Public agencies.   **Public agencies** are authorized by various levels of government. They are controlled and managed financially by the level of government legally authorizing them, whether it is federal, state, or local. Federal health agencies are governed or controlled by the U.S. government. They may be administered through the Department of Health and Human Services. Perhaps the most widely known federal government health

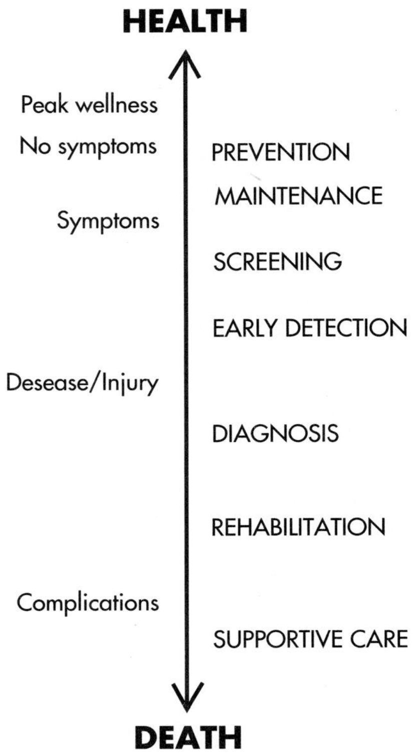

HEALTH

Peak wellness

No symptoms   PREVENTION

                      MAINTENANCE

Symptoms

                      SCREENING

                      EARLY DETECTION

Desease/Injury

                      DIAGNOSIS

                      REHABILITATION

Complications

                      SUPPORTIVE CARE

DEATH

Figure 2-2   The health care continuum.

care agencies are federal hospitals, such as the National Institutes of Health and Veterans' Administration health care facilities. Other federal health agencies include those that provide services to military personnel.

State-regulated government health care agencies (often supported partially by federal funds) are typically available to clients with special needs. These special needs include mental or developmental disorders. Individuals with various developmental disabilities or injuries or diseases that interfere with their ability to hold paid employment can apply for assistance from state divisions of vocational rehabilitation. Vocational rehabilitation counselors assess individual needs for special treatment, education, or training as well as financial assistance. Social service staff employed by various health agencies usually can provide information needed to refer clients to vocational rehabilitation programs.

Other state government agencies are involved in health care indirectly. Nurses need to know which state agencies license and maintain registries of qualified health care providers. These state agencies help ensure that health care providers meet mandatory licensing requirements. The primary function of these regulatory agencies is to protect the public. The state licensing agencies collaborate closely with the state departments that maintain legal definitions of professional practice for various disciplines. The staff of these agencies consult about various situations that might result in unsafe practices. Information about licensing requirements and practice are described in state statutes and administrative codes. These resources are usually available in the reference section of local libraries.

Frequently, legal standards of professional practice at the state level differ significantly from the standards detailed by the professional organizations described earlier. The legal definitions for safe practice of nursing must be followed within a state. These legal definitions frequently differ from state to state. On the other hand, standards of nursing practice delineated by professional organizations are the same nationwide. For example, the American Nurses' Association has established standards of nursing practice that apply to nursing practice in any setting. Some specialty organizations also offer certification. Speciality organizations represent various areas of specialized or advanced nursing practice. For example, specialty organizations have established standards of practice in critical care, rehabilitation, orthopedics, and operating-room nursing. Not all members of specialty nursing organizations are certified. Those who are certified (having met established criteria of nursing knowledge, skill, and/or experience) are expected to meet established standards of advanced nursing practice. Client care managers are also expected to meet the general standards of practice delineated by the American Nurses Association.

Obviously, all nurses must meet all legal requirements for safe practice. In a similar manner, the operation of different types of health care facilities is determined by specific state regulations, which are described in state statutes or administrative codes. If such information is needed, but unavailable within the health agency, it is usually available in local public libraries. These regulations guide organizational operations and define the legal parameters of nursing practice within the various contexts where nurses work. Practicing nurses need to know these parameters. For example, client care managers employed in long-term care agencies are expected to know the specific limits of the various "levels of care" that are provided within the context of state definitions and regulations.

Local public agencies are supervised by locally elected officials who may serve on governing boards. These agencies are frequently county acute and long-term care facilities that receive their primary direction from elected officials; they may receive federal and state funding. An example of such an agency is a county health department that provides therapeutic home care services (largely funded by Medicare and Medicaid programs) and preventive programs designed to meet the various health promotion needs of residents in the specified area. Client care managers are expected to be aware of the availability of county health department options as well as the eligibility requirements for these services.

Closely related to the county health department are locally controlled county long-term care (inpatient) facilities, and departments of social services, housing, and recreation. Depending on individual client needs, client age, and agency requirements, the client care manager may collaborate with these agencies to enable the client to meet basic human needs.

Schools often provide limited health or support services. It is necessary to be knowledgeable about differences in schools and the age groups they typically serve. Local elementary, secondary, and postsecondary schools provide different types of health care services to support the health care programs of children, adolescents, and adults. These agencies are instrumental in helping clients meet their developmental needs or occupational goals.

At the other end of the age spectrum, the county or area office of aging often provides a wide array of supportive services to older people. Such support services include information and referral; nutrition programs, including home-delivered meals; socialization activities; recreation; chore services; assistance in completing forms to obtain health insurance benefits; and special transportation for medical appointments. Though information about these agencies is frequently available in local community resource manuals, social service or other support staff may be excellent sources of current information within a health care agency.

Private agencies.   In contrast to public agencies, **private agencies** have voluntary governing bodies. They are not governed or administered by government employees. Private agencies are not directly publicly funded, although fees for their services might be paid by publicly funded insurance programs. For example, clients served by private agencies may use Medicare or Medicaid insurance benefits to pay for services received. In addition to meeting specific "Conditions for Participation," private agencies are required to meet state licensing requirements and regulations corresponding to the classification of their governing authorities. Private agencies provide health care services needed throughout the health care continuum, as do public agencies.

Private agencies can be further classified as being "for profit" or "not for profit." "For profit," or **proprietary agencies,** have financial gain as one of their primary purposes. "Not for profit," or **nonprofit agencies**, receive tax exemptions but cannot transfer funds acquired in excess of expenses to owners or governing bodies.

Common private health agencies provide either institutionally based or community-based services. Traditional **institutionally based** health care **services** are provided on a 24-hour daily basis, in settings such as hospitals or nursing homes. Traditional **community-based services** are provided on an intermittent basis in settings such as homes or neighborhood health clinics. As health care agencies have become more organizationally complex and competitive, more acute and long-term health care institutions have developed programs to provide community-based services. For example, in addition to traditional inpatient services, an increasing number of acute care facilities provide episodic (intermittent illness-oriented) primary health care, emergency care, and follow-up ambulatory care. Comparable services are often provided in proprietary medical clinics or physician's offices at comparable or lower cost. In addition, these acute care facilities also provide inpatient services, including one-day or extended-stay programs that are very similar to traditional hospital treatment but of a shorter duration. Sometimes, the needed equipment, staffing, or cost determines to whom and where the services are provided. In other situations, the specific requirements of health insurance programs may influence the client to select one setting over another to reduce personal costs.

Depending on the variety of agencies in the region, some acute care facilities also provide other supportive programs, such as screening tests, health education programs, telephone reassurance services, and self-care support group assistance. Some health agencies provide health maintenance services to market or promote a positive image within the community. These contacts with the public are also used to promote access to other hospital services. In accordance with evolving demographic trends, acute care facilities are very involved in providing services needed by chronically ill people. For the most part, these services are of limited duration for specified diagnostic and treatment purposes.

Long-term care facilities sometimes provide a wide variety of services to chronically ill people in addition to the traditional 24-hour daily care. Typically, however, their primary purpose is to provide health and social services to people who reside in the facilities for varying and often indefinite periods of time. In addition, long-term care facilities might provide day care, home care, or respite care programs to reduce the high costs of institutionalization.

Ideally, the client's health and social needs determine participation in selected health care options. More frequently, however, cost reduction efforts undertaken by public or private insurance programs dictate which programs clients participate in or which services they receive. Emphasis is placed on costs and the clients' sources of payment in many current health care contexts. Consequently, nurses need information about various options, about the client's rationale for choices, and about the risks and advantages of selected options. In addition, nurses are expected to accurately document services rendered to meet the requirements of third-party payers such as insurance programs. In this somewhat confusing and demanding routine, nurses incorporate advocacy activities to help their clients obtain and pay for needed care.

SUMMARY

The transition from the industrial era to the information era entailed many societal changes that affected the health care system. Characteristics of the information era include increasing emphasis on self-help, individual choice, and representative participation in decisions affecting oneself. Consistent with these changes, organizational structures are increasingly complex, interconnected, and interdependent on other organizations on a global level.

Economic interests are influencing technological and political trends. Within the health care arena, government regulations and financing mechanisms are shifting emphases from individualized quality care to reducing length of stay. Through professional organizations, providers of care are involved in establishing standards of care used to evaluate the services provided.

The context of health care shapes nursing practice. Entry-level staff nurses use their knowledge of the various types of health care agencies available to help clients plan for follow-up care and to provide continuity of cost-effective and efficient care. The agencies that commonly comprise the external health care system are likely to be multipurpose in nature and receive funding from several sources. These agencies are designed to address the needs of clients of various ages throughout the health continuum. Staff nurses are expected to use information about these agencies to help clients select options for providing continuity of care. They are expected to have access to current information about available services from many different sources in and outside of the agency where they practice. To plan continuity of care, the staff nurse must identify available options within the limits of the client's financial resources.

APPLICATION EXERCISES

    a. Compare the changes occurring within the health care system related to the information era with those previously associated with the industrial era.

    b. Describe how changing social roles of women affect human resources available to the health care system and recipients of its services.

    c. Your client is a three year old male who was admitted with fractures likely caused by child abuse. The client's parents are currently unemployed and have no health insurance. What types of agencies need to be involved in providing follow-up after the client is released from your agency?

    d. Your client is an 87-year-old female who was admitted because of dehydration and malnutrition. She is unable to describe her daily routines or her caretakers. She vaguely describes a nephew's family. Which types of agencies might be involved in providing follow-up care and protective services?

e. Discuss whether Medicare is more likely to be involved in financing institutionally or community-based services? Give reasons for your answer.

REFERENCES

Estes CL: Long-term care is mainstream. Why separate it from acute care? *Perspect Aging* 19(4):4–8, 1990.

Kyle BAS, Pitzer SA. A self-care approach to today's challenges, *Nurs Manage* 21(3):37–39, March, 1990.

Lee JL: The historical method in nursing. In Sarter B, editor: *Paths to knowledge: innovative research methods for nursing,* New York, 1988, National League for Nursing.

Naisbitt J, Aburdene P: *Megatrends 2000: ten new directions for the 1990's,* New York, 1990, Avon Books.

Nornhold P: 90 Predictions for the '90s, *Nurs 90* 20(1):34–41, 1990.

Raymond C: Global migration will have widespread impact on society, scholars say, *Chron Higher Ed* 37(2):A6, September 12, 1990.

Sinclair VG: Potential effects of decision support systems on the role of the nurse, *Comput Nurs* 8(2):60–65. (February, 1990).

Smeltzer CH: The impact of prospective payment on the economics, ethics, and quality of nursing, *Nurs Ad Q* 14(3):1–10. (Spring, 1990).

Toffler A: *The third wave,* New York, 1980, Bantam Books.

U. S. National Center for Health Statistics, Public Health Service: Charting the nation's health trends since 1960, DHHS Pub. No. (PHS) 85-1251, 1985, Hyattsville, Md.

chapter three

SUPPORTING THE ORGANIZATION

OBJECTIVES

Completing this chapter should enable you to:

1. Describe how all departments of a health care agency work together to meet its stated purposes.
2. Use communication protocols to foster effective working relationships within the health team.
3. Participate in establishing nursing policies.
4. State reasons nurses need to accept and support client care goals.
5. Participate in continuous quality improvement and assurance processes.
6. Describe common types of nursing service delivery patterns.
7. Explain the scope of practice and responsibilities of entry-level nurses, using position descriptions.
8. Describe how classification systems are used to identify client needs and allocate nursing resources to meet them.

KEY CONCEPTS

agency
    interdepartmental policies
    stated purposes
    philosophy
    organizational chart
    policy
    procedure
    departmental philosophy
communication protocols
telephone etiquette
continuous quality improvement and
    quality assurance
      structure

      processes
      products
patterns of nursing service delivery
    case method
    functional nursing
    team nursing
      modular nursing
    primary nursing
    case management method, alternative
      practice model
position description
classification system

███████ MEETING CLIENT AND AGENCY GOALS

As indicated in Chapter Two, the nurse uses knowledge of current trends affecting health care delivery to understand the context of nursing practice. As a client care manager, the nurse is in a pivotal position to help clients meet their needs. The responsibility of coordinating services needed by clients places the nurse in a very influential organizational position. The success of the health care organization depends on the nurse's effective coordination of clinical client care services. At the same time the nurse enables the **agency,** or health care organization, to meet its goals. The nurse who does not support the internal organization does not serve clients well. However, the goals of the health care organization need to be distinguished from individual client health care goals.

It is paramount to remember that health care organizations and the profession of nursing exist to serve clients; clients do not exist to serve health care organizations. In modern health care settings, the nurse is expected to focus primarily on client goals, in accordance with the American Nurses' Association (ANA) Code for Nurses. This nursing responsibility includes providing client care and mobilizing organizational resources when needed (Nelson, 1988, pp. 140–141). At times, client care wrongly becomes secondary to maintaining staff routines. Priorities should not be misaligned in such a way that, for example, nursing staff adhere to nursing unit schedules first and place client needs second. Client advocacy frequently requires the nurse to communicate with various levels of the organization and departments to clarify client options. As an advocate, the nurse pursues client goals until they are met through coordination of organizational resources. In advocacy activities, the timeliness of the nurse's activities is critical.

In today's evolving health service organizations, clients need experiences to convince them that they are nursing's first priority! This chapter is designed to help the staff nurse understand the major components of the client care manager's role in supporting the internal organization of the health care agency. Supporting the agency in this way helps it achieve its goal of meeting client needs. Departmental functions, methods used to promote interdepartmental communication, common methods of organizing nursing services, and methods of communicating with varying levels of the organization will be discussed.

The nurse is expected to know the various stated purposes of the health care agency in meeting individual client needs. The nurse should also know what the individual client's needs are, where on the health care continuum these needs can best be met, and how the client's goals relate to agency purposes. The nurse uses this information to determine care priorities and discharge plans. The nurse also uses this information to help clients select specific options based on the nature of their individual health needs, personal resources, and financial considerations.

Identifying Agency Objectives

An agency's **stated purposes** are reflected in its philosophy, programs, and services it provides to meet them. A **philosophy** is a general description of beliefs, key concepts or ideas, values and purposes. Frequently, information on philosophy is readily available in administrative or personnel manuals.

Each health care agency has both stated and assumed objectives concerning its governance and fiscal management. These objectives directly relate to the agency's clients. It is important, for example, to know whether the agency is "for profit" or "not for profit" and whether the organizational system is centralized or decentralized. This information is used to establish the agency's routines and policies and to develop procedures to resolve potential ethical issues on behalf of clients.

Policies and procedures.   Written descriptions of departmental roles and functions are a reflection of the organizational chart. Each department develops a system of meeting its responsibilities which varies with the department's functions and size. The system is maintained by policies and procedures written to guide staff.

The formal **organizational chart** often is illustrated in administrative manuals. This chart describes the formal divisions of the organization's work into departments. As mentioned in Chapter One, the organizational chart depicts lines of authority and patterns of decision making used by the organization to accomplish its goals. It describes the relationships of various departments to each other.

A **policy** is a general description of the required agency approach to achieving agency goals in an expedient manner. For example, an admission policy commonly describes an agency's intent not to discriminate on the basis of age, color, creed, disability, ethnicity, or gender. Another policy might be that admission documentation be completed within 24 hours. A **procedure** on the other hand, is a specific process needed to complete a task, such as a procedure for inserting a sterile urinary catheter or the steps to follow in preparing a client for a myelogram.

Typically, **interdepartmental policies,** as expressed in administrative manuals or written policies, describe how the various divisions of staff relate to each other to accomplish the agency's goals. These policies are the highest level and are broad in scope.

Nurses can usually access their **departmental philosophy** and associated policies and procedures in reference manuals located on each nursing unit. The nursing department's philosophy describes the beliefs, values, assumptions, purposes, and goals of the nursing staff that contribute to meeting the agency's goals. Nurses review these materials to learn about their client care coordination responsibilities. As new technology and equipment are introduced, revisions in policies and procedures are communicated to staff, often both verbally and in writing. At other times, revisions in federal or state regulations associated with publicly funded health care programs stimulate revisions in nursing policies and procedures. As a basis for coordinating client care activities, nurses are expected to know current policies and procedures of the nursing department and where to locate information about other policies that affect client care.

WORKING WITH OTHER DEPARTMENTS

To coordinate client care activities, the nurse uses information about departmental functions and services and interdepartmental policies and procedures. This information enables the nurse to request needed services on the client's behalf and to communicate concerns to other departments when clients present special needs not addressed by agency routines. For example, the nurse needs to know the various types of nutritional services provided by the dietary department to enable the client to receive a general or therapeutic diet. It is important that the nurse follow procedures when requisitioning them. The nurse also communicates special nutritional needs to the nutrition department if the client has food intolerances, preferences, allergies, or restrictions related to health needs or other therapies, such as drug therapy. In addition, the nurse is expected to inform the client of special dietary programs required for diagnostic tests and to help the client adhere to them.

Within the context of clinical client care management, the nurse is expected to know the primary functions of each department. In addition to nursing department protocols, the nurse is expected to follow interdepartmental policies and procedures to provide services to individual clients. Again, these policies and procedures are operational descriptions of the health care organization's division of work. The nurse is expected, for example, to understand nursing responsibilities related to preparing the client for surgical procedures and prescribed therapies. Policies may not always be written, and written documents may not always be current, but nurses are expected to know what the policies and procedures are and adhere to them to support the organization's division of work. In addition, the nurse is expected to know the client's priorities and to determine if and when policies and procedures require modification to address those priorities.

If information about agency policies and procedures is not adequate to enable the nurse to meet client needs, such as the need to withhold medications prior to a diagnostic study, the information must be obtained. It may be necessary, for example, to contact the department where the study is to be performed as well as the client's attending physician for clarification. These efforts should be documented in the client's clinical record to avoid duplicating clarification efforts and to provide for follow-through to prevent unnecessary delay in the client's diagnostic procedures.

FOSTERING EFFECTIVE COMMUNICATION

An essential part of the staff nurse's role in managing client care is to relay accurate information about client needs, responses, and plans to various members of the nursing and interdisciplinary health team. Nursing staff are available throughout the client's stay. Consequently, the client care manager accepts responsbility for coordinating the client's care with nursing team members so that the client is prepared and available to other departments as scheduled. When these goals cannot be met, the nurse is expected to communicate with others in a timely manner to assure that the client's needs are ultimately satisfied. The nursing student is expected to have developed basic verbal and communication skills prior to being assigned the responsibilities of a client care manager.

Communication Protocols

Communication protocols include customary manners of addressing others face to face, by telephone, and in writing. These protocols are designed to meet the needs of each party involved, and include common considerations of courtesy, information, and follow-through. Applying basic principles promotes effective communication by increasing the likelihood that messages sent will be received and comprehended as intended. The beginning staff nurse uses knowledge of the communication process in each of the core roles.

To communicate without employing common courtesies reduces effectiveness by decreasing the receiver's ability to actively listen and to accurately receive messages sent. To communicate effectively, the sender designs the message so that it can be readily understood by the receiver, using appropriate words, tone of voice, and gestures. Proper medical terminology can be used to increase accuracy, but in practice, paraphrasing such terminology can increase the receiver's comprehension of the message. Because words are symbols that often have different meanings in different contexts, feedback is needed to assure that messages sent were perceived accurately. The communication process should be repeated as often as necessary to assure that the messages sent were perceived by the receiver as the sender intended them.

Common communication mistakes result when words or their abbreviations are used as if they have the same meanings for both senders and receivers when in fact, they do not. Nursing staff members with different educational credentials or experiential backgrounds are at risk for communication mistakes because they might not be using a common language. Observing behavioral cues and seeking feedback to monitor the perceptions of receivers in face-to-face situations promotes effective communication.

Similarly, errors may occur when members of different disciplines use words that have different meanings in different fields. Common nursing situations require staff nurses to anticipate interdisciplinary communication needs to ensure effective coordination. For example, nurses often discuss client needs face-to-face with members of the health care team and complete requisition forms sent to other departments to meet special needs. To communicate effectively, the nurse must determine what information is needed by other departments. Before communicating with other health team members, the nurse tries to anticipate what basic information other departmental staff members use to address the client's needs. Often, the nurse must collect and organize the information beforehand. After the information is communicated, the nurse documents it to avoid duplication of nursing effort and to provide a record for follow-through.

Information about the client's current status is needed by other health team members. Nursing staff caring for the client have current information about individual clients and their responses to treatment. Nursing staff communicate this information to the interdisciplinary team to enable them to provide services in an effective and efficient manner. To the extent possible, clients are expected to assume responsibility for making decisions about their diagnostic and treatment programs, so they need to know what those plans are and the expectations placed on them. The staff nurse is expected to assume responsibility for assisting the client to follow through on the interdisciplinary treatment plan.

Face-to-Face Communication

Staff nurses need to communicate effectively with co-workers in face-to-face situations. Some nurses find face-to-face communications relatively difficult and prefer other ways of relaying information (e.g., in writing, by computer, or by telephone). In face-to-face situations, the nurse needs to be sensitive to the receiver's circumstances. If the recipients do not percieve the messages as important due to the competing demands placed on them, they may not be ready or able to receive them when the client care manager sends them. Frequently, a receiver's response to the information, instruction, or request initially may not be favorable. Or a nurse who is feeling rushed might not seek needed feedback to assure that the message received was interpreted accurately. The nurse communicates in many different ways. If the nurse is ambivalent, uncertain, or anxious, face-to-face communications are less likely to be effective. Sometimes, a nurse's behavior (e.g., lack of eye contact, tone of voice, or nonverbal gestures) can be inconsistent with or override the actual verbal message. The nurse needs to be sensitive to the messages sent both verbally and behaviorally. The nurse also should seek feedback from others regarding their perceptions of the messages sent. In face-to-face communications, the sender can readily gather feedback by monitoring the receiver's behavior. Sensitivity to the receiver's responses often increases communication effectiveness.

As mentioned earlier, verbal and behavioral communication skills are critical to client care management. As a nurse gains nursing experience, the need to continue to improve communication skills becomes obvious. The nurse, as client care manager, needs to strive to communicate through words and actions those attitudes and messages that accurately convey the nurse's expectations of others.

Telephone Etiquette

Nurses frequently use the telephone to communicate with various departments in a timely manner. It is important to use telephone etiquette to convey information effectively and efficiently. **Telephone etiquette** consists of guidelines that take into account the needs to both senders and receivers. Using telephone etiquette promotes positive working relationships between departments and staff. When coordinating interdepartmental efforts, the nurse is expected to follow communication protocols and telephone etiquette. The box below presents guidelines for telephone etiquette.

The nurse's telephone communication skills improve with practice. The box at right shows a performance checklist for monitoring telephone etiquette in common clinical situations. This checklist describes behaviors expected of nurses in the client care manager role.

ACTING AS A LIAISON BETWEEN ADMINISTRATION AND THE HEALTH CARE TEAM

Members of the nursing team include directors of nursing, assistant directors of nursing, staffing coordinators, shift supervisors, clinical area coordinators, nursing specialists (such as infection-control nurses or enterostomal therapists), head nurses, and charge nurses. Sometimes, more frequently in long-team-care settings, coordinating client care re-

---

Guidelines for Telephone Etiquette

Be alert:	A cheerful, wide-awake greeting sets the tone of any conversation and communicates that you are ready to help.
Be natural:	Use common terms. Avoid slang and jargon.
Be expressive:	Speak at a normal pace and loudness, but vary the tone of your voice to add life and emphasis to what you say.
Be distinct:	Pronounce your words clearly and carefully. Always speak directly into the telephone receiver. Keep *everything* out of your mouth while you are speaking.
Be pleasant:	Show that you want to help. Personalize your conversation by using the person's name. Try to visualize the caller and speak to her or him—not to the telephone.
Be attentive:	Listen politely. Do not interrupt the speaker.
Follow up:	Determine whether the caller wants to leave a message or if another staff member could return a call. Summarize what you will do.
Be courteous:	Use "please," "thank you," and "you're welcome" when appropriate.

Telephone Etiquette Performance Checklists

Talking with peers and colleagues

Criteria:
- □ Answer the telephone promptly.
- □ Speak clearly and distinctly and at a moderate rate.
  - Identify agency.
  - Identify unit.
  - Identify self.
- □ Establish purpose of telephone call.
- □ Determine if you are an appropriate respondent.
- □ Ask questions to verify message.
- □ Answer questions appropriately.
- □ Offer help by describing specific options.
- □ Promise specific action in follow-up.
- □ Document message if indicated.

Receiving information from other departments

Criteria:
- □ Answer the telephone promptly.
- □ Speak clearly and distinctly and at a moderate rate.
  - Identify unit.
  - Identify self.
- □ Listen carefully to establish purpose of telephone call.
- □ Determine if you are able to respond as needed.
- □ Ask questions to verify message.
- □ Offer to help by stating choices to caller.
- □ Promise specific action as follow-up.
- □ Document message or describe nursing implications of message received.

Sending information to other departments

Criteria:
- □ Gather information needed to make telephone call: anticipate questions.
- □ Call desired telephone number.
- □ Verify identity of respondent.
- □ State purpose of call.
- □ Deliver information.
- □ Ask questions to verify respondent's receipt of information.
- □ Allow respondent to react to the information.
- □ Answer questions accurately.
- □ Promise specific action as follow-up.
- □ Document telephone call if indicated.

quires the nurse to act as a liaison between administrative, interdisciplinary, and nursing care teams. In acute care settings, client care managers often communicate concerns directly to their immediate supervisors within the organization. These supervisors often have varying administrative responsibilities and may be referred to as shift supervisors, "charge" nurses, or clinical area coordinators. Liaison activities help client care managers remain sensitive to evolving client needs by listening to concerns expressed by others on the health team, including the client. By relaying information to administrative staff, the client care manager is assured that administration is aware of the health team's concerns. Participation in liaison activities facilitates client advocacy.

Supporting the Goals of Client Care

Indirectly, satisfying organizational needs promotes individual client interests. Sometimes, however, the administrative staff allow gaps to develop in communicating their expectations to direct service staff (such as nursing assistants) or in giving feedback about effectiveness. Direct service staff (those who work directly with clients) depend upon the organization's division of work for guidance in performing their duties. When the nature of the services clients need changes, staff need administrative help to make the corresponding changes. Staff often modify their responses to client needs when demands of the external health care system change; for example, the pain experienced by terminally ill clients can be controlled by using new techology and drugs, allowing these persons to return to their homes sooner. Frequently, these changes result from new legislation, health care financing methods, technology, or regulatory requirements. As discussed in Chapter Two, these changes affect the types of clients served as well as the methods and equipment used to meet their needs. If direct staff are not informed of changes in a timely manner, they may perceive the lack of communication as a lack of support or interest. In most cases, the goals of the agency and the health team do not change, but the procedures used to meet them do. The client care manager, as liaison, is expected to explain the need for these changes to direct service staff and communicate their expressed concerns to administration. These communications help direct service staff to make the desired changes in procedures and provide administration with feedback about the staff's success in making them.

As a liaison between the health team and administrative staff, the nurse needs to accept and believe in the agency's general goals and individual client care goals. If the nurse does not accept them, both sets of goals are devalued. It is critical that the nurse seek clarification of goals that are vague or seem to be in conflict. Conflicts in goals may arise with the emergence of ethical issues related to various treatment or nontreatment plans, culturally diverse client value systems, or priorities established on the basis of costs. When the nurse becomes aware of conflicting goals, putting them in writing can help the staff appreciate and focus on agency and individual client goals. When conflicts between client care plans and organizational goals arise, the nurse communicates with administrative staff to seek organizational support and needed resources.

The component of the client care manager role that involves liaison activities helps the staff nurse to coordinate organizational resources on behalf of clients. In addition to acting as a liaison between the health team and administrative staff, the entry-level nurse may be involved in quality assurance or improvement processes to support organizational development.

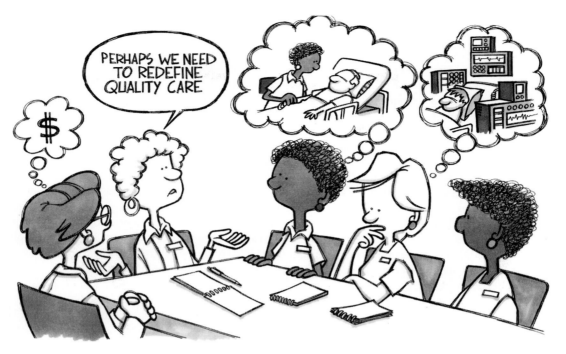

When conflicts between client care plans and organizational goals arise, the nurse communicates with administrative staff to seek organizational support and needed resources.

Participating in Continuing Quality Improvement Processes

Continuous quality improvement (CQI) (formerly known as **quality assurance) processes** are activities designed to monitor and ultimately improve the quality of care provided. Quality improvement efforts are continuous. That is, they are an ongoing component of implementing the agency's philosophy. Client care managers use quality indicators often identified in the agency's standards of care to guide nursing practice.

CQI efforts are integral to the nurse's practice. The standards of care used to monitor quality are usually expressed in a written description of the various components of quality care as defined by the agency's leadership staff. These standards may help nurses determine desired client outcomes, consistent with the agency's stated philosophy and purposes. Participation in CQI activities enables client care managers to provide the input and feedback required to maintain or improve the quality of nursing services provided.

Two forces external to the agency influence CQI processes related to nursing practice in most acute care and some long-term care facilities. The first are the American Nurses Association's (ANA) Standards of Care. The second are the Joint Commission on Accreditation of Healthcare Organizations (JCAHO) criteria.

The standards of nursing care established by the ANA are of primary importance in the design of continuous quality improvement programs. These standards, established by nurses for nurses, represent expected nursing practice or performance criteria. Nursing peers use these standards as performance criteria to evaluate the quality of their practices. They apply to nursing practice in any context. They center on the nurse's use of the nursing process to meet individual client health care needs. These standards may also be used by the judiciary system in settling legal disputes.

Entry-level nurses are probably familiar with these standards since they are frequently used by educators to enable students to acquire the attitudes, knowledge, and skills needed for nursing practice. They are described in most texts used by nursing students to learn the fundamentals of nursing. Ideally, entry-level nurses have thoroughly integrated these standards into their personal nursing philosophies and theories and use them in providing care to individual clients.

The ANA has also established standards that address specialty areas or populations with special needs. Like the general standards, specialty standards are used as performance criteria by nursing peer review organizations in health care settings.

The other external force influencing CQI programs is the criteria for accreditation used by the JCAHO. The JCAHO is a private agency that incorporates medical and nursing practice standards in its criteria for continuous quality improvement efforts. Health care agencies voluntarily request review by JCAHO to receive accreditation or approval of their operations as practicing quality health care. JCAHO has established criteria for all health agency department operations, including nursing. Recently, JCAHO accreditation has been used as one requirement for reimbursement by some third-party payers, since it is used as a measure of the quality of care provided.

CQI programs focus on three primary components: (1) organizational structure, (2) process, and (3) product, or client outcomes. **Structure** refers to the agency's establishment of representative committees and their purposes and related activities. Examples include CQI departments and unit CQI committees. Agency support may include providing staff with the time, equipment, supplies, and operational decision-making authority to make effective use of these committees.

CQI **processes** are the activities of these committees. They design special data collection, analyses, and follow-up recommendations to help the organization improve the quality of care being provided. For example, a group of staff nurses working on a surgical unit, concerned about the incidence of postoperative complications, might collect data on the number of postoperative wound infections. On the basis of their analysis of this data and interpretation of their findings, they would make recommendations as to indicated remedial actions to be taken to prevent or reduce the number of postoperative wound infections.

Frequently, these committees review records and other readily available organizational data to identify key issues and problems. In addition, committee members act as key resource persons to help nurses manage clients' special needs to achieve desired outcomes. The CQI committees work closely with administrative staff to revise policies and procedures to improve the quality of care so it meets various standards.

A CQI process includes all the steps of the problem-solving process, from informing involved persons to eliciting the cooperation needed to follow through. The entry-level staff nurse is expected to participate in CQI programs (Fralic, Kowalski, and Llewellyn, 1991, pp. 40–42). Entry-level staff nurses are expected to provide input about issues, concerns, and problems encountered in providing care; to understand the standards of care involved in the issues identified; and to participate in collecting the necessary data.

To perform these responsibilities, the nurse must understand the structure, processes, and outcomes of these programs in the agency. In addition, the nurse needs to use resources that describe the agency's standards of care and methods used to monitor them. By participating, the nurse can provide input for data generation, collection, and analyses needed to improve the quality of care the agency provides.

Often, if the CQI process relies heavily on historical data, an entry-level nurse is asked to use specified guidelines to document discharge planning in acute care facilities. The nurse should not wait until continuous quality improvement and quality assurance processes reveal problems. That is, clients with similar needs are likely to benefit from a staff review of records, a common method of data collection used to improve the quality of care. This type of review typically benefits clients later.

The **products** of CQI programs are described in terms of the agency's standards of care or desired client outcomes. Documentation of discharge plans and client outcomes is frequently used to measure the products of CQI efforts. Often, CQI activities contribute to the revision of nursing policies and procedures used by staff nurses. These standards refer to behaviors expected of clients with specific types of problems. Frequently, these criteria relate to Diagnoses Related Group (DRG) guidelines and the availability of client and community resources. If CQI programs truly address the issue of quality, they will include clients' perceptions of the care they received in their measurements (Mukherjee, 1989, p. 30).

Establishing Nursing Policies

Many nursing departments organize policy and procedure committees that seek input and feedback from staff nurses. Frequently, a decentralized organization has a nursing department that has its own philosophy and that relies on staff nurse input to maintain policies and procedures affecting practice. Nursing staff representatives serve on committees whose purpose is to revise policies when approaches to care change. Frequently, these committee members attempt to help staff nurses adhere to policies by acting as resource persons to accurately interpret the policies when questions arise. In addition, beginning staff nurses attend in-service programs and conferences to learn about these policies.

NURSING SERVICE DELIVERY PATTERNS

History provides valuable insight into the evolution of various organizational settings (Hannan and Freeman, 1989, pp. 17–27). In a similar manner, insights into the evolution of nursing service delivery patterns may help entry-level nurses to understand their varied use in current organizational settings.

Five common **patterns of nursing service delivery** in current use are
1. the case method
2. functional nursing
3. team nursing
4. primary nursing
5. case management

These models will be discussed with reference to their historical context and factors that promoted their evolution. No single pattern of service delivery is inherently good or bad. Rather, each method must be considerd within the context of the organization and the goals to be achieved with the available resources. Each pattern of service delivery is evaluated according to its effectiveness and efficiency in meeting client needs.

Comparing these patterns of service delivery out of context is like comparing a horse and carriage, Model T Ford, street car, gasoline-powered compact car, and electrically powered van. All of these vehicles are means of getting from one point to another. None of these forms of transportation is good or bad in itself. Rather, each form is best evaluated within its context, considering the extent to which it meets passenger needs and goals with available resources. There are situations where the horse and carriage method of transpora-

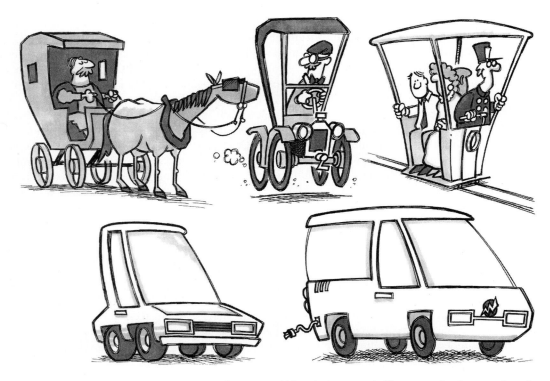

Comparing patterns of service delivery out of historical context is like comparing horse and carriage, model T Ford, streetcar, gasoline-powered compact car, and electrically powered van.

tion is highly valued and popular. Similarly, Model T Fords, streetcars, gasoline-powered compact cars, and electrically powered vans can meet diverse passenger needs. Their popularity has been influenced by their history and perceived effectiveness within the context of the contemporary transportation industry. In a similar way, each of the various patterns of nursing service delivery should be viewed within the context of its historical development and relationships to some of the key forces that shaped its evolution.

The use of each pattern of nursing service delivery will be briefly discussed in the context of its historical development. Many current nursing departments use an adapted combination of several of these models to provide care within an institutionally based practice setting.

The Case Method

The **case method** of nursing service delivery was used by private duty nurses in the early stages of modern nursing. This method involved one nurse providing nursing care needed by an ill client (Donahue, 1985, pp. 338–343). Figure 3-1 illustrates this pattern of nursing service delivery. The nurse worked collaboratively with the client, family, and physician, monitoring the client's condition and providing for the client's basic needs and comfort. The nurse was usually compensated directly by the client or family. Typically, the nurse performed all of the nursing work at the bedside without involvement of a health care organization. The public perception of nurses was based on the experiences of individual clients and families; there were no mass media.

The major advantage of this method was its efficiency since there was no need to com-

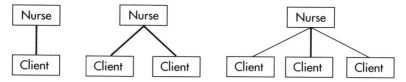

Figure 3-1   The case method.

municate to many staff members over several shifts each day for a number of days. The nurse was familiar with client and family needs since she consistently provided the care. In addition, the nurse was accountable to them since she was paid directly by them.

Functional Nursing

Functional nursing came into common use in the early twentieth century (Donahue, 1985, pp. 441–446) (Figure 3-2 illustrates this pattern of nursing service delivery. Historically, as sanitation concerns grew, there was an increased need for nurses to provide the proper care and environment for ill and injured persons. Functional nursing emphasized the tasks of care. Its pattern of work division was consistent with those of the common military and manufacturing organizations of the industrial era. The nursing staff performed tasks of care in a routine manner; the primary emphasis was on the type of task, and less attention was paid to the nature of the client's needs. For example, one member of the nursing staff would provide drinking water, another would perform personal hygiene tasks, another would administer medicines, and another would give treatments. Typically, the "charge" nurse, more recently known as the head nurse or nurse manager, would assign nursing staff according to their qualifications, abilities, and the tasks to be completed. The head nurse was responsible for coordinating the client's care. Organizationally, the emphasis was on the treatment of diseases or injuries from a medical point of view. Nursing evaluation of client progress was difficult to do and not perceived as important. Nursing documentation of client responses to care was sketchy and not highly valued by the organization. The health care organizations of this era emphasized custodial tasks and delegated medical procedures rather than client care plans. Completion of delegated medical functions was perceived to have high priority in nursing. Consequently, these functions were emphasized in the corresponding organizational structures to divide the work of nurses.

A major advantage of the functional method of care included the correspondence between pattern of work division and the tasks to be done. Staff assignments also corresponded to their qualifications. More clients could be provided basic care with fewer staff.

Team Nursing

Team nursing came into vogue in the 1950s (Donahue, 1985, pp. 446–447). Figure 3-3 illustrates this pattern of nursing service delivery. Several trends supported its popularity. Health care increasingly came under the influence of third-party payers, and more private insurance programs were financed by employers. As a result, the emphasis gradually shifted from custodial services and medical procedures to treatment and goal-directed approaches to care.

Many nursing practice acts included expectations that nursing practice include disease prevention, promotion of health, and restorative care for the ill or injured. Nursing leaders articulated the need for autonomy in the practice of nursing as a profession. The need for nurses to obtain formal preparation in institutions of higher learning was more frequently

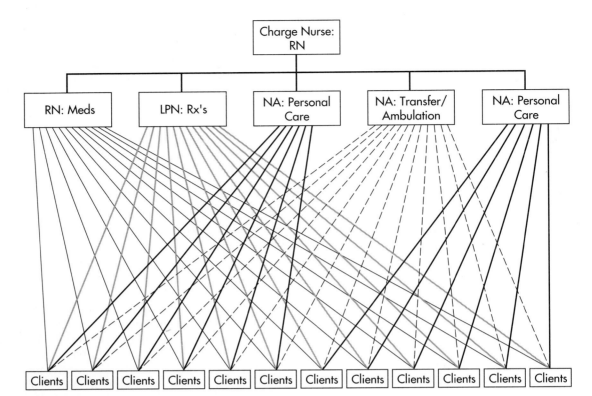

Figure 3-2 Functional nursing.

recognized. Organizational leaders supported this trend by advocating that more nurses obtain formal nursing preparation in institutions of higher learning to meet requirements for licensure; the number of nurses who received such training remained small, however.

During this period, health care organizations had been confronted with a persistent shortage of qualified nurses. Organizational structures were designed to divide nursing work by geographic subdivisions of a hospital (formerly known as wards). The head nurse assumed responsibility for the overall effectiveness of the ward. The head nurse usually assigned nursing "work" according to the qualifications of the staff available to provide for groups of patients. The RNs were assigned to lead the work group, develop nursing care plans, coordinate efforts of the team in implementing care plans, provide care requiring complex nursing skills, and assist the team in evaluating their effectiveness. Faced with the multiple demands of communication, coordination, and evaluation of client progress, RN team leaders frequently noted that nursing care plans were difficult to keep current. Documentation of client outcomes was often incomplete. The use of nursing care plans as references for change-of-shift reports gained popularity as a communication tool to promote continuity of care.

Depending on available staff, nursing team assignments changed with every shift on a daily basis. Many nurses believed that compared to the functional method, using the nursing team method decreased fragmentation of care. Some nurses accepted greater responsi-

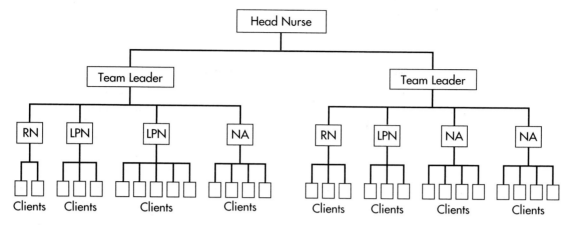

Figure 3-3   Team nursing.

bility for clinical decision making. As clients progressed in their treatment programs, some nursing staff were uncertain about which decisions could be made by various team members. The head nurse assumed the primary responsibility for coordinating client care with other disciplines and organizational departments.

A variation of the team nursing method of service delivery in which the geographic location of clients in the physical setting largely determines nursing assignments is sometimes referred to as **modular nursing.** In this approach, nurses are assigned varying numbers of clients. In addition, they supervise other nursing staff members assigned to care for the same clients. The number and qualifications of staff per nursing module depend on the number of clients and complexity of client needs. A clinical coordinator, head nurse, or supervisor usually is responsible for assignment of staff to each module of clients (Young and Duncan, 1990, p. 97). The RN, as group leader, provides specific directions, assigns client care in each group, and evaluates the effectiveness of the group's efforts. Modular nursing uses characteristics of the floor plan to divide the work involved in providing care for a group of clients. It is intended to reduce nursing efforts (frequently the amount of walking) needed to care for a large number of clients.

A major advantage of team nursing is that the method of work division enables the nurse to broadly apply her knowledge of nursing and influence the care provided to more clients than he or she could care for alone. This method of organization gives the nurse some autonomy in designing care plans to benefit the client. Indeed, team nursing popularized "client-centered care" while also addressing the persistent shortage of highly skilled nurses.

Primary Nursing

As the information era began to establish itself, the complexity and cost of health care increased. High-tech equipment began to be used to process large amounts of data. In the search for cost-effective solutions, greater emphasis was placed upon systematic study of health care issues. Similar ways of processing health care data and managing information were used by many public and private organizations. Complex problems were studied more systematically to identify solutions. The complexity of health care issues was caused in part by competitive forces of the emerging global economy.

The private insurance mechanisms for financing health care needed by employees became increasingly diverse. Government agencies became more involved in financing health care for high-risk populations. Concurrently, regulations affecting health care organizations increased. These regulations reflected the interests of various professional organizations, primarily those of medicine. These organizations, as special political interest groups, advocated that their standards of practice be implemented. Organizational structures of health care agencies became more decentralized, reflecting the increased complexity of health care and interdependencies of external agencies.

Primary nursing evolved as a predominant method of service delivery in acute care health agencies to conserve scarce nursing resources (Marram, Schlegel, and Bevis, 1974, pp. 51–53). Nursing knowledge and skills were need to communicate with various health team members about complex issues involved in client care. Figure 3-4 illustrates this method of nursing service delivery.

To accommodate changes in the division of work involved in providing complex client care, organizational changes were needed. Decentralized organizational structures enabled nurses to readily interact with interdisciplinary health team members. As a result, nurses could more readily participate in clinical decision-making processes on behalf of individual clients. The primary nurse was assigned to provide direct client care, which included personal hygiene, dependent nursing functions delegated by physicians, and independent nursing functions. These independent nursing functions included assessing client status, planning care with clients, teaching clients and families, evaluating client responses within the context of desired standards, and coordinating care with interdisciplinary team members and other organizational departments. Some clients and families reported that they could more readily identify the "primary" nurse accountable for their care. Again, many nurses believed that under the primary system, fragmentation of care was reduced while efficiency increased. Because health organization goals emphasized cost effectiveness, the length of institutional stays decreased, particularly in acute care settings.

Primary nursing made greater use of the nursing skills acquired in basic educational

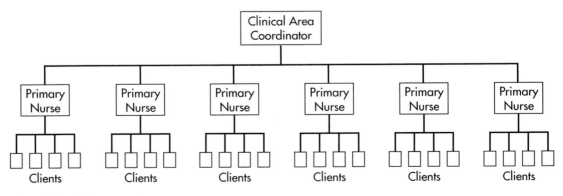

Figure 3-4   Primary nursing.

programs. Proponents of this method of service delivery believed the quality of care was higher compared with other popular methods. Increased nurse satisfaction was believed to reduce the costs of staff turnover and of higher nurse/patient ratios (Freeman and Coronado, 1990, p. 556).

Some primary nurses continued to express frustration with limited time available and the need to maintain current nursing care plans as communication tools when the primary nurse was not on duty. In addition, the acuity levels (quantity and complexity of nursing needs) of client conditions frequently involved marked changes in relatively short periods of time, and these changes in client conditions required corresponding revisions in care plans. This was a problem because many plans written by primary nurses described common routines or standard approaches and didn't account for the possibility of dramatic changes.

Often, during a 24-hour care period, the client received several different methods of nursing service delivery. Most commonly, a pattern of primary nursing service delivery was used on the day shift. A team nursing model was used during the evening shift. A functional method was followed on the night shift due to organizational allocation of scarce nursing resources to meet client needs. Emphasis on cost effectiveness and corresponding client acuity levels increased the demand for highly skilled nursing staff to direct the client's care based upon the client's responses to treatment of multiple disease processes and complex needs for health promotion and maintenance.

Two major advantages of primary nursing were the increased coordination of care by skilled nurses on a continuous basis and the increased accountability of the nursing team to clients and families. Communication between nurse and client usually improved. Care plans were more frequently used to provide for identified client needs.

Case Management

The **case management method** of nursing service delivery emphasizes the assignment of one nurse to plan, direct, and evaluate a client's care throughout the client's stay. Various methods of case management became popular in the late 1980s, not because of dissatisfaction with the primary nursing model, but rather as deliberate response of health care organizations to provide cost-effective care and retain qualified, highly skilled nurses to manage complex care of clients who could not receive adequate care in other, less costly settings.

A variation of the case management method, known as the **alternative practice model,** provided staff nurses with two or more organizational options for nursing practice. This approach to staffing supported the evolution of two levels of nursing practice.

In 1983, the majority of nurses employed in institutional care settings were prepared at the diploma or associate degree levels (ANA, 1985, p. 7). In addition, research findings indicated a need for organizational structures that promoted nurse satisfaction with practice (Jacobson, 1990, pp. 24–26; Kramer, 1990, 67–74). Health care organizations needed to retain nurses in response to the persistent nurse shortage. The demand for adequately prepared nurses to meet complex client needs continued. Greater emphasis was placed upon efficient and effective use of available nursing resources to satisfy complex client needs. The case management method provided nurses with practice options designed to increase work satisfaction and effectiveness.

The case management pattern of nursing service delivery required organizational changes. The evolving organizational structure was determined by both internal and external forces. The case management pattern of nursing service delivery used reflected the agency's response to scarce nursing resources, external financing mechanisms, and the agency's philosophy.

The emerging patterns of nursing service delivery reflect different nursing practice options that utilize different levels of nursing skills available within the agency. The actual division of work in various case management models incorporates elements of primary nursing. Case management models incorporate "a multidisciplinary care process method" (Olivas et al, 1989a, 17). Figure 3-5 illustrates the organization of a common alternate practice model of case management.

It is believed by some that alternate methods of case management organize nursing staff and divide their "work" to meet client needs in an effective (quality) and efficient (cost-effective) manner. In dividing the work, primary consideration is given to the complexity of client needs, including both health promotion and treatment of illness. The available nursing expertise and number of nursing staff are critical to the design of various alternate practice models using a case management pattern of service delivery.

Some case management models, for example, focus on a division of nursing work based upon the assessment of client needs by a qualified (often more experienced) nurse (Tonges, 1989, p. 34). Based on client needs as assessed by the nursing case manager, plans are devised to direct the nursing team in providing care to assure that it meets specified standards of quality. Depending on the context of care, the nursing staff may include varying ratios of registered nurses (RNs), practical nurses (LPNs), nursing assistants (NAs), and critical care technicians (CCTs). The critical care technicians implement plans developed by the nursing case manager when the client is in a critical care unit, whereas RNs, LPNs, and NAs provide care corresponding to the plan when the client is on a convalescent or general nursing unit. Again, this model of case management emphasizes client needs. It is driven by the nursing case manager's assessment of client needs.

Other common case management models of nursing service delivery differentiate nursing practice on the basis of the nurse's educational preparation. That is, the organizational structure is designed so that nurses prepared at the BSN level are nursing case managers. Nurses with diploma or ADN preparation are associate nurses expected to imple-

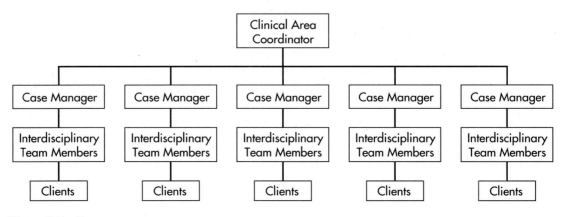

Figure 3-5   Case management.

ment plans of care developed by case managers. LPNs and NAs are assigned as needed to meet client needs. In this way, some believe that the case management method makes judicious use of scarce nursing resources.

In case management patterns of nursing service delivery, the health care organization focuses on varying the use of resources on a case (client)-by-case basis to address requirements imposed on it by government and private insurance financing limitations (Olivas et al 1989b, 13–16). Models of case management used to deliver nursing services are, and will be, thoroughly studied and researched qualitatively and quantitatively. The survival of the case management method is closely related to its effectiveness in satisfying client needs and allocating scarce resources.

The major advantage of the case management method of service delivery is its focus on the complexity of client needs. In addition, it selectively uses scarce nursing resources.

◼◼◼ POSITION DESCRIPTIONS

The entry-level nurse is expected to understand both the philosophy of the nursing department and the organizational pattern or patterns of delivering care within the health care setting. As mentioned previously, the nursing department's philosophy of nursing should be consistent with the purpose of the health agency. The nursing philosophy usually reflects attitudes held by practicing nurses, including their attitudes toward education and research. Consequently, these values and beliefs reflect the organization of the nursing department and its division of the work involved in meeting client needs. The nursing department's organizational chart visually depicts the relationship of nursing staff to client care. **Position,** or job **descriptions** include a list of the duties and responsibilities of nursing staff. In addition, position descriptions indicate the qualifications for each category of nursing staff and to whom each nursing staff member is expected to turn for supervision and guidance.

The position description for the entry-level staff nurse describes the level of organizational decision making expected. It typically indicates to whom the entry-level nurse is to turn for help with organizational management matters and clinical decisions affecting client well-being. Again, the type of facility, the type of clients it serves, and the patterns of nursing service delivery determine the functions of the staff nurse. The pattern of nursing service delivery reflects the organization's expectations of the nurse, influencing how the nurse relates to others in the nursing work group and the interdisciplinary health care team.

Current position descriptions for entry-level staff nurses employed in many long-term care facilities, for example, outline expectations of modified team nursing, in which elements of team nursing and primary nursing are combined. In many acute care facilities, position descriptions for entry-level staff nurses incorporate expectations of an associate nurse in which modified primary nursing and case management methods of nursing service delivery are used. All entry-level staff nurses are responsible for reviewing the descriptions of the nursing position for which they are employed. This helps assure that the nurse understands her or his responsibilities toward clients, nursing staff, and interdisciplinary team members.

To understand the scope of nursing practice expected, the entry-level staff nurse needs to pay close attention to several aspects of the position description. The position description usually describes the expected use of the nursing process and responsibilities for assessing client responses, analyzing client data to formulate nursing diagnoses, establishing written care plans, and revising care plans on the basis of client outcomes and responses to treatment. It is critical that nurses understand the extent of their responsibilities to communicate client needs to interdisciplinary staff and to provide the necessary feedback about client responses. In addition, the nurse needs to comprehend the extent of expected involvement in teaching clients about routine and complex self-care regimes. The nurse needs to know the scope of practice expected of the entry-level staff in the nursing department to avoid gaps in care or duplication of efforts.

CLASSIFICATION SYSTEMS

With the increasing complexity and costs of care, the need for accurate, reliable information about client care from staff nurses has also increased. Indeed, entry-level staff nurses employed by health agencies providing institutionally based services are expected to participate in collecting such information and regularly monitoring the reliability and validity of the classification system in use.

Purposes and Uses

What is a classification system, and why is it used? A **classification system** is a method of regularly collecting information about the nursing needs of clients to provide adequate staff for a specific time period. This system may be referred to as "acuity levels" at some acute care agencies. Information from the classification system is often used to plan for adequate staffing, budgeting, billing for services, and continous quality improvement processes. To satisfy these varied purposes, it is critical that the data collected be consistently accurate. Staff nurses are usually expected to use information about their assigned clients to provide the data needed for the classification system. They are often required to record this data permanently in client records. Staff nurses need a basic understanding of the elements of classification systems to enable them to produce the needed data and document it accurately.

Essential Components

Accurate and dependable classification systems have six basic parts (De Groot, 1989a, p. 30). These six basic parts are: (1) critical indicators [concepts used to describe essential features of quality care] that accurately describe all of the important parts of nursing care; (2) a way to measure critical indicators so that the data accurately reflect the amount and type of care each client needs on each shift on every nursing unit; (3) a way to judge the adequacy of staffing ratios; (4) a way to monitor the accuracy of data obtained by the system; (5) a way to compute staffing requirements; and (6) a way to check the suitability of the critical indicators over time.

Critical indicators are the foundation of a classification system, and they must accurately reflect the many dimensions of client care. The critical indicators of nursing care reflect the nursing department's philosophy. When complete, these descriptive concepts measure all components of nursing care provided to all the types clients served by the health agency. These measuring tools quantify by categorizing and rating all varieties of client needs and the degree of nursing expertise required to address them, rather than merely listing specific activities and tasks done by nursing staff.

To quantify client needs accurately and consistently, these needs are defined according to the perceptions of agency staff. The definitions must have the same meaning for all staff nurses who rate client needs and related nursing expertise. That is, all nurses need to use a common definition for every measure of a client's needs. In addition, for purposes of consistency, each staff nurse needs to rate critical indicators in the same way. To gain a common understanding of these measuring tools, it is helpful if nurses understand how the agency's classification system was developed. Such background information helps nurses understand critical distinctions in the categories of client needs and the nursing skills needed to address them.

To promote consistency in quantifying client needs, each staff nurse needs to categorize and rate nursing care as it is provided on the unit. Such quantification often requires staff nurses to distinguish between the routine and nonroutine care provided by various members of the nursing staff on different shifts. The staff nurse should understand that the classification system is used by all nursing units to enable the nursing department to calculate overall requirements for nursing staff. Understanding the relationship of the needs of clients on the unit to the context of the total nursing department helps the nurse rates client needs more accurately.

Thus, a reliable classification system produces data that accurately measure client needs. Repeated monitoring of the accuracy of data obtained from staff nurses on each unit with varied types of clients is necessary. Staff benefit from feedback about their accuracy and from in-service programs that keep them informed of system modifications.

In acute care settings, the data produced by staff nurses are converted into staffing requirements on a shift-to-shift basis. Usually, the calculations of staffing requirements are done by computers programmed according to the specifications of the agency's classification system. Calculated staffing requirements guide the distribution of nursing resources, which include both the number of staff and their levels of nursing skills and qualifications. In this way, both the quantity and quality of nursing expertise are matched with client needs.

As a nursing management tool, a classification system is only as good as the data provided by staff nurses. It is critical that all levels of nursing staff be committed to maintaining the classification system (De Groot, 1989b, p. 26). Regular efforts are necessary to assure that staff nurses receive adequate orientation to the system. Changes in client needs must be accurately addressed by the definitions used to measure the critical indicators. From time to time, client records might be reviewed to check on the accuracy of the classification of client needs. Such monitoring is particularly important if persistent shortages of nursing staff occur.

This facet of the client care manager role is so critical to an agency's success that it is frequently included in the entry-level staff nurse's position description. The data provided by the staff nurse's use of the agency's classification system is also frequently incorporated into quality assurance processes. Indirectly, using the agency's classification system may contribute to monitoring the quality of care.

◼ SUMMARY

The entry-level staff nurse is expected to understand how all departments within the health care organization work together to enable the agency to achieve its objectives. The nurse uses this information to communicate with the interdisciplinary health team and coordinate organizational resources on clients' behalf. To foster effective working relationships within the health team, the nurse follows communication protocols and uses telephone etiquette.

The staff nurse may contribute to establishing and maintaining nursing policies and procedures by involvement in liaison activities between administrative and direct service staff and participation in continuous quality improvement programs. To support the internal organization, it is essential that meeting client needs be the staff nurse's first priority. It is also important that the nurse serve as a client advocate when conflicts arise concerning policies, procedures, or agency interests.

The nurse needs to understand common patterns of nursing service delivery to determine the scope of practice intended by position descriptions for various categories of nursing staff. Background information about the classification system used at the specific agency helps the nurse accurately rate client needs so that nursing resources can be effectively and efficiently used to meet client needs.

APPLICATION EXERCISES

a. Describe how your agency's organizational chart reflects how its departments work together to achieve its purposes? How would you change it to increase its accuracy and clarity?

b. Discuss the pros and cons of using computerized interdepartmental and interpersonal communications to satisfy the need for current, accurate information between various parties? Would written protocols increase communication effectiveness between departments?

c. Identify the specific pattern of nursing service delivery used on the unit to which you have been assigned. Is it consistent or in conflict with the agency's formal organization?

d. Review the position description of the entry level nurse at your agency. Does it explicitly describe components of the nurse's role as a client care manager?

e. Classify an assigned client, using your agency's classification system. Did your rating agree with the staff nurses's rating? How is the consistency and accuracy of this classification system monitored? By whom?

REFERENCES

American Nurses' Association. Facts about nursing 84–85, Kansas City, Mo, 1985, American Nurses' Association.

De Groot HA: Patient classification system evaluation, part I: essential system elements, *J Nurs Adm* 19(6):30–55. (June, 1989a).

De Groot HA: Patient classification system evaluation, part II: system selection and implementation, *J Nurs Adm* 19(7):24–30, (July/August 1989b).

Donahue MP: *Nursing, the finest art: an illustrated history,* St. Louis, Mo, 1985, C.V. Mosby.

Fralic FF, Kowalski PM, Llewellyn FA: The staff nurse as quality monitor, *Am J Nurs* 91(4):40–42. (April, 1991).

Freeman BA, Coronado JR: A supportive clinical practice model, *Nurs Clin North Am* 25(3):551–560. (September, 1990).

Hannan MT, Freeman J: Organizational ecology, Cambridge, Mass, 1989, Harvard University Press.

Jacobson E: Three new ways to deliver care, *Am J Nurs* 90(7):24–26, (July, 1990).

Kramer M: Trends to watch at the magnet hospitals, *Nurs 90* 20(6):67–74. (June, 1990).

Marram GD, Schlegel MW, Bevis EO: Primary nursing: a model for individualized care, St. Louis, Mo, 1974, C.V. Mosby.

Mukherjee R: The quality of life: valuation in social research, Newbury Park, Calif, 1989, Sage Publications.

Nelson ML: Advocacy in nursing, *Nurs*

Outlook 36(3):136–141. (May/June, 1988).

Olivas GS, Del Togno-Armanasco V, Erickson, JR, Harter S: Case management: a bottom-line care delivery model, part I: the concept, *J Nurs Adm* 19(11):16–20. (November, 1989a).

Olivas GS, Del Togno Armanasco V, Erickson JR, Harter S: Case management—a bottom line care delivery model, part II: adaptation of the model, *J Nurs Adm* 19(12):12–17. (December, 1989b).

Tonges MC: Designing hospital nursing practice: the professionally advanced care team (ProACT) model, part 1, *J Nurs Adm* 19(7):31–38. (July/August, 1989).

Young S, Duncan B: From primary to modular nursing, *Nurs Manage* 21(5):97. (May, 1990).

MANAGING TIME PURPOSEFULLY

Completing this chapter should enable you to:

1. Explain the differences between effectiveness and efficiency.
2. Describe four categories of client care priorities.
3. Describe principles of priority setting that staff nurses use when managing care of a group of clients.
4. Rank the nursing priorities of a group of clients for a specified time period.
5. Describe the principles of work organization.

KEY CONCEPTS

effectiveness

efficiency

categories of priority nursing needs of individual clients

    first-order priority

    second-order priority

    third-order priority

    fourth-order priority

ranking priority nursing needs

    urgency

    timeliness

planning to meet priority nursing needs of a group of clients

    flexibility

    creativity

principles of work organization

TIME: A VERY PRECIOUS RESOURCE

The client manager's time is a very precious resource. Time is money. To waste time is to waste money. Each nurse is expected to manage time purposefully every day on every shift. This chapter addresses the many different principles that client care managers apply to assure that their time is spent effectively and efficiently.

THE DIFFERENCE BETWEEN EFFECTIVENESS AND EFFICIENCY

What is the difference between **effectiveness** and **efficiency?** Effective use of time entails doing the right things. It depends on the nurse's assessment and analysis of client needs. Efficient use of time entails doing things right. It depends on the nurse's work organization and ability to complete nursing activities smoothly without using excessive effort, time, or resources. Purposeful time management requires that each nurse select the right activities to attend to and complete them correctly without waste.

Beginning and intermediate nursing courses provide opportunities for nursing students to practice using the nursing process. Students assess the client's health status, diagnose the client's health problems, and formulate plans to carry out nursing interventions. When the nurse's assessments, diagnoses, and plans are appropriate, the nurse is likely to be effective. That is, the nurse is likely to do the right things to assist the client.

To be efficient, the nurse provides client care without wasting time, equipment, supplies, or effort. Efficiency refers to the smoothness with which the care is performed without compromising effectiveness. Efficient care conserves effort and minimizes interruptions. With practice, the nursing student usually becomes more efficient in performing nursing procedures. Obviously, the nurse is not managing time purposefully if inappropriate nursing care is performed efficiently or if appropriate nursing activities are performed but take excessive time, resources, or effort.

To be effective and efficient, the client care manager assesses each client needs at the beginning of the shift, ranking needs in order of priority and setting out to meet them accordingly. Actually, as a nurse gathers information about each client he or she ranks the priority of nursing needs immediately and makes a mental note of the ranking to set priorities for an assigned group of clients. After completing the initial assessments of individual clients, the client care manager is in a position to prioritize needs for the total group.

PRIORITY NURSING NEEDS OF INDIVIDUAL CLIENTS

Staff nurses are expected to judge the urgency of common client situations and to automatically respond in a timely manner to assure that each client's needs are met. Common situations encountered by staff nurses are judged in terms of their urgency. The major **categories of priority nursing needs of individual clients** used to rank their urgency are presented in the box below.

Priority Ranking of Individual Client Needs

First-order priority client need

An immediate threat to client's survival or safety.

Second-order priority client need

Actual problems for which the client or family have requested immediate help.

Third-order priority client need

Actual or potential problems that are unrecognized by the client or family.

Fourth-order priority client need

Anticipated actual or potential problems for which the client or family will need help in the future.

First-Order Priority Nursing Needs

First-order priority nursing needs are threats to a client's immediate survival or safety. For example, a client with an obstructed airway has a first-priority nursing need. The airway obstruction threatens the client's immediate survival. A client who is about to fall faces a threat to immediate safety. The client urgently needs nursing intervention to prevent injury. If this need is unmet, the fall may cause additional first-priority needs. First-priority needs demand immediate nursing intervention.

Second-Order Priority Nursing Needs

Second-order priority nursing needs relate to actual problems for which the client or family has asked for immediate help. These actual problems frequently relate to comfort. For example, relief of pain, nausea, or full bladder or bowel often requires urgent nursing responses to prevent client problems from becoming worse. To minimize the urgency of these needs may put the client at risk physiologically, psychologically, and emotionally. If the nurse does not respond promptly, the client's confidence in the nurse is likely to be threatened and the health of their working relationship may suffer. The nurse must respond to second-order priority nursing needs as soon as possible.

Third-Order Priority Nursing Needs

Third-order priority nursing needs concern actual or potential problems unrecognized by the client or family. These needs require close monitoring by nursing staff, since neither the client nor the family can be relied upon for help in managing them. For example, a client who is not aware of the side effects of drugs received is usually at greater risk than a client who is aware of the side effects. Sometimes third-order priority nursing needs involve clients experiencing cognitive dysfunction such as sedation. Other common situations involve potential complications of diseases or treatments. The nurse monitors the client's situation until nursing needs related to the actual or potential problem are met.

Depending on the nature of the client's situation, the nurse might teach the client or family about the condition in an attempt to reduce the urgency of the need for the nurse's watchfulness. Satisfying third-order priority nursing needs often involves teaching the client or the client's family to provide self-care or to reduce the need for nursing care. Third-order priority needs are characterized by relative urgency. To prevent complications or injury, the nurse manages actual or potential problems on the client's behalf.

Fourth-Order Priority Nursing Needs

Fourth-order priority nursing needs involve actual or potential problems that the client or family may need help with in the future. These concerns often relate to the client's need for continuity of care within the facility or in preparation for discharge. For example, the nurse may help the client learn about self-care and treatment procedures long before leaving the health care agency. These needs often include teaching plans for managing anticipated discomforts, nutrition, skin integrity, or elimination problems. Teaching plans are often limited by the learner's readiness and ability to use new knowledge and skills within the time available during the length of stay. The nurse also tries to enable the client to make alternative plans for anticipated continued care should anything go wrong. Written instructions are often used to help the client and family recall essential facts and related instructions. To the extent possible, the nurse assists clients and families to perform actual care to assess their capabilities, instead of asking them to verbally describe the care.

Thus, in **ranking priority nursing needs,** the nurse assesses the client's condition and responses to health problems and their treatment. This ranking is performed with the antici- pated length of stay and requirements for continued care taken into consideration. The prior- ity ranking often relates to predictable consequences of not meeting the client's needs, the perceived **urgency** of preventing such risks, and the client's and family's resources to pro- vide the indicated care. **Timeliness** is of the essence when responding to priority nursing needs. The less time, the higher the priority! That is, the nurse typically has less time to ad- dress more urgent needs and more time to plan to meet nursing needs that are less urgent.

PRIORITY NURSING NEEDS OF A GROUP OF CLIENTS

Staff nurses use several principles in planning **to meet priority nursing needs for a group of clients.** These principles are commonly understood and treated as basic assump- tions by experienced nurses. With practice, beginning staff nurses can learn to apply these principles while providing care efficiently without compromising effectiveness.

To plan for meeting the nursing priorities of a *group* of clients, the nurse needs to know both the needs and the priorities of each *individual* client. This is not to imply that the nurse does not respond to client needs until all individual client needs are assessed. Rather, the nurse completes these assessments as soon as possible while addressing first- and second-priority needs in a timely manner. Every nurse develops a unique pattern of se- quencing nursing activities to assure that each client's condition is assessed and priorities are identified early in the shift. To identify which clients need assessment first, the nurse uses information from the change-of-shift report and the agency's classification system to help identify the client's acuity level (need for nursing resources). When initial nursing as- sessments are completed, the nurse spontaneously ranks individual clients needs in terms of priority or urgency.

To determine the priorities of care needed by a group of clients during a specified time period or shift, the nurse considers a number of factors. First, to help promote appropriate use of resources, the nurse thinks about the amount of time and skills required to do the nursing activities. For example, clients who need complex dressing changes, protective iso- lation, or encouragement to increase self-sufficiency in completing personal hygiene mea- sures often require more nursing time and skill than those who do not. At the same time, the nurse tries to match client needs with available resources—the number and qualifica- tions of staff. The number and type of available staff are frequently related to the agency's classification system and the acuity and predictability of clients' needs. In addition to edu- cational credentials, some nursing staff have unique skills and talents that when matched with client needs bring out the best in both client and nurse.

Depending on the purpose of the agency, the nurse may also consider the need to make provisions for each client's continued care or discharge preparations. If the client's needs are simple (predictable), as determined by the client's diseases, treatments, and re- sponses, the nurse matches them with less complex nursing services. That is, the needs of such clients are likely to be satisfactorily addressed with care provided by LPNs and NAs. These needs are also frequently addressed by nursing routines, policies, and procedures. Typically, repeated nursing assessments and related interventions by an RN are needed less frequently when the client's acuity level is low or the client is physiologically stable.

When the client's needs are more complex, often because the client's physiological status is less predictable, the nurse often plans to provide the care. this is to assure that more frequent assessments and corresponding interventions are made. If the client's care depends on various diagnostic study results and requires considerable interdisciplinary collaboration, the staff nurse frequently provides the needed nursing attention. Suppose the nurse anticipates that clinical laboratory study results will be used to identify a client's likelihood of continued internal bleeding and to determine the need for further diagnostic workup. The staff nurse often cares for this client to reinforce the diagnostic plan and to lessen the client's anxiety. This plan enables the nurse to teach the client to adhere to to various interdisciplinary requirements and to help complete the diagnostic process and follow-up, which might, in this example, include blood transfusions.

By evaluating each client's needs and matching them with corresponding resources, the nurse addresses the priorities of the group of assigned clients. While matching client needs with available nursing staff, the nurse considers what the staff needs to do. The nurse also considers the equipment, routines, policies, and procedures involved in each individual's care during the shift.

Flexibility

The nurse is expected to be flexible, when possible, in response to priority client needs. For example, client and staff preferences are incorporated in nursing responses. To provide for unpredicted client needs, the nurse allocates nursing resources so that nursing staff capable of making complex assessments of client needs are continuously available. To provide such flexibility, RNs must be available to meet client needs throughout the shift, including during staff coffee and lunch breaks. This approach provides for adequate nursing responses to the first- and second-order priority needs of clients during these times.

Flexibility in responding to priority needs requires that the nurse remember each client's primary goals. The goals are often described in terms of the client's symptoms, responses to treatment, or preparation for continued care in another setting. By keeping the

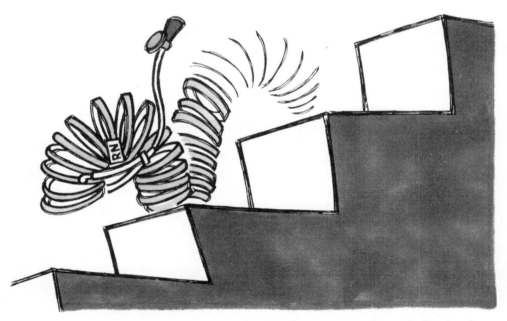

Flexibility in responding to priority needs requires that the nurse remember each client's primary goals.

goal clearly in mind, the nurse can consider other options that might better fit the client's preferences and needs.

The nurse determines which policies, procedures, and routines best meet the client's needs. The nurse also helps the client understand the available options. For example, the nurse assesses the effectiveness of approaches being used to alleviate postoperative pain, including the client's use of the patient-controlled analgesia equipment. If the client is not obtaining adequate relief, the nurse looks for other causes of discomfort, such as anxiety, atypical response to the analgesic, or evidence of postoperative complications. Based on repeated assessments, the nurse provides other comfort measures to reduce anxiety, teaches the client about anticipated progress, and collaborates with other disciplines to manage potential complications.

The beginning staff nurse is expected to understand how various routines promote continuity of care. For example, various client responses to postoperative routines are often described in the change-of-shift report. The client's responses to treatment are also described. The nurse is expected to modify routines if they do not help the client meet specific goals. For example, postoperative coughing and deep breathing exercises need to be modified if the client is unable to perform them due to discomfort. The timing of these exercises might be scheduled to coincide with the client's response to analgesia. By focusing on the client's responses and progress, routines can be used flexibly to enable clients to reach their goals. As clients progress, different routines can be emphasized to reinforce attention to priority needs.

Creativity

In addition to incorporating flexibility, the beginning staff nurse is expected to use **creativity** in responding to the priority needs of assigned clients. Clients usually have limited abilities to complete the activities of daily living. These limitations are often emphasized to the detriment of the client's actual abilities. To avoid reinforcing negative expectations, the nurse emphasizes the client's strengths. To preserve client autonomy and independence, the nurse creatively encourages each client to use remaining abilities and skills rather than focusing on disabilities. Frequently, such creativity requires the nurse to help the client alternate periods of activity with rest periods to promote self-care and to control symptoms. Or, the nurse might offer the client choices in various aspects of self-care, such as the sequencing self-care activities or methods of performing treatments, when possible. Such approaches are used to maximize client control and decision making when real choices are available.

In addition, the nurse encourages client and family participation in care. Client and family involvement helps motivate them to learn about the changes needed to facilitate their adjustment to the circumstances. This helps avoid compromising the client's autonomy or independence any more than absolutely necessary. Some client choices require the nurse to collaborate with other members of the health team to coordinate the client's treatment program.

With practice, priority setting for a group of clients enables the nurse to spontaneously rate the urgency of nursing attention needed to meet individual needs. This information is used to allocate available nursing resources. Through continued effort, the nurse learns to modify nursing routines, interpret policies, and perform procedures to address priority needs in a timely manner. In addition, the complexity of client needs guides the nurse's response so that appropriate nursing skills are consistently available to address first- and second-order priority needs.

The nurse strives to emphasize client's abilities and strengths without ignoring disabilities or vulnerabilities. That is, strengths are emphasized to encourage clients to continue their chosen lifestyles. Limitations or vulnerabilities are given attention but are not the primary focus.

Nurses collaborate with other members of the health team to incorporate client choices in treatment programs. In this way, nurses act as client advocates.

PRINCIPLES OF WORK ORGANIZATION

The acuity levels of many clients needing nursing care in acute and long-term care settings can be overwhelming if nurses do not have an effective method for organizing their work. Using **principles of work organization** may prevent the nurse from feeling overwhelmed and promote feelings of success. Entry-level staff nurses are expected to use principles of work organization to manage time effectively and efficiently. The box below lists principles of work organization. This section discusses how these common principles of work organization are used in the nursing context.

Determine Short- and Long-Term Goals of Assigned Clients

To reach a destination, you need to know where it is. Then the journey can be made in single steps. In a similar manner, staff nurses need to know the short- and long-term goals for each of their assigned clients. Short-term goals are client outcomes desired within specified time periods, such as a shift, day, or week. Sometimes, they refer to a particular phase of hospitalization, such as the immediate postoperative period or the first week of residence at a long-term care facilty. Rarely are all short-term goals identified on a nursing care plan, though many are frequently described in terms of quality assurance standards of care. For example, nursing assessments are done to detect potential postoperative complications; their frequency depends on individual client responses.

Long-term goals might be the desired outcome of a client's hospitalization or of a month's stay in a long-term care facility. These goals relate to the client's priority needs; when they are satisfactorily met, the client's response reflects desired progress. Once the nurse knows the client's short- and long-term goals, it is possible to identify priorities and evaluate the client's progress.

Principles of Work Organization

Determine the short- and long-term goals of assigned clients.
Make a "Things To Do List" and rank each activity.
Estimate how much time is needed to complete various activities.
Set limits by saying no to unreasonable assignments.
Eliminate unnecessary steps or work.
Reserve time to respond to unexpected demands. Plan to "free up" time of a more skilled staff member to provide for unexpected demands placed on the work group.

Make a "Things To Do List" and Rank Each Activity

With an overview of the work to be done, the nurse should jot down the essential tasks facing the work group (DuBrin, 1986, pp. 70–71). When the nurse cares for one client, it is less difficult to remember the various activities that need to be done to complete the care. When the nurse is assigned several clients, however, it is more difficult to remember all the activities that need to be done throughout the entire shift. Consequently, to complete a work assignment, the nurse makes a "Things To Do List" at the beginning of the shift. Activities may be added to this list throughout the shift as they come up. Such a list enables the nurse to efficiently recall activities that need to be done to meet client needs. Sometimes nurses use a nursing worksheet to help organize their activities. Figure 4-1 illustrates a nursing assignment worksheet that might be used as a "Things To Do List."

Ranking activities. The nurse ranks each item on the "Things To Do List" in accordance with its importance or the order in which activities are to be done. Ranking these items takes only a short time, but the gains from spending concentrated thought early in the shift are invaluable later, especially since nursing practice entails multiple distractions and interruptions (Mackenzie, 1972, p. 42). With practice, the nurse designs a unique "Things To Do List," ranks the importance of each nursing activity spontaneously, and fits the activity into a unique pattern of activities. However, until work organization skills are well developed, the nurse needs to take time early in the shift to rate the desired sequence of completing activities on the list. Four suggestions may help in the sequencing of a "Things To Do List."

First, consider items that have specific time limits in terms of addressing client needs.

Client	Room	VS/Time	Meds	Rx	Special Needs/Observations
TD	107 A	TDR @ 8-12	730 800 1130 1300	Incentive Spirometry I & O	Assess breath sounds; reinforce activity restrictions
CM	108 B	BP, TRR @ 800	800 1200	I & O I & @ 1100 1500	Encourage fluids; Reinforce teaching plan in prep for D/C
LR	109 A	BP, TPR @ 800 1200	800 1300	Drug I & O change in AM	Assess breath sounds monitor adherence to fluid restrictions
AP	109 B	TPR @ 800	900	PT @ 1000 1400	Monitor use of crutches, safety of transfers

Figure 4-1   Nursing assignment.

For example, the nurse cannot prepare a client for discharge from the agency if the client has already gone. If some clients gain more benefit from physical therapy if they receive analgesia beforehand, these clients need to receive analgesia sufficiently in advance of their treatment.

Second, compile the client care worksheet or "Things To Do List" at the beginning of the day, while or immediately after receiving the change-of-shift report. Developing it at this time helps the nurse recall details and specific tasks that promote doing the right thing when it needs to be done. This approach to immediate recall of details is likely to increase effectiveness and efficiency.

Third, analyze the "Things To Do List" to identify activities that are scheduled due to agency policies or routines developed for the sake of all involved (Bernhard and Walsh, 1990, p. 90). That is, note which activities need to be done "on time" to enable health team members to maintain efficiency. Identify the activities that can be done at your own discretion. Then, plan to "work around" those scheduled activities—for example, intravenous antibiotics as scheduled, and while you are with the client identify what else might be done. This approach often helps decrease fragmentation of client care as well as footwork. It also should help you make good use of the time consumed by scheduled activities. For example, by gathering equipment and supplies needed for an individual client after you have done your initial assessment rather than before, you might avoid bringing what you don't really need and interrupting your care to get what is needed but not available.

Fourth, try to estimate how much time is needed to complete the various activities in your assignment. Include longer amounts of time for activities with which you have little or no experience. In addition, identify the activities with which you will need help from another staff member. Such activities often take more time since you must plan and coordinate your efforts with the schedule and efforts of one or more persons.

When your initial "Things To Do List" is developed with others on the nursing team and with clients you can begin to plan when to do what. Such planning helps to gain the cooperation of others and to identify any "impossible" plans early so they can be changed to make them feasible.

As you proceed throughout the shift, check off completed activities to reinforce your success and progress. Refer to the list at regular intervals. Check it to see what else you had planned to accomplish. Add activities that have high priority but that you had not anticipated earlier. Use of a current "Things To Do List" will help you feel successful in managing time purposefully.

Developing time management skills is a continuous process. Practice estimating how much time you need to complete various assigned client care activities. Notice what type of activities consume more time than you expected and what types of interruptions delay your completion of various nursing tasks. You may find that you frequently attend to several clients' needs concurrently and yet respond to various demands efficiently. The smoothness with which you complete your assignment will increase as you learn to monitor your assigned clients regularly throughout your shift (Davis and Thomas, 1989, p. 92). You will gain confidence as you identify client needs that respond to preventive nursing measures. You will also learn about the amount of time needed to respond to unanticipated activities that require your attention.

Set Limits By Saying No To Unreasonable Assignments

Keeping a time log for several consecutive days may help you distinguish between reasonable and unreasonable assignments. Unreasonable assignments are those that cannot be done with the available resources and time (Cushing, 1986, pp. 389–390). Figure 4-2 is an example of a form that might be used at two or more intervals to help you identify your patterns of time management throughout a workday. Comparing your data at intervals will help you distinguish assignments that merely need improvement from those that are unreasonable. Analyze your patterns of response to reasonable client care assignments and determine which aspects of each assignment required more time or resources than you had anticipated. If you are unable to monitor and respond to your clients' needs adequately, your clients are in danger. By continuously looking for improvements in time management, you will develop a clear understanding of which assignments are reasonable, given the available staffing, and which are unsafe for clients and staff.

It is important to remember that no amount of education, good will, or practice will enable you to complete unreasonable client care assignments. Unreasonable assignments often reflect inadequate staffing, which can occur for many reasons and place impossible demands upon you. With the persistent shortage of qualified nurses, some beginning staff nurses may be given unreasonable assignments. If after careful analysis of your assignment, you think your assignment reflects understaffing, you have an immediate obligation to inform your supervisor on behalf of your assigned clients (Fiesta, 1990, pp. 22–23).

You need to explain in detail to your supervisor the reasons you believe you are understaffed (Mallison, 1987, p. 151). Saying "I won't have enough time to do all the care my clients need" is not as helpful as describing what the actual client needs are. For example, "I have three clients that need continuous careful monitoring of vital signs, three others receiving blood transfusions who need careful watching, and another client is expected to be admitted within the hour." You need to proceed with your assignment to the best of your ability if adequate staffing is unavailable and you believe you have the necessary skills to provide the needed care but not enough time to do so (Nurse's Reference Library, 1984, pp. 124–129). It is important to describe in detail why you think the assignment is unreasonable (Cushing, 1988, p. 1635–1637).

You also have a responsibility to inform your supervisor if you think your assignment exceeds the limits of your educational preparation and clinical expertise. Take time to discuss the situation with your supervisor to identify alternate options. If the situation is not remedied, you will need to decide your next course of action and whether to continue your employment. Make your concerns known throughout every level of the organization. Keep a written log of actions you have taken to find solutions to inadequate staffing.

You will need to determine how you will say no to unreasonable assignments (Knippen and Green, 1990, pp. 6–7). To not recognize unreasonable assignments due to inadequate staffing is to accept compromised standards of sound nursing practice and to jeopardize your clients' safety and well-being.

Eliminate Unnecessary Steps or Work

As you strive to improve time management skills, it is necessary to eliminate unnecessary steps or nursing activities. Again, it is critical that efforts to increase efficiency not compromise effectiveness. To reduce footwork, assemble needed equipment and supplies before entering client care areas to do specific nursing procedures. It takes a very short time to mentally review a procedure and identify needed equipment and supplies when you are in the client's room completing your initial assessment. Noting your findings can help you assemble needed equipment, avoid contaminating unneeded supplies, and avoid interruptions in procedures due to lack of supplies or equipment.

Another method of promoting efficiency is to reduce fragmentation of an individual's

TIME LOG

Date: _____

Time	Activities	Comments
6:30		
6:45		
7:00		
7:15		
7:30		
7:45		
8:00		
8:15		
8:30		
8:45		
9:00		
9:15		
9:30		
9:45		
10:00		
10:15		
10:30		
10:45		
11:00		
11:15		
11:30		
11:45		
12:00		
12:15		
12:30		
12:45		
1:00		
1:15		
1:30		
1:45		
2:00		
2:15		
2:30		
2:45		
3:00		
3:15		
3:30		
3:45		
4:00		
4:15		
4:30		

Totals: Direct client care activities: _____

Planning activities: _____

Staff conferences: _____

Documentation activities: _____

Telephone communications: _____

Socialization: _____

Breaks and lunch: _____

Figure 4-2 Time log: analysis of time management patterns.

care. Reduce fragmentation by grouping similar activities done at the bedside. A nurse can, for example, gather needed information, monitor symptoms and client responses, administer treatment, and assist with personal hygiene activities during one contact with a client. Grouping procedures means fewer interruptions for the client, allowing him or her to rest. If the client's care is expected to take considerable time, the nurse might block off time in the work plan and make provisions to assure that other clients' needs are addressed during that time. This approach may require planning with peers or co-workers to provide the necessary coverage, but it benefits both clients and time management.

To manage time well, it is best to complete one task before beginning another. In a similar way, it is best to complete the nursing tasks for one client's care before starting with another client. Usually, clients appreciate the reduced fragmentation and reduced waiting for assistance. Furthermore, it is usually less difficult to recall detailed observations of a client's assessment if it is documented right after it is done, rather than waiting until the end of the shift.

Collaboration with co-workers avoids or reduces duplication of staff efforts. It ensures that everyone involved in the client's care knows exactly what is expected in terms of the nursing assignment. Clients who must repeat requests for help or reiterate information for assessments several times bear the burden of duplication or gaps in staff efforts. Client confidence in such staff efforts cannot be sustained if duplicated efforts or gaps occur repeatedly.

To judge the success of your time management efforts, evaluate the extent to which your plans and use of nursing routines met your clients' needs. By listening to what clients and their significant others say or questions they ask, a nurse can identify needs for modification of nursing routines and ways to eliminate duplicated efforts and unnecessary steps. In addition, it is helpful to ask co-workers for feedback about the plans used to provide the needed care. Such information often provides helpful insight into the interrelationships important in effective and efficient use of resources.

Plan For Unexpected Demands

As mentioned earlier, since a number of unpredicted client needs arise during a shift, it is necessary to plan to provide for them. Initially, you may need to allow more time to deal with unpredicted situations. Later, as you become more experienced with the agency's routines and variations in clients' needs, there should be fewer unpredicted needs. To manage these needs, whenever possible plan to "free up" a more skilled team member, preferably an RN, to respond to unexpected demands placed on the work group. A more skilled worker can be expected to respond to a greater variety of client needs than a less skilled one. A more skilled worker should also be more flexible and creative in responding to a wide variety of client needs. This flexibility will enable more members of the work group to carry our their plans to complete their work assignments. Although it may appear to be preferential treatment, this approach actually promotes increased satisfaction and positive feelings about staff work assignments.

These principles of work organization will assist the entry-level staff nurse to manage time purposefully. To provide effective care, however, it is critical that the client care manager understand what needs to be accomplished with the assigned group of clients. That is, effective time management relies on an accurate assessment of the client's conditions, analysis of needs, and formulation of nursing plans, including short- and long-term goals.

Purposeful time management also requires the nurse to allocate nursing resources to match assessed client needs. Consistent delegation of client care according to nursing staff skills and qualifications within the context of the agency's position descriptions promotes efficiency. (Principles of proper delegation will be discussed further in Chapter Twelve.) With the shortage of qualified nurses, it is important to maximize the effectiveness and efficiency of available staff members.

By repeated use of a time log, the entry-level staff nurse can gain insight into realistic work assignments and expectations for accomplishing them. Frequently, nurses omit rest or lunch breaks to complete various aspects of client care. Although well-intentioned, such patterns of time management often reduce the nurse's effectiveness. Nurses are aware that to prevent fatigue and excessive physiological stress, they must include breaks in their work schedule and stick to them. Ultimately, such an approach preserves the nurse's resources and avoids neglecting oneself to the detriment of clients.

Time management skills are learned approaches, not inherited characteristics. Work organization skills develop from careful attention to determining what needs to be done in a specified time period, and how it can best be accomplished with the available resources: staff, equipment, supplies, and time. Both clients and nurses benefit from continuous effort to improve time management.

SUMMARY

The client care manager's time is a very precious resource. Client care managers are expected to manage their time purposefully when providing care to an assigned group of clients. Time management requires commitment to both effectiveness and efficiency; that is, staff nurses are expected to do the right things for clients and perform them without excessive use of time, energy, equipment, or supplies.

Priority client needs require urgent nursing attention. These priority needs of individual clients can be ranked in four basic categories: (1) threats to immediate survival or safety; (2) actual or potential problems for which the client or family have asked for immediate help; (3) actual or potential problems unrecognized by the client or family; and (4) actual or potential problems for which the client or family needs help in the future. Timeliness is of the essence when the client care manager responds to priority nursing needs. The more urgent the client need, the less time the nurse has to respond to the client's needs. More urgent needs rank as higher priorities.

Staff nurses follow several principles when planning to meet the priority needs of a group of clients. The nurse must focus on the primary goals of clients to provide flexible and creative responses. In addition, client strengths and abilities should be emphasized without neglecting disabilities or vulnerabilities. The effective nurse promotes client and family participation in decisions that affect them. Nurses collaborate with the interdisciplinary health team to incorporate client choices in treatment programs.

Staff nurses apply a variety of principles of work organization to address assigned client needs. After determining short- and long-term goals, effective nurses compile a "Things To Do List" early in the workday and refer to it often to assure that priority client needs are met. They estimate time needed to complete various client care activities to plan with others and avoid interruptions and delays. If inadequate staffing jeopardizes client well-being, staff nurses report unreasonable assignments to supervisors to obtain the needed help. To promote efficiency, client care managers strive to eliminate unnecessary steps and work by planning activities based on nursing assessments, clustering activities with one client before beginning care of others, and collaborating with others. By repeated analyses of a time log, nurses can gain insight into patterns of time management that reduce their effectiveness. Though sometimes diffcult, development of purposeful time management skills is a continuous process. Both clients and nurses benefit from the use of these skills.

APPLICATION EXERCISES

a. Observe a staff nurse's activities during the first hour of a shift. List six sources of information the nurse used to complete nursing assessments to increase effectiveness.

b. Observe a staff nurse's activities during the last hour of a shift. List six techniques the nurse used to increase efficiency in completing nursing assignments.

c. Review previous client care assignments that you completed within the last month. Give an example of each category of nursing priority as described in this chapter. Be prepared to give reasons for your selections.

d. Describe three examples of creativity involved in adapting nursing routines to increase the quality of client care.

e. Application of principles of work organization is a very individualized activity. Describe at least one principle of work organization that you use or know of that is not described in this chapter.

REFERENCES

Bernhard LA, Walsh M: *Leadership: the key to the professionalization of nursing,* ed 2, St. Louis, 1990, C.V. Mosby.

Cushing M: Staffing: sometimes a no-win situation, *Am J Nurs* 86(4):389–390. (April, 1986).

Cushing M: Refusing an unreasonable assignment, Part 2: strategies for problem solving, *Am J Nurs* 88(12):1635–1637 (December, 1988).

Davis GA, Thomas MA: *Effective schools and effective teachers,* Needham, Mass, 1989, Allyn and Bacon.

DuBrin AJ: *Essentials of management,* Cincinnati, 1986, South-Western Publishing.

Fiesta J: The nursing shortage: whose liability problem? Part II, *Nurs Manage* 21(2):22–23 (February, 1990).

Knippen JT, Green TB: Knowing how and when to accept responsibility, *Supervis Manage,* 35 (10):6–7, October 1990.

Mackenzie R: *The time trap: how to get more done in less time,* New York, 1972, AMACOM.

Mallison MB: Protesting your assignment, *Am J Nurs* 87(2):151. (February, 1987).

Nurse's Reference Library: *Practices,* Springhouse, Pa, 1984, Springhouse.

MANAGING CLIENT CARE

chapter five

DEVELOPING MANAGEMENT SKILLS

OBJECTIVES

Completing this chapter should enable you to:

1. Describe basic nursing competencies required to develop the client care management skills expected of entry-level staff nurses.
2. Describe the relationship of other core nursing roles to the client care manager role.
3. Compare the nursing process with the management process.
4. Describe how client care managers use the nursing process.
5. Describe a client care manager's typical day.
6. Describe how client care manager routines may vary with organizational patterns of nursing service delivery, during evening or night shifts, and with the personal strengths of individual nurses.

KEY CONCEPTS

core nursing competencies
core nursing roles
   provider of care
   member within the discipline of nursing
   manager of care

nursing process
management process
typical client care management routines
variations in client care management routines

BUILDING ON BASIC NURSING ROLES

Key elements of the client care manager role were introduced in Chapter One. The relationship of basic nursing competencies to the client care manager role is described in this chapter.

Core nursing competencies are required of all entry-level nurses. These competencies are the learned skills and attitudes that are integral to practicing nursing safely. The basic or core nursing competencies described in this chapter were delineated by groups of entry-level staff nurses and supervisors of such nurses (Wywialowski, 1987). These competencies will be described within the parameters of the **core nursing roles** common to all entry-level nurses, as described by the National League for Nursing (Council of Associate

Degree Programs, 1990, pp. 3–12). These core roles are **provider of care, member within the discipline of nursing,** and **manager of care.** Nurses prepared at the baccalaureate level may take on additional nursing roles, such as communicator, client teacher, and investigator. In accordance with their broader liberal education, they are prepared to "evaluate research findings for applicability to nursing practice" and participate in community health programs "to meet the emerging health needs of the general public in a changing society" (Council of Baccalaureate and Higher Degree Programs, 1987, p. 2).

Providing Client Care

As a **provider of care,** the entry-level staff nurse is expected to develop a knowledge base pertinent to nursing practice. The nurse uses the nursing process to apply this knowledge as a basic strategy for clinical decision making. In addition, as a provider of care, the entry-level nurse performs various nursing procedures to meet client care requirements.

The entry-level nurse's knowledge base includes information about
1. Normal anatomy and physiology and its relationship to diseases and dysfunction.
2. Psychology, sociology, and spirituality as they relate to human needs.
3. Pharmacology as it relates to responsible administration of medicines. This includes drug actions, side effects, and indicators of toxicity.
4. Aging processes related to changes in self-concept and physiology.
5. Behavioral manifestations of diseases.
6. Nursing implications of normal nutrition and diet therapy.
7. Hydration.
8. Oxygenation.
9. Information about common normal and abnormal lab values and related symptoms.
The entry-level staff nurse needs to be able to locate information about lab values with which he or she is unfamiliar. In addition, the entry-level staff nurse is expected to use the client record and other general resources of information available on nursing units.

Entry-level nurses are expected to use the nursing process to make clinical decisions that they can readily defend. The nursing process consists of five phases: assessment, analysis, planning, implementation, and evaluation. Entry-level staff nurses are expected to view the client holistically. That is, they are to view the client as a unique person with varied physical, psychological, spiritual, and social needs. Each nursing assessment includes a health history, data about subjective and objective symptoms, data about current health status and functional abilities, and information about the client's participation in self-care.

Adequate analysis of assessment data by beginning staff nurses includes
1. Identifying health problems and formulating nursing diagnoses
2. Identifying interdisciplinary approaches needed to address client needs
3. Listing the client's health problems
4. Ranking the client's needs in order of priority and acuteness
The nurse is expected to analyze the nature of the client's responses and distinguish between dependent and independent nursing functions as collaborative problems or nursing diagnoses arise. In addition, the entry-level nurse is expected to use information from the agency's system of classification or level of care to estimate the client's acuity and complexity of nursing needs.

Beginning staff nurses are expected to plan client care. The nurse helps the client set realistic goals and develop discharge plans within the context of the interdisciplinary approaches and available agency and community resources. That is, the nurse helps the client to understand his or her own health needs, identify realistic short- and long-term goals, and plan to use available resources to meet them. As a conclusion to these activities, the nurse writes a nursing care plan to communicate with other members of the nursing and health care team.

As a provider of care, the beginning staff nurse carries out the client's plan of interventions. While performing various nursing procedures, the nurse is expected to apply principles of restorative nursing and encourage clients to participate in the rehabilitation process. Based on the treatment plan, the nurse is expected to monitor the client's responses and to propose alternative approaches. Depending on the nature of the health care agency and the client's health needs, the nurse performs various procedures to help the client meet basic human needs. For example, the nurse uses methods of infection control to administer parenteral therapy, oxygen therapy, and skin and wound care. To meet long-term goals, the nurse is expected to involve family members in the client's care.

Another integral component of the provider-of-care role relates to the nurse's evaluation of the client's responses. Evaluation efforts involve comparing the client's responses with quality assurance criteria and desired client outcomes. The nurse's evaluation is expected to result in a clinical decision to continue or revise the plan of care based on current nursing data. The client's progress is measured and judged in terms of indicators (measures) of client progress.

Entry-level staff nurses are expected to use communication skills in various ways while providing direct client care. That is, nurses communicate with clients, families, nursing staff, and the interdisciplinary health team. Nurses are expected to modify their communication for clients with sensory deficits, language barriers, and speech deficits. In addition, they should use terminology that enables clients and families to comprehend information about health needs and treatment.

Nurses are also expected to communicate in a manner that enables all members of the nursing and interdisciplinary health teams to comprehend the terminology used. At the same time, they should comprehend the terminology used by others. These skills include both written and verbal techniques.

Fulfilling Role Obligations as a Member Within the Discipline of Nursing

Another core nursing role is that of a **member within the discipline of nursing.** Entry-level staff nurses are expected to exhibit a sense of professionalism. That is, they should accept responsibility for adhering to ethical codes of conduct, which includes maintaining confidentiality and accepting points of view that differ from their own. They should demonstrate self-respect as well as respect for others. These attitudes enable them to provide for the client's dignity and quality care regardless of the type of payment the client uses to finance health care. Entry-level nurses should expect continuous change and prepare to adapt. They should be receptive to constructive criticism and suggestions for improving their nursing practice. They serve as role models to other members of the nursing team.

In addition, beginning staff nurses must be able to interpret legal issues involved in health care. For example, they are expected to practice within the parameters of state licensure laws and nurse practice acts, ANA standards of practice, and institutional quality assurance standards. They are expected to comply with their employing agency's policies and procedures. In addition, they should adhere to "patient" rights guidelines and state laws requiring informed consent and reporting of child or elder abuse or neglect.

Entry-level staff nurses are expected to demonstrate accountability for their nursing actions. This competency requires them to accept responsibility for their own actions and those of their subordinates. To remain competent, entry-level staff nurses should participate in life-long learning programs. This includes continuing and in-service education programs and other activities that promote personal growth. At times, these activities enable entry-level staff nurses to identify developing ethical issues and available alternatives to resolve them.

Managing Client Care

As described in Chapter One, the **manager of care** role requires nursing skills needed to coordinate the services received by a group of clients during a specific time period, usually an eight-hour workday. It is generally more complex than and builds on the other two core nursing roles.

In summary, entry-level staff nurses are expected to acquire the core nursing competencies inherent in provider-of-care and member-within-the-discipline-of-nursing roles. These competencies provide a foundation of nursing skills that beginning staff nurses expand on to develop competencies expected of managers of care.

◼ RELATIONSHIP OF MANAGER ROLE TO OTHER CORE ROLES

Every entry-level staff nurse is expected to demonstrate competency in all three core nursing roles. As described in Chapter One, client care management skills are essential for success as a beginning staff nurse. The other two core nursing roles that beginning staff nurses are expected to be competent in are provider of care and member within the discipline of nursing.

In reality, the three core nursing roles are interrelated. That is, depending on the nature of the practice setting and client needs, the nurse enacts varying degrees of the interrelated roles concurrently, rather than separately from each other. While the nurse provides client care, for example, he or she also enacts varying degrees of the manager-of-client-care and member-within-the-discipline-of-nursing roles in any setting. Generally, the nature of the client's needs and the context of practice guide which nursing actions are taken. The nursing roles emphasized also depend on the nature of client needs and the pattern of service delivery in a specific context. For example, entry-level staff nurses employed to provide care for critically ill clients emphasize the provider-of-care role, while those employed in long-term care settings caring for less acurately ill clients often use client care manager skills more extensively.

Typically, students learn to practice nursing by developing less complex skills and proceeding to more complex skills. Accordingly, as students' nursing skills develop, they practice in increasingly complex situations.

Since the core nursing roles are interrelated, students develop varying degrees of the skill inherent in each role as they gain practical experience. Indeed, refining the skills needed for competency in each of the core roles is a continuous process. However, many of the nursing skills used to provide care and meet obligations as a member within the discipline of nursing are less complex than those used to manage client care. To successfully manage client care in common nursing situations, the entry-level staff nurse builds on the less complex skills needed to provide client care and to fulfill obligations as a member within the discipline of nursing.

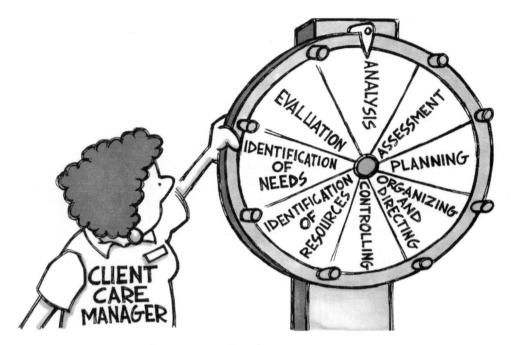

The client care manager performs many nursing roles.

COMPARISON OF NURSING AND MANAGEMENT PROCESSES

The nursing student builds on previous nursing skills to develop more complex client management skills. As described previously, nursing students learn to use the **nursing process** to apply knowledge needed to provide care. This process consists of five phases: assessing, analyzing, planning, implementing, and evaluating. Though these phases are typically listed in this order, in reality, the nurse might engage in any of these activities at any point in time, depending on the circumstances. For example, the nurse admitting the client to a nursing unit spends considerable effort assessing client needs. On the other hand, the nurse assisting the client with personal hygiene activities might be involved in implementing, evaluating, and planning activities to correspond to the client's response to treatment.

Basically, the **management process** is used to meet client needs in an efficient and effective manner with available resources. The management process consists of five phases: (1) identification of needs, (2) identification of resources, (3) planning, (4) organizing and directing, and (5) controlling. See the box at right for a comparison of phases of the nursing process with those of the management process.

For the client care manager to address client needs, these needs must be clearly identified. Often they can be readily prioritized, based on the purposes and objectives of the health care agency. That is, the client care manager determines very specifically what nursing services each assigned client needs during the workday and identifies group priorities. Without determining what services the group of assigned clients needs, the client care manager cannot establish what resources are needed.

The assessment of the nursing service needs of an assigned group of clients is closely related to the client care manager's need to identify available resources. Usually, entry-level staff nurses obtain information about community and agency resources from orienta-

Phases of the Nursing Process and the Management Process

Nursing process	Management process
Assessment	Identification of needs
Analysis	Identification of resources
Planning	Planning
Implementation	Organizing and directing
Evaluation	Controlling

tion, in-service, and continuing education programs and from internal communications from various departments within the agency. In addition, a staff nurse assigned the care of a group of clients is informed about the number and type of nursing staff available during the shift. The nurse obtains preliminary information about client needs and available resources when receiving the change-of-shift report.

The planning phase of client care management should begin immediately after client needs and available resources have been identified. Additional planning may be needed throughout the shift, depending on the success of the initial plan, the changing needs of the assigned group of clients, and the availability of resources. For example, the priorities of clients' needs might change, or the client care manager might be requested to "share" staff with other managers or nursing units as overall agency needs change. Obviously, when establishing a plan for matching agency resources with client needs, the client care manager attends to specific time constraints of scheduled activities, routines, and required treatments. Realistic plans reflect the client care manager's awareness that staff cannot be in more than one place at a time. The client care manager does not, for example, plan to administer complex treatments for one client in one room while preparing another client for a diagnostic procedure in another room at the same time.

The entry-level staff nurse is expected to organize and direct the use of available resources in the best interest of assigned clients. That is, on the basis of assessed client needs, the client care manager attempts to provide staff with an overview of client priorities and plans to meet them. The client care manager seeks input from other staff when planning activities that affect them. In addition, the client care manager assigns care and directs staff to assure that specific needs are addressed in a timely manner. While providing direction, the client care manager might offer specific instructions to address individual client approaches or adhere to agency protocols for providing safe, effective care. For example, a client care manager might request that a co-worker adjust a plan of care to incorporate special family needs in preparation for discharge, or adhere to a specific procedure to assure control of infections. The client care manager uses very complex communication and teaching skills when organizing and directing activities. The skills needed to manage others will be addressed in more detail in Unit III.

As a provider of care, the staff nurse evaluates the extent to which desired client outcomes are met during the shift. To address this controlling function, at intervals throughout the shift the client care manager seeks feedback from co-workers regarding their success in completing care plans for clients. Careful attention is given to the feedback received to determine whether care plans need revision or adjustments in the use of available resources are needed. In this way, the client care manager monitors the progress of the client and of the work group in addressing priorities in a timely manner. Depending on the conclusions drawn, the client care manager revises the plan or redirects the use of resources to meet identified priorities.

Another facet of controlling the process of client care involves evaluating the overall management plan for the shift. It is important that client care managers provide positive feedback to co-workers about their efforts to implement the management plan. It is also important to provide accurate information about client needs and outcomes that need continued attention. The client care manager communicates progress in meeting desired client outcomes when giving a change-of-shift report. This information is used to help client care managers on the following shift to identify the current needs of an assigned group of clients. More information about change-of-shift reports is provided in Chapter Seven.

As discussed earlier, the phases of the management process might occur in any order. The phase of the management process that is emphasized depends upon the context and needs of the assigned group of clients. If clients' needs are less predictable due to physiological instability, for example, more emphasis might be placed on planning allocation of highly skilled staff. If the assigned clients are physiologically stable, more emphasis might be placed on evaluating the extent to which clients are achieving desired outcomes in accordance with established standards of care.

Client care managers combine the skills needed as a care provider with those needed to mobilize agency resources to care for a group of clients. The client care management process also requires that the entry-level nurse use more complex skills, including setting priorities for a group of clients on the basis of assessed need; communicating with and teaching clients and co-workers in a timely manner; planning the use of available resources within the constraints of established schedules and routines and changing client needs; and evaluating the work group's success in meeting desired client outcomes.

CLIENT CARE MANAGER ROUTINES

During a typical workday, a client care manager follows a series of routines that promote effectiveness and efficiency. As mentioned previously, the client care manager's approach to caring for a group of assigned clients incorporates nursing skills inherent in each of the three interrelated core nursing roles. **Typical client care management routines** for an eight-hour day shift are listed in the box at right. Client care management routines commonly include the following sequence of activities.

At the beginning of the workday (7:00–7:30), the client care manager receives a change-of-shift report for assigned clients. On the basis of this report, the client care manager completes a preliminary assessment of these clients' needs (7:30–8:00). These activities might include reviewing available clinical information and conferring with co-workers. Finishing these tasks permits the client care manager to complete assigning client care activities to appropriate co-workers. During the same period, scheduled drugs and treatments are administered as prescribed before meals or with meals.

After clients have received meals (8:00–9:30), the client care manager typically administers drugs to be given after meals and per agency schedules. In addition, the nurse uses this time to complete detailed assessments of acutely ill or unstable clients and provides comfort and personal hygiene measures. Often, changes in medical plans are noted

Typical Routines of a Client Care Manager

7:00–7:30: Receive change-of-shift report.

7:30–8:00: Complete preliminary assessment of assigned client needs; complete assigning client care to co-workers; administer scheduled drugs and treatments before meals and with meals.

8:00–9:30: Administer drugs to be given after meals and per agency schedules; complete detailed assessments of acutely ill clients and provide comfort and personal hygiene measures; note changes in medical plans and other interdisciplinary diagnostic or treatment programs.

9:30–10:00: Administer scheduled drugs and detailed assessment of stable clients; provide comfort and personal hygiene measures; implement exercise treatments.

10:00–11:30: Obtain feedback from co-workers regarding progress and special needs; complete all personal hygiene routines; provide assistance to co-workers and plan to receive assistance from others for complex procedures; administer drugs before meals; involve clients in routine health education programs.

11:30–13:00: Take lunch break and "cover" for co-workers while they are on break; monitor unstable clients; assist clients with meals; administer scheduled drugs and those to be given with meals.

13:00–14:00: Monitor client progress; provide comfort measures, promote client rest periods; administer drugs to be taken after meals and as scheduled.

14:00–14:45: Monitor unstable clients; seek feedback from co-workers; complete care plan revisions and documentation not completed earlier; organize data for change-of-shift report; involve clients in health education programs.

14:45–15:30: Give change-of-shift report.

during this time, as are those made by the interdisciplinary team needed to complete diagnostic and treatment programs.

At midmorning (9:30–10:00), the client care manager often administers scheduled drugs and completes a detailed assessment of stable clients. These activities are often done while the nurse is with these clients to provide comfort and personal hygiene measures. Sometimes the client care manager implements exercise treatments at this time.

If the client care manager shares responsibility with co-workers for some of the assigned clients, the manager obtains feedback about their progress and special needs (10:00–11:30). Conferring with co-workers enables the nurse to assist them and to plan to receive help from others for complex procedures. The nurse also administers drugs before meals. In addition, the nurse might involve clients in routine health education programs.

During the lunch hour (11:30–13:00), the client care manager takes a lunch break and "covers" for co-workers while they are on break. Specific efforts are made to monitor unstable clients, assist clients as needed with meals, and administer scheduled drugs as well as those to be given with meals.

After meals (13:00–14:00), the client care manager continues to monitor client progress. While visiting clients, the nurse provides comfort measures and promotes client rest periods. The nurse typically administers drugs to be taken after meals and as scheduled.

Before the change of shift (14:00–14:45), the client care manager monitors the conditions of unstable clients. In addition, the manager seeks feedback from co-workers to update the care plans. During this time, the nurse completes documentation not completed earlier. These activities help the nurse organize data for giving the change-of-shift report. This time might also be used to involve clients in health education programs.

At the end of the workday (14:45–15:30), the client care manager gives the change-of-shift report to oncoming staff who are assigned his or her clients. To the extent possible, the client care manager uses data gathered during the shift to relay information about client needs. These routines are similar to those used on other shifts.

VARIATIONS IN CLIENT CARE MANAGEMENT ROUTINES

Variations in client care management routines occur frequently. Client care managers might vary their routines throughout each workday due to different organizational patterns of nursing service delivery, changes in client care routines associated with evening and night shifts, and changes in client needs and associated goals. In addition, they adjust their typical routines to correspond to individual personal strengths, patterns of work organization, and use of time management skills.

As mentioned earlier, the pattern of nursing service delivery used relates to the nature of client needs, available staff, and agency purposes and goals. For example, nurses using the primary nursing method of service delivery might spend more time communicating with peers than with subordinate staff. This is so because the clients' needs might require more skilled attention due to the increased acuity levels more common in hospitals. In comparison, staff nurses using team nursing often spend more time communicating with subordinates. Often these clients are less acutely ill but consistent detailed attention to implementing established individual client care plans is required. Nurses involved in functional nursing methods of service delivery might spend more time earlier in the workday assuring that each task is assigned to available staff. They are more likely to emphasize providing the bare necessities of care and to pay less attention to identified individual client outcomes.

Client care management routines also vary according to the daily activities of clients and of other departments. For example, compared to day shift client care managers, evening shift managers spend less time feeding clients and performing related mealtime routines. Evening workers may devote more time to communicating with families and to teaching programs. The evening hours are often more compatible with visitors' lifestyles, which incorporate employment demands and personal preferences. Nurses working during evening shifts often use less time to communicate with representatives of other disciplines. However, they might use more time to communicate concerns to others through other shifts, in written form, or by interdepartmental methods.

In contrast, nurses working during the night shift often focus on monitoring client responses and promoting comfort in ways that do not interfere unnecessarily with sleep. Accordingly, as appropriate, they avoid unnecessary contact with clients. Their contact with representatives of other disciplines is usually minimal. Staffing mix and routines may change to reflect these client needs and priorities. Fewer interdisciplinary team members are available on other than an emergency basis, and almost nobody appreciates being awakened to discuss nonurgent concerns. Less time is likely to be spent on the routine administration of medicines. In fact, many agencies establish drug administration schedules to minimize involvement of night staff and disruption of typical sleeping hours. Interdepartmental communications for routine revision of care plans are rare. Indeed, nurses who frequently work the night shift must provide and seek feedback from nursing staff and the interdisciplinary team about client care to assure that priority needs are addressed. This feedback promotes follow through of individual treatment plans.

These common patterns of night-shift communication can place greater demands on staff working this shift to be assertive and extremely well organized. Often night-shift nurses are expected to complete all of the special diagnostic procedures and treatments in a timely manner to avoid interrupting the client's sleep. In addition, they are required to communicate current information about client needs to other departments in the early morning hours. Often less time is available to complete routine documentation before giving the change-of-shift report.

The staff nurse is expected to apply nursing process skills throughout each shift. However, routines corresponding to the basic human needs of clients (such as nutrition, rest, and interaction with others) influence priorities and clinical decision making. Opportunities for communicating with clients, families, and interdisciplinary health team members affect how the nurse responds to evolving needs.

The entry-level nurse is expected to respond to client needs in a timely manner on any shift. However, each nurse has a combination of unique strengths that influence her or his effectiveness as a client care manager in different contexts. For example, some nurses are more effective as primary nurses, providing care to acutely ill clients who need close monitoring. Others thrive on the social interactions involved in supervising subordinates caring for more physiologically stable clients. Some nurses have analytical skills that make them very effective planners. Others are especially good at formulating detailed assessments to guide their work organization and use of available resources. Ultimately, a client care manager's effectiveness in enabling clients to meet desired outcomes in a timely manner is what counts.

SUMMARY

Core nursing competencies basic to entry-level nursing practice are used to fulfill the obligations of three core nursing roles. These core roles, which are common to all entry-level staff nurses, are provider of care, member within the discipline of nursing, and client care manager. In practice, these roles are interrelated. The nurse emphasizes a specific role depending on the client's priority needs within a specific organizational context.

Typically, client care managers develop their skills by building on skills used as providers of care and members within the discipline of nursing. In addition, they combine application of the nursing process with the process common to management. Consequently, they mobilize resources of the nursing and interdisciplinary health team to meet the health needs of an assigned group of clients during a specified time period.

Just as the nurse may use any phase of the nursing process at any point in time, he or she might also be involved in any phase of the management process. Consequently, the client care manager's typical routines incorporate the mobilization of agency resources to address established clients' needs and evaluation of the effectiveness of the group's efforts. A client care manager's typical day requires a plan that focuses on clients' needs and sensitivity to needs of co-workers. Typical routines vary with evolving priorities of clients' needs, with different patterns of nursing service delivery within organizational contexts, with the changes in emphases of different shifts, and the personal strengths of entry-level staff nurses.

APPLICATION EXERCISES

a. Describe the differences between core nursing competencies and core nursing roles.
b. Make a chronological list of nursing courses you have completed. Indicate which client care management competencies you developed in each. Compare your findings with those of your peers.
c. Make another chronological list of nursing courses you have completed. Indicate which core nursing roles were emphasized in each. Compare your findings with those of your peers.
d. Keep a log of your use of time for two clinical days. Compare your findings with the typical routines of a client care manager described in this chapter.
e. Observe a client care manager for a shift. Describe the typical routines for this nurse and how they increase effective and efficient use of available resources. Compare this client care manager's routines with those discussed in this chapter.

REFERENCES

Council of Associate Degree Programs: *Educational outcomes of associate degree nursing programs: roles and competencies,* New York, 1990, National League for Nursing.

Council of Baccalaureate and Higher Degree Programs: *Characteristics of baccalaureate education in nursing.* New Yorks, 1987, National League for Nursing.

Wywialowski E: A study to determine skills expected of entry-level staff nurses using the DACUM method. A MARP report presented to Nova University, Fort Lauderdale, Fl, July 1987.

chapter six

IDENTIFYING AND RESOLVING CONFLICTS

OBJECTIVES

Completing this chapter should enable you to:

1. Differentiate constructive and destructive conflict.
2. Identify symptoms of conflict.
3. Classify common types of conflict encountered by entry-level staff nurses.
4. Describe how personal beliefs, values, and biases might contribute to conflict.
5. Describe causes of conflict between nurses and clients.
6. Describe causes of conflict between members of the nursing team.
7. Describe causes of conflict between nurses and other health team members.
8. Describe techniques that staff nurses use to resolve destructive conflicts.

KEY CONCEPTS

conflict   intergroup
  types: interpersonal
    constructive   symptoms
    destructive   sources
    intrapersonal   conflict resolution process

IDENTIFYING CONFLICT

The fast-paced and diverse work demands of common nursing practice settings provide fertile territory for conflict. The cultural diversity of staff and clients frequently contributes to conflict as well. Entry-level staff nurses are expected to identify and resolve conflicts that interfere with client care. This chapter is designed to provide insight into sources of conflict and strategies that might be used to resolve them.

A **conflict** exists when individuals, acting in their own best interests, participate in activities that generate tension. The tension results from significant disagreements or incompatible interests and activities (Gibson, 1986, p. 47). The differences are important to the individuals involved and can interfere with mobilizing resources to achieve common goals. A conflict can be caused by almost anything and result in disagreement and produce stress.

Culturally, many nurses have learned to perceive all conflict as negative (Gibson,

1986, pp. 48– 49), but conflict can be constructive. In fact, **constructive conflict** should be nurtured because it stimulates desired change. In contrast, **destructive conflict** causes stress and interferes with the quality of client care provided, work satisfaction, and the effectiveness of communication between co-workers. Entry-level staff nurses are expected to identify destructive conflict and implement strategies to reduce or eliminate it. They are also expected to respond appropriately to constructive conflict.

Intrapersonal Conflict

Conflict can be intrapersonal, interpersonal, or intergroup (Douglass, 1992, p. 170). **Intrapersonal conflict** is conflict that occurs within the individual when he or she tries to engage in incompatible activities. For example, a nurse might choose to work overtime to complete a work assignment and therefore be unable to attend to scheduled commitments with family or friends. Entry-level nurses often experience intrapersonal conflicts. This type of conflict requires the nurse to use problem-solving skills to help set personal priorities and goals.

Intergroup Conflict

Intergroup conflict often arises between groups with differing values and goals. Intergroup conflict often occurs between nursing groups working different shifts or between interdisciplinary staff assigned a client with complex needs. Entry-level nurses experience intergroup conflict from time to time. This type of conflict frequently involves more than one shift, work group, or combination of health team members, however, and often indicate potential systems problems (i.e., problems within the health care organization). These conflicts are typically addressed by first line (nursing unit managers) or higher levels of management instead of client care managers. Administrative staff strive to manage intergroup conflicts so as to nurture organizational development.

Interpersonal Conflict

Interpersonal conflict is conflict that occurs between individuals. Interpersonal conflicts occur when tension results from differences between two or more people, often people presumed to be working toward common goals. Entry-level staff nurses frequently encounter interpersonal conflict as they supervise the work of LPNs or NAs who hold different perceptions of client care needs and how they might be provided. Entry-level staff nurses are expected to identify and try to resolve interpersonal conflicts existing between two or more people during a specified work shift. Conflict resolution techniques often includes communication with the administrative staff to manage the conflict. This might evolve into a systems change process. The advocacy role of the staff nurse as a liaison between administration and the health team was described in detail in Chapter Three.

Symptoms of conflict frequently include frustration, anger, and missed or ineffective communication. As mentioned earlier, conflict produces stress, which can consume valuable staff resources and energy. Prolonged conflict frequently produces continued stress, which is very costly in terms of "wear and tear" on valuable human resources. Health problems such as hypertension, heart disease, muscular tension, and headaches frequently result from long-term conflict. Learning to differentiate between positive and negative stress and learning when to intervene is a fine art. The goals of conflict resolution include nurturing desired changes while avoiding destructive conflict (i.e., conflict that interferes with providing quality care and erodes valuable human resources). If a conflict results in improved client care, work satisfaction, or communication among health team members, it may be justified.

SOURCES OF CONFLICT

Sources of conflict vary widely. Frequently they originate in the personal beliefs, values, and biases of individual staff, clients, or family members. When these covert (hidden) sources of conflict are combined with ineffective or missed communications, destructive conflict is likely.

Recognizing Personal Beliefs, Values, and Biases

An entry-level staff nurse soon learns about the numerous sources of conflict when observing the behaviors of coworkers. Behavior reflects basic beliefs about human nature or motivation, and these beliefs vary widely from person to person. Individual perceptions about the people's capacities, for example, are often described in conversation. One person may say "If you don't expect much, you avoid disappointment"; another will say "I never cease to be amazed by what people can do, given half a chance." Due to their differences in basic beliefs, these people might come into conflict when faced with demanding situations.

Personal values are reflected in individual attitudes. Attitudes influence how people

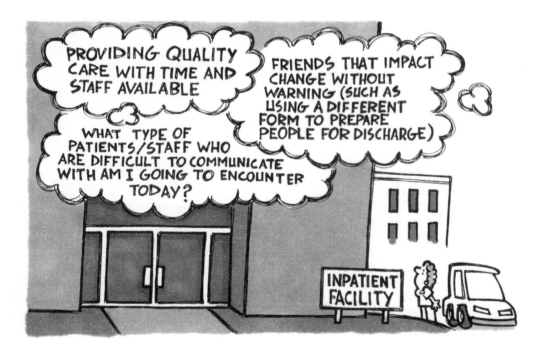

Sources of conflict vary widely.

perceive the demands of the workplace and often contribute to conflict. For example, individuals differ in how they perceive their employment activities and how they "make a living." These perceptions affect the types of employment they accept and how they communicate with co-workers. Differences based on personal values may be a source of conflict in work settings that require flexibility and a focus on the needs of others. One employee may be primarily concerned with "making a living" while another is trying to provide the best possible care. Staff nurses are expected to recognize such conflicts and work toward resolving them so that client needs are satisfactorily addressed.

Personal biases, when unrecognized or unchecked, can also contribute to conflict. They can contribute to negative feelings by communicating nonverbal messages that are perceived as devaluing the worth of others. For example, one co-worker's lack of eye contact might convince another that he is being ignored or that the co-worker is unfriendly when in fact, the coworker is merely trying to focus on the client's symptoms and needs. To relate effectively with co-workers, beginning staff nurses need to be aware of personal beliefs, values, cultural differences, and biases. This will help avoid ineffective communication in stressful situations and behaviors that clients might perceive as insensitive.

Gaining Insight Into Individual Client Differences

Clients, too, have personal beliefs, values, and biases. Consequently, nurses need to confirm with the client their interpretations of client behavior to communicate effectively. For example, the nurse might interpret the client's facial expression as evidence of tension. By confirming this interpretation with the client, the nurse might learn that the client is feeling tense due to discomfort or frustration related to limitations of self-care, or boredom related to lack of involvement in diversional activities. As nurses confirm their interpretations, they gain insights into the client's personal beliefs, values, and biases.

Conflicts may arise when individual client goals differ from those of the predominant culture. Differences between individual client goals and those anticipated by the nurse usually become apparent during the assessment and planning phases of care. A client, for example, might select health care options on the basis of religious beliefs different from those held by the nurse. A client might place greater value on mystical powers than on health professional's interventions to preserve human life, resulting in refusal to accept common medical procedures. Such conflicts, if they are not recognized and managed constructively, could lead to infringement of the client's right to refuse treatment.

In a similar manner, a client's ethnic background might result in responses that do not fit the nurse's expectations. For example, a client might not eat certain types of foods because he or she is unfamiliar with them. If not discussed with the client, this behavior might be incorrectly interpreted as a lack of appetite. If nurses are insensitive to a client's ethnic preferences, routines are often not adjusted to meet individual needs. Special attention is required in the initial assessment and continued evaluation efforts to assure that differences in the spiritual and ethnic backgrounds of clients are addressed.

The family dynamics of clients with different religious and ethnic backgrounds can complicate communication processes. Members of some ethnic groups do not share the predominant American cultural norms and patterns of communication and decision making. For example, the "breadwinner" of a client's family might expect to make all major decisions about how money and family resources are used. Such patterns of decision making among family members need to be recognized and incorporated in strategies to establish plans for continued care. Otherwise, implementation of discharge plans might be very difficult or unworkable.

Gaining Insight Into Differences in the Personal and Professional Beliefs of Co-Workers

Consistent with ANA Standards of Nursing Practice, entry-level nurses are expected to provide care on the basis of assessed client need. This standard of practice does not allow nurses to provide the client care that they would personally prefer. Rather, nurses are expected to provide client care consistent with a plan mutually agreed on with the client.

Sometimes, a nurse's professional experiences caring for clients with various diseases and types of illnesses can color subsequent perceptions of the needs of clients experiencing similar illnesses. A nurse can be sensitized or emotionally affected by client situations, especially those involving intense pain or suffering. Experience might also influence a nurse's personal perceptions of death. These types of emotional response can influence the nurse's ability to remain objective in determining the client's best interest. Personal perceptions should be separated from professional perceptions. The nurse needs to distinguish his or her personal perspectives about illness and death from the professional perspective involved in providing care to clients, who have their own varying perceptions of illness and death. That is, the nurse is expected to respond to assessed individual client perceptions and responses. The nurse is not in a position to choose for others what the clients want done on their behalf.

Similarly, nurses need to be sensitive to expressed personal perceptions of co-workers. Co-workers are likely to have had similar experiences, but they will have affected each of them differently (Arnold, Mills, and Willoughby, 1988, pp. 40– 49). As client advocates, nurses are expected to help co-workers recognize when personal experiences and preferences conflict with those of clients. Particularly when situations involve intense emotions (such as following serious injury or death or during intense discomfort) special effort is needed to separate personal desires and professional responsibilities.

This is not to suggest that compassion be eliminated in the interest of objectivity. Compassion is an integral part of nursing care. Compassionate nursing effort focuses on client perceptions and needs instead of self-interests. Appropriate nursing actions minimize conflict.

Distinguishing Client and Family Expectations

Another source of conflict the entry level nurse is expected to manage involves differences between the expectations of clients and their families. Though the client and family usually have similar spiritual beliefs and ethnic traditions, the adjustment process to illness often differs from family member to family member. In addition, the client's adjustment is likely to present different needs than the adjustment of family members.

Clients who live with a long-term health problem experience and adjust to varying degrees of loss. The duration and intensity of the adjustment experienced by the client varies. Stages of adjustment to loss of body function or health correspond to those described by Crate and by Kübler-Ross (Crate, 1965, pp. 72– 76; Kübler-Ross, 1969, pp. 38– 137). The box at top of p. 84 compares the stages described by these two theories. An individual client's success in progressing from one stage to the next depends on the client's physiological status and the availability of psychological, social, and spiritual resources. Since the

---

Comparison of Cate's and Kübler-Ross's Theories

Crate's model of the adaptation phases of individuals to illness	Kübler-Ross's model of adjustment stages of individuals to death and dying
1. Disbelief	1. Denial and isolation
2. Developing awareness	2. Anger
3. Reorganization of relationships with others	3. Bargaining
4. Resolution of loss	4. Depression
5. Identity change	5. Acceptance

---

family is usually the primary care giver, clients are expected to adjust their dependencies to family resources. In other words, the client is expected to adjust to changing family resources as well as lost or decreased body function.

While the client strives to adapt to long-term loss of health and ability to meet the demands of daily living independently, family members cope with a realignment of priorities, use of time, and resources. Hasselkus (1988, pp. 60–70) described the various stages of family adjustment to a member with a long-term health problem. The box below lists stages of family care-giver adjustment. Each family member, depending upon the extent of

---

Stages of Family Care Giver Adjustment

In-hospital

They know best—Family care givers believe the professionals know best.
Coming up with the reasons—Family care givers search for causes of the client's illness.

Discharge time

Critique and modification—Family care givers try to do what they are "supposed to do" but change approaches to fit personal capabilities and perceptions.
Figuring it out together—Family care givers work in parallel with professionals.

On their own

Teaching the professional—Family care givers decide what the client needs and how to get it.
Sharing what works—Family care givers develop their own special knowledge and seek to "teach the professionals" about what "works" for the client.

Adapted from Hasselkus BR: Rehabilitation: the family caregiver's view, *Top Geriatr Rehabil* 4(1):60–70, 1988.

support he or she provides to the client, adjusts at his or her own rate. As Hasselkus described, both client and family attempt to adjust to demands placed upon them by health care providers. When the health care provider's perspective differs from that of the client or family, conflicting expectations often arise. Both the client and family usually try to cope with these conflicting expectations as they adapt to long-term health problems.

As client care manager, the nurse is expected to assess both the client's and family's progress and to monitor how effectively they are using resources. If conflicts arise that interfere with their progress, the nurse promotes communication processes that clarify perceptions and reduce misunderstandings. In addition, the nurse might initiate referrals and mobilize other agency resources to provide needed support. For example, in addition to regularly monitoring the client's progress, the nurse might refer the client and family to self-help groups and other social and pastoral services.

In summary, many sources of conflict involve ineffective communication processes. Nurses can contribute to conflict by failing to recognize personal beliefs, values, and biases. The assumption that others hold the same beliefs, values, and biases leads to communication errors in sending and receiving messages. Language barriers between people of different cultures also contribute to misinterpretations of speech and behaviors. Frequently, communication patterns are complicated by less interaction caused by language barriers, when more is actually needed. In addition, differences in cultural patterns and family decision-making processes can complicate the nurse's efforts to provide for continued care. Clients and families do not adjust at the same rate. Conflicts may arise when client and family needs change frequently.

Conflict is often associated with ineffective communications. Besides retaining a client-centered focus, the entry-level nurse is expected to identify when destructive conflicts exist. The client care manager should also be familiar with specific approaches to resolve conflict, to prevent such situations from interfering with the effectiveness of the client's care.

Using Communication Techniques to Resolve Conflicts

Obviously, if the client care manager encounters conflict frequently, he or she can be overwhelmed by prolonged stress. As providers of care, however, nurses have developed communication skills that enable them to assess client needs and evaluate responses to care provided. The nurse recognizes that lack of anticipated progress in meeting desired client outcomes could be an indication of conflict. If the client situation indicates potential for ineffective communications, several techniques can be used to determine if a conflict exists. The box at the top of p. 86 describes the **conflict resolution process.** It includes the following steps:

First, separate facts from opinion. Collect information about the facts of the client's situation or what actually happened. *Listen* to how the people involved describe their perceptions. Determine if the perceptions of the client and care giver overlap or differ. Pay attention to the terminology used. Which concerns are difficult to discuss or are not discussed at all? Try to identify reasons for the opinions presented. Does the client understand his or her predominant health problem? Has the client received the information needed to participate in priority setting? Do you or does the staff member recognize existing language barriers or misinterpretations of behavior? Were any inappropriate assumptions made?

Second, identify the specific problem. Describe the conflict in your own words. Try to

Conflict Resolution Process

1. Separate facts from opinion.
2. Identify the specific problem.
3. Seek suggestions and ideas from those involved.
4. Select the solutions that settle the disagreement.
5. Note the consequences of the solution.
6. Evaluate your success in resolving the conflict.

locate the source of the conflict and how those involved have responded. What is the underlying source of the disagreement? How have the participants contributed to ineffective communication processes?

Third, seek suggestions and ideas from those involved. To the greatest extent possible, attempt to settle the conflict in such a way that it results in a win-win situation for all involved. Avoid blaming participants for the conflict. Rather, emphasize the problem-solving process, beginning with the positive value of their ideas about potential solutions. Because their perceptions have contributed to the conflict, discussing possible solutions can help you gain further insight into their beliefs, values, misinterpretations, and biases. If feasible, make a mental note of the words the participants use to describe their ideas. Think about the various possibilities and their acceptability to the involved persons.

Fourth, select the solutions that settle the disagreement. This step is not easy. Often, the solution selected is not a suggestion from one of the participants, but rather a combination of ideas from participants on both sides of the disagreement. If the conflict is deeply rooted organizationally, you will probably be limited to a temporary solution. You should inform those involved of your intention to discuss the situation with your supervisor. Typically, you can expect your supervisor to support your efforts. Explain to the participants the expectations related to the solution. Request that the participants attempt to carry out the solution to the best of their ability.

Fifth, note the consequences of the solution. Observe the reactions to those involved in the conflict. Note their attitudes as well as their behaviors. Do you believe each of the participants gained from the conflict resolution process, or did they perceive the solution as a lose-lose or win-lose situation? If you believe that some participants perceive the solution as a "lose" situation, the conflict may not be completely resolved. Expect to spend more effort to maintain or improve the communication process.

Sixth, evaluate your success in resolving the conflict. Recall that when you identified the conflict, you believed that the existing ineffective communication or disagreement was interfering with the client's care. Have your efforts increased the likelihood that the client will progress toward desired outcomes in a timely manner? Has communication improved among those involved in the conflict?

In general, efforts to improve communication when conflicts arise are well spent. Client care managers, though frequently under stress from multiple conflicts in a fast-paced work environment, are highly motivated to improve the quality of care provided. When conflicts are complicated by intergroup disagreements, and organizational involvement is indicated, client care managers might reasonably "sink their heels in for a long haul." Conflict management leading to organizational change is often a very lengthy process. As client care managers refine the communication skills used in conflict resolution, their value to clients, employing agencies, and the nursing profession increases as well.

SUMMARY

Entry-level staff nurses are expected to identify and resolve interpersonal conflicts that interfere with client care. Conflict is stressful, but it can be helpful. Common symptoms of conflict include frustration, anger, and missed or ineffective communication. Prolonged conflict can result in health problems.

Staff nurses are expected to distinguish between destructive and constructive conflict. Constructive conflict resolution leads to organizational development. Destructive conflict decreases quality client care, work satisfaction, and the effectiveness of communication between workers.

To resolve conflicts that interfere with quality client care, nurses need to be sensitive to differences in personal beliefs, values, and biases of staff, clients, and families. Nurses also need to monitor the various phases of adjustment to health problems of clients and their families. Various illnesses involve intense pain or suffering and can influence the nurse's ability to remain objective in determining the client's best interest. Insensitivity to these issues can result in effective communication and potential destructive conflict. To comply with Codes of Conduct, nurses must provide care consistent with assessed client needs, choices, and preferences.

To resolve conflict, six steps are suggested. They are (1) separate facts from opinion, (2) identify the specific problem, (3) seek suggested solutions from those involved, (4) select the solution that settles the disagreement, (5) note the consequences of the solution, and (6) evaluate success in resolving the conflict.

APPLICATION EXERCISES

a. The assigned staff nurses on the day and evening shifts have expressed differing opinions about the intensity of a client's pain and its etiology. The client's family reported their concerns about the client's need to "wait" for two hours on the evening shift before receiving "something for pain." Identify the type of conflict involved in this situation, its symptoms, and its source.

b. Describe likely consequences if facts are not separated from opinions when attempting to resolve a conflict.

c. Describe the likely consequences if the specific problem created by a conflict is not identified when attempting to resolve it.

d. Describe the difficulties likely to occur when the disagreeing parties are not involved in identifying possible solutions. Discuss the likely sequence of events in resolving a conflict if a win-lose situation is allowed to occur.

e. Resolution of a conflict may or may not occur. Describe how meeting desired client outcomes helps to evaluate success in conflict resolution.

REFERENCES

Arnold L, Mills J, Willoughby TL: Nursing assistants' attitudes toward dying patients in a long-term care facility, *Top Geriatr Rehabil* 4(1):40–49. (September, 1988.)

Crate M: Nursing functions in adaptation to chronic illness, *Am J Nurs* 65(10):72–76. (October, 1965.)

Douglass LM: The effective nurse: Leader and manager, ed 4, St. Louis, 1992, Mosby—Year Book.

Gibson D, Theory and strategies for resolving conflict, *Occup Ther Ment Health* 5(5):47–62. (Winter 1985/86).

Hasselkus BR: Rehabilitation: the family caregiver's view, *Top Geriatr Rehabil* 4(1):60–70. (September, 1988).

Kübler-Ross E: Death and dying, New York, 1969, Macmillan.

chapter seven

RECEIVING AND GIVING CHANGE-OF-SHIFT REPORTS

OBJECTIVES

Completing this chapter should enable you to:

1. Describe the purposes of change-of-shift reports.
2. Describe how specific nursing service delivery patterns influence who gives the report to whom.
3. Describe advantages of oral and taped change-of-shift reports.
4. State reasons why the change-of-shift report focuses on client needs during the next shift.
5. Describe the format for presenting individual client information.
6. Describe methods for organizing the information in a change-of-shift report.
7. List the types of information that can be omitted from the report without neglecting the purposes of the report.

KEY CONCEPTS

continuity of care
change-of-shift report
  form
  style
  purpose
  summaries of individual client
    progress
communication tools
  Kardex
  sequencing
  client assignment work sheets
  flow sheets

progress notes
variations in change-of-shift reports
form and style advantages
  taped
  face-to-face
preparations
components
  client identification
  medical plan and progress
  nursing plan and progress
omissions

GETTING ACQUAINTED WITH CHANGE-OF-SHIFT REPORTS

Client care managers receive and give change-of-shift reports to provide for **continuity of care.** Staff focus on exchanging information about each client's status, current care plan, responses to current care, and what needs further nursing attention to provide consistent follow-through. The **form** and **style** of the **change-of-shift report** depend upon agency policies and preferences of nursing unit work groups (Monahan et al, 1988, p. 80; Reiley and Stengrevics, 1989, pp. 54–56; Richard, 1989, pp. 63–64). The form of the report varies somewhat with the nursing service delivery pattern and the preferences of involved staff. Though the forms of change-of-shift reports vary, the face-to-face and taped forms are most common, and this chapter focuses on these types.

The registered nurses assigned responsibility for care of individual clients typically give the reports, although some patterns of service delivery require associate nurses, who might be LPNs, to report on their assigned clients under the supervision of the RN. The RN finishing a shift typically gives the change-of-shift report to his or her counterpart beginning a shift. The reporting nurse bears a legal responsibility to communicate all facts relevant to the continuity of care of her or his assigned clients. With practice, client care managers learn to efficiently exchange information about their assigned clients' care that meets the needs of the oncoming shift. To give an effective report, the client care manager provides information to oncoming staff that is pertinent, current, and accurate.

The Purpose of Change-of-Shift Reports

The major **purpose** of the change-of-shift report is to provide for continuity of care. A method of imposing order on seeming chaos, the report is a regularly scheduled, structured information exchange. It consists of **summaries of individual client progress** for each client assigned to an RN. Its primary purpose is to effectively and efficiently exchange information between groups of nursing staff about client responses and changes in treatment programs. As described by Wolf (1988, p. 238), "Change-of-shift report was a scheduled, three-times-a-day opportunity for nurses to come together to discuss nursing care and patient progress." Though the report does not include all the details contained in clinical records, it provides accurate, current summaries of individual client progress.

Organizing the Information Exchange

The information exchange has several key features. Typically, nurses use several **communication tools** to gather the needed information. In most inpatient settings, nurses use the **Kardex** as a communication tool, which when kept current, contains summaries of the clients' statuses as well as treatments and care plans. A typical Kardex is a written description of a client's personal care needs, as well as individualized treatment goals and related desired outcomes, and nursing interventions; it often includes a list of prescribed drugs and medical treatments. Sometimes, the nurse giving the report will update details on the Kardex during the change-of-shift report to efficiently maintain its currency as a primary resource for exchanging information between nursing work groups.

The **sequence** of client summaries in the report is often organized to correspond to the work assignment of the reporter. For example, if two RNs working nights each cared for a group of clients, one nurse would give report on those he or she was assigned to care for while the other provided nursing supervision of the entire unit. When the first RN had completed giving change-of-shift report, the other RN would give the report, while her or his counterpart "covered" the unit. Sometimes, the reporter organizes the report to correspond to groups of clients assigned to individual staff members on the next shift.

Typically, the nurse giving the report starts at the beginning of a Kardex and continues sequentially to its end, which helps the staff who are listening to anticipate when individual client summaries will be presented.

If the Kardex is not used, the nurse giving the report often uses a **client assignment work sheet** or a form that lists the clients assigned to her or his care. In addition, the nurse might use **progress notes** or **flow sheets** used to monitor a client's condition as sources of reliable information. Using this method, the nurse giving the report may use clinical records to provide additional details.

The change-of-shift report focuses on information about the anticipated needs of individual clients within the next 24 hours. The reporting nurse describes client care events that occurred during the previous shift and nursing activities anticipated during the next shift. The information exchange helps the nurse receiving the report monitor individual client signs and symptoms of disease, discomforts, and their management. The reporting nurse describes client progress in completing laboratory studies and diagnostic tests and related specimen collections. In this way, the change-of-shift report prepares nursing staff to carry out dependent functions efficiently.

In addition, nursing responses to individual client's needs are included, as are those of other interdisciplinary team members. The change-of-shift report includes discussion of medical and nursing actions aimed at resolving actual or potential client problems.

The information provided in the report helps the nursing staff anticipate activities needed to coordinate the client's care during the next shift. Sometimes, the reporting nurse describes "unfinished" nursing activities to enable staff on the next shift to complete needed client care.

VARYING THE CHANGE-OF-SHIFT REPORT

Client care managers **vary** the **change-of-shift report** form and style to efficiently and effectively communicate between shifts. Each **form and style** of the change-of-shift report offers **advantages.** The form and style of the reports vary with agency policies and nursing work group preferences. The pattern of nursing service delivery and the nature of the client's health needs also affect how nurses exchange meaningful information.

Modifying the Change-of-Shift Report According to the Pattern of Nursing Service Delivery

The organizational method used to divide the work of caring for a group of clients affects who the nurse reports to and how the change-of-shift report is given. When the functional method is used, the RN from the previous shift usually reports to the RN responsible for the direct care of a group of clients within the nursing unit. If subordinate staff attend the report, the reporting nurse typically addresses a broader range of concerns, so that the oncoming nurse uses less time to explain the special care needed by individual clients. Consequently, the report may take longer at first, but less time is needed later in the shift to assure that subordinate staff know the details of the care they are expected to provide. Sometimes, RNs report only to RNs to save time and to provide continued availability of subordinate nursing staff to clients as the report is being given. When this is done, the client care manager responsible for groups of clients is expected to "give report" to the subordinate staff to assure appropriate follow-up for changing client needs.

The pattern of change-of-shift reporting might be similar when the team nursing

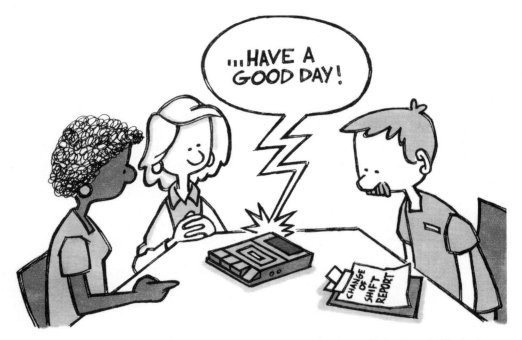

Client care managers vary the change-of-shift report form and style to efficiently and effectively communicate between shifts.

method is used. If the clients' conditions are stable and corresponding nursing services are established, considerably less communication is needed. However, if client conditions are changing significantly from shift to shift, the team leader or client care manager typically benefits from having all members of the oncoming shift attend the RN report from the previous shift. This approach reduces the amount of time and communication required to make timely changes in the nursing care provided. In such situations, the team leader monitors individual client conditions more closely and seeks feedback from subordinate staff more frequently. This change in clinical nursing management routine enables the nurse to evaluate client progress, determine if changes are needed, and provide supervision in a timely manner.

As discussed in Chapters Two and Three, trends in health care financing have resulted in increased client acuity levels in both acute and long-term care settings. Consequently, many health care organizations have attempted to use primary nursing to respond to the changing needs of their clients. When the primary nursing method is used, RNs assigned the direct care of individual clients on the previous shift typically give change-of-shift reports to RNs assigned the care of the same clients on the next shift. Often, client assignments do not correspond to geographic locations or Kardexes. Primary nurses report directly to RNs assigned direct client care on the next shift. That is, a primary nurse might give a change-of-shift report to several different nurses, one at a time, according to their specific assigned clients. In fact, several change-of-shift reports might be given concurrently by primary nurses. This method of exchanging information by change-of-shift reports typically takes less time than that required to have one nurse report to all primary nurses on the oncoming shift until all clients have been addressed.

Tape-Recorded vs. Face-to-Face Change-of-Shift Reports

Sometimes the individual nurse **tape records** the change-of-shift report before the next shift is scheduled to receive the report. This consumes less time by avoiding the interruptions common in face-to-face reports. By avoiding the distractions of answering questions, it also helps the nurse to be more systematic and thorough. The break in concentration caused by answering questions can result in omitting significant information. Interruptions also make listening to the report more difficult, since the oncoming shift cannot as readily anticipate when specific individual client summaries will be presented.

Taped reports may increase the reporting nurse's sense of control over the process of giving the change-of-shift report. This increased sense of control helps some nurses to organize the report more effectively. In addition, the nurse who has taped the change-of-shift report can complete other nursing activities while the next shift listens to the report.

Other nurses prefer to give **face-to-face** change-of-shift reports. This permits the reporting nurse to answer specific questions asked by oncoming staff. The content of the report can be varied somewhat according to the information needs of oncoming staff and whether they have had prior experience with individual clients. This approach could increase the effectiveness of the change-of-shift report as a method of exchanging meaningful and pertinent information. In addition, it could reduce the amount of time needed to give and listen to the change-of-shift-report, while still providing sufficient details. It provides flexibility in reporting to a number of different nurses of the next shift. Nurses receiving the face-to-face report are only asked to listen to reports on their assigned clients, not on all those cared for by the reporting nurse. The face-to-face style of reporting allows greater flexibility in sequencing and pacing the exchange of information to match varied staff needs and client care assignments between shifts.

Varying the Form and Style of Change-of-Shift Reports

Client conditions determine nursing responses. If client conditions change frequently, requiring considerable collaboration with interdisciplinary staff, the change-of-shift report includes details of these changes. These changes are first documented in various parts of the clinical record. Rather than use the Kardex as the primary reference for a change-of-shift report, the nurse might refer directly to the client's clinical chart. This approach enables the nurse to provide detailed information without duplicating it on other work sheets often used to organize information prior to giving the report.

In a similar manner, the nurse might use medication or treatment flow sheets in the clinical record as the primary reference when reporting about a client's signs, symptoms, and discomforts. Using these records in this way permits the exchange of detailed information about the timing and effectiveness of treatments provided and about patterns of the client's discomforts. This information helps the nursing staff evaluate whether the treatment plan should be continued or reviewed by the attending medical staff.

Focusing the Change-of-Shift Report

The client care manager giving a change-of-shift report soon learns that the listeners' interest must be maintained. The listeners want to be informed about their assigned clients' conditions and what, if any, special care they need to provide. Consistent with their desire to complete their assignments in a timely manner, the listeners need to understand the nursing goals for each client and how their efforts will help clients meet these goals. All information exchanged during the change-of-shift report is provided to help the oncoming nursing staff. To consume valuable staff time addressing other concerns or discussing situations with which they are already familiar is neither a helpful nor a productive use of time.

Almost without exception, oncoming staff appreciate a clear, concise change-of-shift report. They are not interested in listening to reports that repeat information they already have, such as descriptions of routines. Rumors or gossip about client circumstances can bias staff perceptions. Opinions and value judgments detract from quality client care. Descriptions of staff activities that do not contribute to increased understanding of client conditions, needs, or treatment are irrelevant. Excluding these types of communications enhances the quality of the change-of-shift report and the effectiveness of the reporter.

███████ RECEIVING A CHANGE-OF-SHIFT REPORT

Preparing to Receive a Change-of-Shift Report

To promote efficiency, client care managers make **preparations** to receive a change-of-shift report. At the beginning of a shift, the client care manager usually senses the "mood" of the nursing unit and gathers information about the number of clients and the number and type of staff available to provide care. The client care manager reviews data specific to the the nursing unit, such as the number of clients on the critical list or classified as having high acuity; the number of clients to be admitted, transferred, or discharged during the shift; and which clients have unique needs—for example, those in the immediate postoperative period, those receiving blood transfusions, and those connected to special monitoring devices. These data are used to evaluate the adequacy of available staff and to assign responsibility for each client's care to individual staff. Subsequently, once groups of clients are assigned to individual RNs, the client care manager can begin to compile work sheets and the "Things To Do Lists" mentioned in Chapter Four.

Prior to receiving a change-of-shift report, the client care manager begins to organize her or his assignment. Depending on the type of service delivery pattern, the client care manager completes an assignment sheet that includes the names of various staff members under her or his supervision. Figure 7-1 illustrates a client care assignment worksheet that might be used in a functional or team nursing setting. If in a primary nursing or case management system, the client care manager begins to transcribe her or his assignment onto client care work sheets. Figure 7-2 illustrates a client care worksheet that might be utilized by staff using the primary nursing method.

The client care manager also begins a "Things To Do List" that identifies tasks to be completed during the shift, in addition to assigned nursing care. This might include requests for special equipment or supplies; special correspondence, such as transfer forms; or responses to requests for information from other departments, such as requests from the medical records department for additional information. The "Things To Do List" could also include similar tasks that might be delegated to subordinate staff.

To the extent possible, time prior to the beginning of change-of-shift report can be used to write identifying client information on assignment work sheets. This gives the nurse more time to make written notes while listening to the report, without needlessly delaying the report's progress. This also promotes efficiency by reducing the amount of time used to give and receive the report.

Receiving the Report

Prior to beginning the report, the client care manager confirms that all oncoming staff expected to receive the report are present. If necessary, the sequencing of the presentation

CLIENT CARE ASSIGNMENT SHEET

Date _____   Shift _____   Nurse Leader_____

Unit A: RN_____ /Assignment: Breaks: Mealtime:

      LPN_____ /Assignment;   Breaks: Mealtime:

NA:_____ /Assignment: NA: _____ /Assignment:
Breaks: Mealtime: Breaks: Mealtime:

NA:_____ /Assignment: NA: _____ /Assignment:
Breaks: Mealtime: Breaks: Mealtime:

Unit B: RN _____ /Assignment: Breaks: Mealtime:

      LPN _____ /Assignment;   Breaks: Mealtime:

NA:_____ /Assignment: NA: _____ /Assignment:
Breaks: Mealtime: Breaks: Mealtime:

NA:_____ /Assignment: NA: _____ /Assignment:
Breaks: Mealtime: Breaks: Mealtime:

Unit C : RN_____ /Assignment: Breaks: Mealtime:

      LPN_____ /Assignment;   Breaks: Mealtime:

NA:_____ /Assignment: NA: _____ /Assignment:
Breaks: Mealtime: Breaks: Mealtime:

NA:_____ /Assignment: NA: _____ /Assignment:
Breaks: Mealtime: Breaks: Mealtime:

Fig. 7-1   Sample client care assignment form (functional or team method).

of the individual client information is noted, to enable staff to anticipate information about their assigned clients. This approach helps reduce the need for interruptions and repetition.

As the report is given, the appropriateness of the client care assignments can be checked. That is, the client care manager can note whether all clients and specific activities are assigned appropriately to staff members. Principles for assigning client care appropriately are described in detail in Chapter Twelve. The name and location of each client can also be noted to avoid errors related to client transfers within the unit or to other units within or outside the agency.

CLIENT CARE ASSIGNMENT SHEET

Date _____   Shift _____   Nurse Leader_____

Primary Nurse: Primary Nurse: Primary Nurse:

    Mealtime: Mealtime: Mealtime:

    Breaks: Breaks: Breaks:

Primary Nurse: Primary Nurse: Primary Nurse:

    Mealtime: Mealtime: Mealtime:

    Breaks: Breaks: Breaks:

Fig. 7-2   Sample client care assignment form (primary nursing method).

While listening to the report, the oncoming client care manager makes notes of key information about individual client conditions, progress, and responses to treatment that relate to the care needed during the next shift. To the extent possible, interruptions or distractions should be minimized. Questions should be asked if the information received in the change-of-shift report is unclear. Questions designed to obtain information about an individual client should be addressed before proceeding to the next client summary.

▄▄▄ GIVING A CHANGE-OF-SHIFT REPORT

Preparing to Give a Change-of-Shift Report

To prepare to give a change-of-shift report for the first time, the client care manager reviews agency policies and whether the nursing unit has any guidelines for their form or style. The client care manager could confer with the first-line nursing manager (immediate supervisor) of the unit, who is often an excellent resource for insight about staff expectations about the style and substance of change-of-shift reports.

To maximize the efficiency of the information exchange, the nurse should plan to organize data gathered during the process of caring for assigned clients. Often, these data are collected for individual clients and in chronological sequence. For example, some information received in the prior change-of-shift report is recorded on work sheets for use while providing care and also for the exchange of information at the end of the shift. This allows the nurse to compare data from a previous shift to evaluate client progress or lack of progress, which may indicate need for further medical evaluation. Data collected by the nurse in the process of completing an assignment are often initially recorded on a work sheet and then entered into the clinical record as care is provided throughout the day.

Typically, the client care manager uses the Kardex and assignment work sheets as the primary references to give the change-of-shift report. Depending upon the nature of the flow sheet, progress notes, and the process of documentation within the nursing unit, portions of the client's clinical record might be referred to while giving the report. To the extent possible, copying of data for the change-of-shift report is minimized to avoid errors.

The RN plans to give a report for each assigned client to the RN assuming responsibility for each client on the next shift. If working in collaboration with an LPN as an associate nurse, the RN participates in the shift report to assure that all relevant facts needed to provide continuity of care are communicated.

Presenting Individual Client Information

The substance of the change-of-shift report generally consists of summaries of individual client progress. Each summary includes three **components:** client identification, medical plans, and nursing plans.

Client identification.   **Client identification** is the first component of the individual summary. To the extent possible, the client care manager begins the change-of-shift report promptly as scheduled. Often general information about the nursing unit is given to help focus oncoming staff's attention. When beginning the report, each client should be identified by name as well as room and bed numbers. The next shift is informed if the client is not presently on the unit (i.e., if the client is in the recovery room or radiology department).

The medical plan.   The **medical plan** is the second component of the individual client summary. To provide a broad perspective about the client's current health status, the admitting diagnoses and other major diagnostic or surgical procedures are noted, as are the dates they were performed. Some agencies require that the client's attending physicians be mentioned, particularily if standing orders (routine medical directives) are in effect.

To identify collaborative concerns, pertinent information about the medical plan are typically discussed next. Physician's "orders" that have been discontinued or been carried out in preparation for special procedures during the next shift are included. New orders to be implemented during the next shift are also indicated.

To help the next shift to plan for administering intravenous infusions, types of solutions and the medications added are described. The rate of the infusion and the time that the current bag is scheduled to be completed are also indicated. To confirm the infusion schedule and to help the staff plan for timely addition of the next bag, the amount of solution currently remaining is given.

The client's response to treatment is discussed, including any untoward effects that merit special nursing attention. The client's emotional response to her or his condition and medical plan are described. If the client's symptoms are being medically managed by PRN medications, the drugs that were administered are named and their effectiveness is described.

The client's progress in completing special procedures and diagnostic studies is also described. The nurse explains which specimens have been obtained and which need to be collected during the next shift. In addition, if a client did not take any medicines as prescibed, receive a treatment, or keep an appointment, the reasons are given.

The nursing plan.   The third component of the individual client summary is the **nursing plan.** Several aspects of the nursing care plan pertinent to its continuity are included. *Personalized* nursing approaches used to enable the client to progress are described, including, for example, use of special equipment, supplies, or special pacing of activities. If the client does not tolerate the prescribed diet or cannot ingest prescribed fluids orally, this information is also provided.

The client's behavioral responses to his or her health status and treatment are summarized. For example, if the client's behavior reflects denial, anger, frustration, or depression, it is briefly described without using negative labels. The focus should be on enabling the staff to help the client achieve his or her goals.

Also described are nursing observations of vital signs, activity levels, and intake and output that pertain to the client's disease, postoperative course, and current status. New problems or concerns are identified. If new client outcomes have been added to the plan, they are briefly described, as are the approaches planned to meet them.

The client care manager also incorporates information about interdisciplinary plans and efforts. The client's response to special resources, referrals, and teaching programs attempted or in progress is described.

Omissions.   The previous discussion of the content of typical change-of-shift reports might seem to suggest that they exclude nothing. In fact, as alluded to earlier in this chapter, several common types of information about clients can be omitted. These **omissions** include descriptions of nursing routines, such as "A.M. or P.M. care." Personal opinions or value judgments about client conditions, behaviors, or lifestyles can distract staff from client goals and are omitted to avoid wasting valuable staff time. Indeed, discussion of client idiosyncrasies not relevant to nursing care can be ignored in the client's best interest.

When giving face-to-face reports, allow a brief period after completing a client summary for staff to ask questions. If the change-of-shift report is taped, whenever possible make yourself available to answer questions of staff on the next shift to promote continuity of care.

Overall, the communication skills used to exchange information to provide for continuity of care improve with practice. By using the Kardex and notes on assignment work sheets, entry-level staff nurses learn to give clear, concise, accurate summaries of client progress. By presenting information in a logical uniform manner, the client care manager helps the next shift to comprehend the change-of-shift report.

■ SUMMARY

Client care managers receive and give change-of-shift reports as a method of exchanging information to provide for continuity of care. The form and style of these reports depend upon agency policies, patterns of nursing service delivery, nursing unit guidelines, the preferences of members of the work groups, and the nature of the clients' needs. Frequently, common nursing communication tools such as Kardexes, flow sheets, progress notes, and related portions of clinical records are used to help organize the information exchanged during reports.

Both tape-recorded and face-to-face change-of-shift reports can be given. Each style has its advantages. The specific style used depends on the needs of those giving the report and those receiving it. Client care managers are expected to prepare for giving and receiving the report to promote an efficient and effective exchange of information. They complete assignment work sheets and "Things To Do Lists" to help them organize their activities and assure that the details of client care are provided.

The substance of change-of-shift reports includes identification of clients and their locations, medical plans, and nursing plans. All pertinent information needed to provide for continuity of care between shifts is incorporated into these reports. Discussion of personal opinions about client lifestyles or value judgments can bias staff perceptions and detract from care. They are omitted to promote standards of care in the client's best interest and to avoid wasting valuable staff time.

With practice, entry-level staff nurses can learn to give clear, concise, accurate, and pertinent change-of-shift reports. By exchanging information between shifts in a logical, systematic manner, client care managers promote continuity of quality care.

■ APPLICATION EXERCISES

a. Describe methods used to communicate client progress between nursing staff on your assigned clinical unit. Identify communication methods that supplement the change-of-shift report. Identify any communication methods that duplicate components of the change-of-shift report.

b. Make a grid consisting of a list of the components of a change-of-shift report and a list of a group of clients. After listening to a change-of-shift report on each client, indicate which components were included. Note whether the information contained in omitted components was readily available elsewhere to the staff nurses.

c. Individual staff nurses use different sequences when giving change-of-shift reports. Identify individual differences that promote effectiveness or efficiency in providing continuity of care.

d. You are assigned to a busy unit using a modified primary nursing pattern of service delivery. A typical staff nurse assignment involves 5-8 clients; the receiving staff nurse expects to spend no more than twenty minutes "in report." Describe what you would do to prepare and organize information prior to giving a change of shift report on your three assigned clients.

e. While receiving a change-of-shift report, prior to its completion, the topic drifts to the personal lives of colleagues attending report. State what you would do. Give reasons for your actions.

REFERENCES

Monahan ML, Bacha H, Phelps C, Whatley H: Change of shift report: a time for communication with patients, *Nurs Manage* 19(2):80. (February, 1988).

Reiley PJ, Stengrevics SS: Change-of-shift report: put it in writing! *Nurs Manage* 20(9):54–56. (September, 1989).

Richard JA: Walking rounds: a step in the right direction, *Nurs* 89:63–64. (June, 1989).

Wolf, RZ: *Nurses' work, the sacred and the profane,* Philadelphia, 1988, University of Pennsylvania Press.

chapter eight

TRANSCRIBING PHYSICIAN'S "ORDERS"

Completing this chapter should enable you to:

1. List the essential components of a physician's "order."
2. Describe each type of physician's "order."
3. Describe differences between verbal and written physician's "orders."
4. Describe the legal requirements for a verbal "order."
5. Compare a verbal"order" received in a face-to-face communication with one received by telephone.
6. Describe the legal ramifications of agency policy regarding physician's assistants' "orders."
7. Describe the principles of transcribing physician's "orders."
8. Describe the steps involved in transcribing physician's "orders" in the proper sequence.
9. Describe common errors made in transcribing physician's "orders."
10. Describe methods used to avoid errors in transcribing physician's "orders."
11. Describe the indicated communications with families when a client's condition changes.

KEY CONCEPTS

transcription process
physician's "order"/prescription
  essential components
  types:
    standing
    PRN
    one time only or limited
    STAT
  style
    written

verbal
  face-to-face
  telephone
physician's assistants' "orders"
principles in transcribing physician's
  "orders"
steps in the transcription process
common errors
communicating changes in client conditions

UNDERSTANDING THE CLIENT CARE MANAGER'S FUNCTION

The entry level staff nurse, as client care manager, coordinates interdisciplinary team efforts to address the diverse health care needs of individual clients. As part of this function, client care managers transcribe physician's "orders." This competency relates to dependent nursing functions. Depending on the agency's purpose and staffing, some of the activities required to translate written prescriptions into the agency's services might be delegated to a unit clerk. Generally, however, a nurse is accountable for the **transcription process,** as indicated by her or his signature when transcription of the "orders" is completed. Prior to signing the "order," the nurse reviews the medical prescription to ensure that it is appropriate—that the physician's "order" is complete and consistent with the client's condition and with agency policies and procedures. The nursing activities associated with transcribing physician prescriptions or directives for diagnosing and treating diseases are often complex, requiring effective communication with many different members of the interdisciplinary team. Consequently, client care managers benefit from fostering effective working relationships within the team by using communication protocols as described in Chapter Three. In addition, transcribing physician "orders" requires client care managers to comply with agency policies and the procedures involved in implementing these prescriptions.

Though nurse practice acts vary from state to state, they often implicitly describe dependent nursing functions. That is, they often refer to the independent functions of physicians related to diagnosing and prescribing treatment for diseases explicitly outlined in medical practice acts. Transcribing and implementing physicians' "orders" involve nursing actions relying on medical functions. Dependent nursing functions are those nursing responsibilities and activities related to medical diagnosis and treatment of diseases, including related interdisciplinary functions. They are dependent nursing functions because the diagnosis and treatment of diseases are the province of the physician upon whom the nurse depends for instruction. For example, the nurse depends on a physician's "order" to guide body fluid replacement to specify the amount and type of fluids. Independent nursing functions are those responsibilities and activities for which nursing is solely accountable. For example, the nurse is accountable for assessing the client's risk for pressure sores and prescribing preventive interventions. Recall that nursing focuses on the human responses of individual clients to their health conditions (American Nurses' Association, 1980, p. 9).

Much of a client care manager's time and effort is devoted to meeting responsibilities associated with dependent functions. Often nurses think that their dependent nursing functions only involve implementation of physician "orders." However, other disciplines also legally prescribe treatment activities. For example, respiratory therapists frequently prescribe various breathing techniques to improve or maintain adequate ventilation. Physical therapists often prescribe exercise routines to be implemented by nursing staff to aid the client's mobility. Clinical psychologists prescribe behavioral therapies designed to enhance the client's coping skills.

Physician's "orders," though broader in scope, are prescribing actions needed to diagnose and treat the client's symptoms or diseases. To be consistent with the client's legal rights, physician's "orders" might more appropriately be labeled medical prescriptions, directives, or remedies (Manthey, 1989, pp. 26–27). However, in the interest of communicating efficiently, the term "orders" will be used in this chapter, since it is still commonly used in nursing contexts.

ESSENTIAL COMPONENTS OF PHYSICIAN'S "ORDERS"

Many types of physician's "orders" are given to direct interdisciplinary staff efforts needed to implement medical remedies. Consequently, a physician's "order" needs to clearly indicate what is to be done, when, and how. Physician's "orders" vary depending on how they are given (i.e., in writing, verbally, or by telephone); why they are necessary (i.e., to meet an agency requirement, to meet the client's dietary or activity needs, to complete diagnostic procedures, or to administer drugs); and when they are to be implemented (i.e., STAT; one time only or time limited; PRN; or continued until further notice). The physician's "order" must clearly answer the questions who, what, when, and how. For example, if the physician's "order" is given to direct drug therapy, it needs to name the drug and specify the dosage, route of administration, and the frequency it is to be given.

The **essential components** of a physician's "order" depend on the nature of the medical directive. To be complete, the physician's "order" must be dated, indicate what the medical plan is, and direct when and how it is to be carried out. Who carries out the directive depends upon the agency's purpose, services, and organization of functions or division of work. To communicate effectively and efficiently, the physician's "order" is frequently written, using abbreviations approved by the agency. In addition, it needs to comply with agency policies and procedures. If specific agency policies or procedures are to be modified when staff implement the "order," the deviation needs to be explicitly indicated. In this way, the "order" legally authorizes staff to address special client needs. For example, if the client is not to receive routine bowel preparations prior to a specific diagnostic procedure, this change is indicated by a physician's "order." Figure 8-1 illustrates a set of complete physician's "orders."

TYPES OF PHYSICIAN'S "ORDERS"

To respond to physician's "orders" in a timely manner, client care managers distinguish four basic **types**. A **standing** "order" (represents the physician's routine) remains in effect until it is discontinued or changed by another "order," generally one written by the same physician. Frequently, physicians express preferences in managing common health needs of their clients. For example, a surgeon may prefer that her clients be intermittently catheterized if they are unable to void twelve hours postoperatively. This preference must be in writing, must comply with agency requirements, and must be entered on the client's record, to be implemented when needed. If it is not, the nurse is not legally authorized to implement the surgeon's preference.

A **PRN** "order" is an order to be carried out when the client needs it. This type of "order" often refers to drugs or treatments designed to promote client comfort. Like a standing "order," it remains in effect until it is discontinued or changed by another "order."

A **one-time-only** or **limited time** "order" is carried out only once or for a specified number of days, or doses, after which the "order" is automatically discontinued. Often controlled substances and antibiotics are discontinued because the agency has a policy limiting the number of doses or time the "order" for the drug can be in effect without further medical evaluation. Depending upon the client's progress, the nurse might confer with the physician to determine whether a particular limited medical directive should be continued. If so, then another physician's "order" is written to indicate this change.

A **STAT** "order" is to be carried out immediately. Such an "order" is often written in an emergency and requires urgent nursing attention. STAT "orders" are transcribed first when they are listed within a set of physicians' "orders." They are communicated to involved interdisciplinary health team members as soon as possible so that urgent client needs are addressed in a timely manner. Figure 8-2 illustrates a set of various types of physician's "orders" that might be written to respond to a client with diverse medical needs.

The client care manager is expected to interpret the varied symbols used to communi-

HEALTH CARE FACILITY
Main Street
USA

Mrs. Alice Jones, age 87

Addressograph Plate to Print Below This Line

PHYSICIAN'S

PROGRESS AND PRESCRIPTION RECORD

Date		Date	
2/1/92	*Admit to general medical services*	2/1	*87 year old ♂ c̄ HX of N & V*
	STAT Med Profile 1		*falls and dizziness for 3 days.*
	v.s. q 4 H		*Lives alone at home.*
	clear liquids as tolerated		
	Bedrest with BRP		
	EKG		
	Chest x-ray		
	IV fluids : 0.45 Nacl at 100 cc/hr;		
	* add 20 meg kcl to every other liter*		
	Weigh in AM		
	I & O.		
	* G. Brown, M.D.*		

PHYSICIAN'S ORDER SHEET	PROGRESS SHEET

Fig. 8-1   Set of physician's "orders."

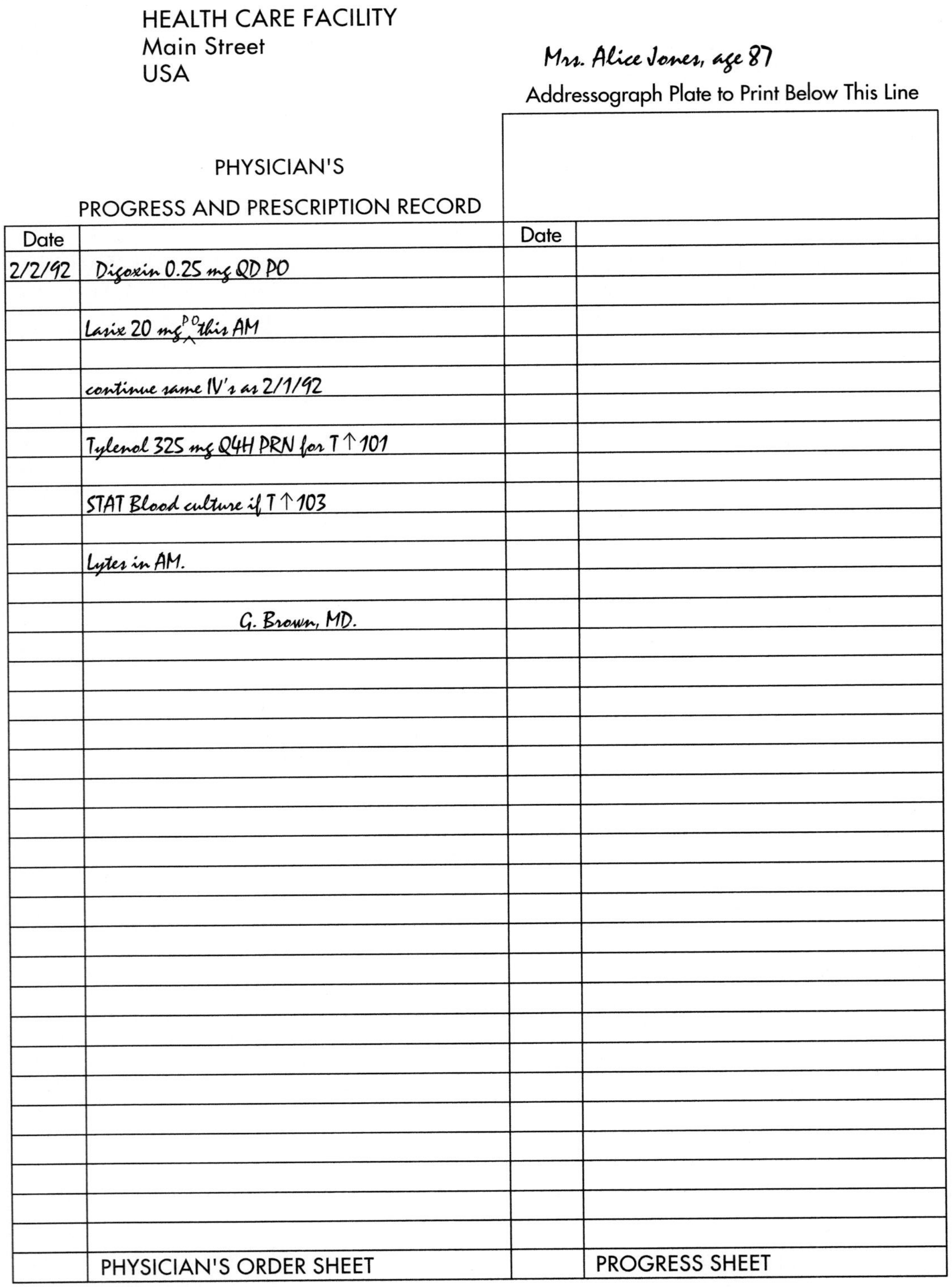

HEALTH CARE FACILITY
Main Street
USA

Mrs. Alice Jones, age 87

Addressograph Plate to Print Below This Line

PHYSICIAN'S

PROGRESS AND PRESCRIPTION RECORD

Date		Date	
2/2/92	*Digoxin 0.25 mg QD PO*		
	Lasix 20 mg PO this AM		
	continue same IV's as 2/1/92		
	Tylenol 325 mg Q4H PRN for T ↑ 101		
	STAT Blood culture if T ↑ 103		
	Lytes in AM.		
	G. Brown, MD.		
	PHYSICIAN'S ORDER SHEET		PROGRESS SHEET

Fig. 8-2.   Various types of physician's "orders."

cate the medical directives efficiently and effectively, regardless of the type of "order." Accordingly, the client care manager uses lists of abbreviations approved by the agency to assure a consistent interpretation. If at any time the physician's "order" is unclear or inconsistent with the safety of the client, the client care manager needs to seek clarification from the physician who wrote the directive. If the physician confirms the "order" but implementing it would jeopardize the client's safety, the nurse needs to discuss the medical directive with her or his immediate supervisor. Legally, the nurse is responsible for the consequences of her or his actions, even though directed to perform them by a physician (Creighton, 1981, p. 111; Nurse's Reference Library, 1984, pp.541–547). The nurse documents the client's condition as well as actions taken to resolve the question about the appropriateness of the physician's "order." Obviously, the nurse needs to communicate effectively and apply steps of conflict resolution to assure that the client's needs are met.

STYLES OF PHYSICIAN'S "ORDERS"

The **style** or form of physician's "orders" varies. Sound nursing practice requires that all physician's "orders" be written in ink on the appropriate form of the client's clinical record. However, most physician's "orders" are initially entered into the client's clinical record by physicians. Occasionally, client care managers enter physician's "orders," received only from those authorized to give them, into the clinical record to address client needs in a timely manner.

Written "orders" are needed to direct the medical plan. This type of "order" is dated, written on the appropriate agency form, and signed by the physician. In many agencies, the physician may also give a **verbal** "order" to a nurse authorized by the agency to receive it. Most often, these nurses are RNs who are responsible for evaluating the appropriateness of the "order" within the context of the client's condition and treatment plan. To promote efficiency, the client care manager requests that the physician write the "orders" that are described in **face-to-face** conversations (Maher, 1989, p. 39). Receiving verbal "orders" for the convenience of physicians is generally not an effective use of the nurse's time (Regan Report, 1986, p. 2). However, in situations where the client's needs are urgent, sometimes the client is better served by the nurse writing the medical directive on the appropriate agency form.

The physician might also give a verbal "order" by **telephone** in accordance with agency policy. When medical directives are communicated verbally, the nurse needs to repeat the "order," with all its essential components, to confirm it. At the same time, the nurse needs to determine the appropriateness of the "order"—whether it is consistent with the client's condition and safety. The nurse seeks clarification if the medical directive is unclear or dubious. Then the nurse enters the verbal "order" on the physician's "order" sheet, beginning with the date, time of day, and medical directive, followed by the approved agency designation for telephone "orders," the physician's name, and the nurse's signature and title. Often, agency policies require that the physician countersign the "order" on her or his next visit or within twenty-four hours.

Many agency policies distinguish face-to-face verbal "orders" from those received by telephone; others do not. Many agencies specify abbreviations to be used to differentiate face-to-face "orders" (e.g., v.o. for verbal "order") from those received by telephone (e.g., "t.o." for telephone "order") when they are entered in the client's clinical record by the nurse.

Verbal "orders" received and written by authorized nurses need all the essential components of "orders" written by physicians. They are transcribed and implemented in the same way as those written by physicians. They need to be countersigned by the involved physician according to agency policy.

"ORDERS" WRITTEN BY PHYSICIAN'S ASSISTANTS

Physician's assistants are extensions of physicians. That is, they perform dependent medical functions. Their educational preparation might vary in length from nine months to five years. Their actual practice depends on the needs of their supervising physician. Generally, they are certified, instead of licensed. Their scope of practice varies with the physician to whom they are responsible. To safeguard the quality of care provided to clients, many states and agencies do not permit physician's assistants to write medical directives since their educational preparation and certification vary widely.

As mentioned earlier in this chapter, the scope of nursing practice includes dependent nursing functions that encompass implementing medical directives needed to diagnose and treat disease. The client care manager's duty to implement medical directives given by physician's assistants varies with state nursing practice acts and specified agency policies. Before implementing a **physician's assistant's "order"** the client care manager needs to know what constitutes a valid physician's "order" according to the agency's policy. Often the policy directs the client care manager to implement the "order" if it is countersigned by the responsible physician.

The nurse needs to be mindful that everyone is legally accountable for his or her own actions. If the physician's "order" complies with agency requirements but is unsafe or is inappropriate to meet the client's needs, it is not carried out.

PRINCIPLES UNDERLYING THE TRANSCRIPTION PROCESS

The process of transcribing physician's "orders" incorporates several communication strategies. These strategies are designed to efficiently document medical directives to specific members of the interdisciplinary team responsible for implementing them. Several **principles of transcribing physician's "orders"** are followed to maximize communication efficiency and minimize errors.

First, the "order" must be clearly understood (Creighton, 1989, pp.18–19; Cushing, 1986, pp. 1107–1108; Langdon, 1984, pp. 23–25). The client care manager needs to know enough about the agency, services, departments, and staffing to be able to determine which department and member of the interdisciplinary team are expected to carry it out. In addition, the client care manager needs to know enough about the purpose of the "order" and its follow-through as it relates to the client to judge its safety and appropriateness (Cushing, 1990, pp. 29–30, 32). For example, is the client's current condition such that the "order" is a reasonable response to symptoms, concerns, and actual or potential health problems? That is, does the "order" fit? In addition, does the "order," when implemented, place the client at unreasonable risk? For example, some types of bowel preparations might place an already dehydrated client at increased risk. If questions arise about the reasonableness, fit, or safety of the "order," they must be answered before the "order" is implemented.

Second, every component of the "order" must be legible. Every component must be written clearly enough that the reader can accurately interpret every symbol. If it is not, each component that is not legible needs to be clarified. The client care manager does not have the privilege of guessing or making assumptions about what symbols were intended in the "order." To do either places the client at risk. The client care manager needs to pay particularly close attention to the exact symbols and letters used to communicate drug pre-

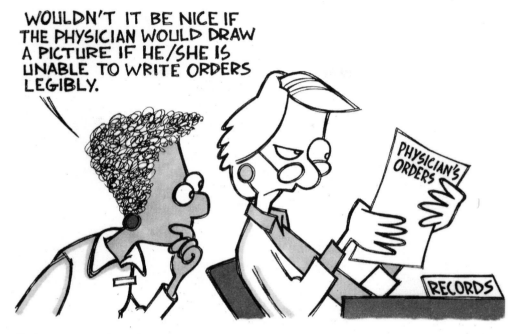

Each component of the physician's "orders" should be written clearly enough that the reader can interpret every symbol used.

scriptions to avoid errors related to the incorrect drug, dosage, route, or frequency. Numerous reports in the nursing literature describe the hazards of interpreting drug "orders" (Cohen, 1991, pp. 48–49).

A physician's "order" is often a combination of abbreviations and symbols. As mentioned earlier, most agencies have approved abbreviation lists to help assure that common abbreviations and symbols have the same meaning for all the people using them. This helps reduce misinterpretation of physician's "orders." In addition, the meaning of the abbreviations in the physician's "order" needs to be interpreted within the context of the client's medical needs. Some abbreviations can have very different meanings, depending upon the context in which they are used. For example, "HS" might mean "half strength" or "at hour of sleep." The intended meaning of the abbreviation depends upon the client's condition, health needs, and the other essential components of the physician's "order." If all the symbols are not interpreted as intended in the entry, the "order" will not be implemented safely.

Third, the "order" must be communicated to others exactly as it was entered by the physician in the client's clinical record. This strategy promotes accurate interpretation of the physician's "order" by those responsible for carrying it out. When communicated in writing, the symbols are duplicated exactly, without interpretation. "Orders" are copied exactly on the Kardex or requisition forms. Each symbol and word is spelled exactly as it was initially entered. Some agencies use carbonless copy paper to avoid errors in duplication of "order" entries that need to be routinely transmitted to other departments, such as the pharmacy.

Fourth, transcription procedures vary among agencies. The client care manager needs to use the symbols required by the agency policy to assure consistency in interpretation. For example, some agency policies require the nurse to use check marks to indicate "orders" that have been transcribed; others might require that one line be drawn around the set of "orders" transcribed by the nurse.

Fifth, transcription procedures vary with the type and nature of the physician's "order." For example, if the "order" relates only to nursing, it will be communicated to the involved staff members and written on the Kardex. If it involves drug or fluid therapy, it might be transmitted directly to the pharmacy, using the duplicate carbonless copy, and also entered in the appropriate location on the Kardex. If it involves requisitioning diagnostic studies, it might require a signed consent form, scheduling, and special client teaching and preparations. Specific requisition forms may need to be completed with the client's name and identification numbers, and appropriate notations may need to be made on the Kardex to inform all departments involved in the "order's" implementation.

In a similar manner, computerization of physician's "orders" requires different responses needed to implement them as compared to noncomputerized "orders." These differences relate to checking accuracy instead of writing the "order" exactly as written. The transcription process varies depending on the agency's interdepartmental communication methods. Generally, the system requires that specific notation be made regarding when the "order" was entered and when it was communicated to those responsible for carrying it out. It also identifies the person involved in any special transcription procedures.

STEPS IN THE TRANSCRIPTION PROCESS

To avoid errors in communicating physician's "orders" to others, a specific sequence of **steps in the transcription process** is recommended. Not completing these steps increases the potential for error in transcribing "orders."

First, *read the complete set of orders.* This review provides an overview of the medical plan and of changes in the current plan. It provides information about the urgency of the "orders" and about what will need to be done to implement them. If clarification is needed prior to further implementation of the medical directive, the client care manager is legally required to obtain it (Guarriello, 1984, pp. 19–21; Rhodes, 1990, p. 193; Tammelleo and Gill, 1984, p. 1314).

Second, *collect all necessary forms.* This approach saves time, increases your efficiency, and reduces the need to interrupt your concentration on the task at hand. It also helps you avoid distractions that increase the potential for errors of omitting or duplicating more than one requisition for a specific "order."

Third, *complete all requisition forms for diagnostic tests, treatments, and supplies.* This approach may increase your recall of special requirements for specific studies, such as permits, preparations, equipment, supplies, client teaching, and compliance with restrictions on diet, activities, elimination, etc. It maximizes the time available to obtain needed specimen containers, equipment, and supplies needed to prepare the client for the study and avoids delays in completing the procedures. In addition, the client's name can be added to all requisition forms, saving time and avoiding errors related to client identification.

Fourth, *if indicated, write the physician's "order" on the Kardex exactly as it was entered in the client's clinical record.* This helps to keep the Kardex current, which is crucial to its usefulness as a handy reference tool for staff. More detailed information is available in the client's record. The entry helps staff recall important components of the client's medical plan and progress in the diagnostic and treatment processes.

Fifth, *complete the communication process needed to implement medication orders.*

To complete this step, the client care manager needs to know the agency's drug administration procedures and to complete the necessary forms. This ensures that every drug prescribed is transcribed and administered in a timely manner and documented properly. For example, the drug administration procedure of some agencies requires the nurse to record all STAT drugs on "medication administration records" located in the client's clinical record. Other agencies require nurses to record STAT drugs on a "Medix" form located within the nursing Kardex to become a part of the client's clinical record after the client's discharge. Routine drug administration procedures might differ from those for administering "once only" drug prescriptions. The client care manager needs to comply with the agency's drug administration procedures to transcribe such "orders" accurately and to assure the necessary follow-through.

The fifth step might involve sending requisitions or the "order" sheet to the pharmacy, or contacting the department by telephone if the client needs the drug urgently. In addition, it might require that the medication "order" be verbally communicated to other nursing staff members, so that the change in the medical plan can be implemented as soon as possible. This helps the staff to incorporate the change into their work plans for the shift.

Sixth, *place telephone calls as needed to complete the physician's "orders."* As much as possible, to promote efficiency, physician's "orders" are communicated through regular computer entry or by routine forms. This method of communication reduces unnecessary interruptions of work flow of all departments receiving information (Rocereto and Maleski, 1984, p. 19). Routines promote efficiency as well as accuracy. Of course, if the client's need cannot be satisfactorily met using routine communication methods, use of the telephone is appropriate. For example, routine dietary changes can be communicated by completing forms and forwarding them in a timely manner. If the client has special needs not readily communicated in this way, conferring with the dietary staff by telephone is necessary.

Seventh, *recheck each step to assure accuracy and thoroughness.* Client care managers encounter many interruptions and distractions in providing care. To avoid omitting entries or details associated with specific "orders," a specific effort to check accuracy is worthwhile. This promotes accuracy in transcribing physician's "orders" and reduces avoidable human errors that place the client at unintended risk.

Eighth, *"sign off" your completion of transcribing the set of physician's "orders."* This step legally confirms your completion of the transcription process. It informs others that these medical directives have been communicated to those who carry them out. It is important to delay signing off on physician's "order" until the transcription process is complete. Otherwise, your signature might result in omitting "orders" that were incompletely transcribed. Figure 8-3 depicts a common method of confirming completion of the transcription process.

The policies of many agencies require the nurse to indicate the date and time the "orders" were transcribed and sign her or his full name, and title in a specific color of ink. This helps readers differentiate the physician's "order" from the person transcribing it. If a computer is used to communicate physician's "orders," the nurse is often required to enter identification, date and time this information. If questions about the transcription of the orders arise, a specific person can be contacted in reference to them. The box on p. 111 summarizes the steps in the transcription process.

AVOIDING COMMON ERRORS

As in so many situations in health care, avoiding **common errors** in transcribing physician's "orders" is much easier than correcting them. For example, verbally communi-

HEALTH CARE FACILITY
Main Street
USA

Mrs. Alice Jones, age 87

Addressograph Plate to Print Below This Line

PHYSICIAN'S

PROGRESS AND PRESCRIPTION RECORD

Date		Date	
2/2/92	TS ✓ *Digoxin 0.25 mg QD*		
9:00 A			
	TS ✓ *Lasix 20 mg P O this AM*		
	TS ✓ *continue same IV's as 2/1/92*		
	TS ✓ *Tylenol 355 mg p.o. Q4 PRN for T↑101*		
	TS ✓ *STAT BLOOD Culture if T↑103*		
	TS ✓ *Lytes in AM*		
Smith RN	*G. , Brown, MD.*		

2/2/92
9³⁰
A

PHYSICIAN'S ORDER SHEET		PROGRESS SHEET	

Fig. 8-3.   Confirming completion of the transcription process.

Transcription Process

1. Read the complete set of orders.
2. Collect all necessary forms.
3. Complete all requisition forms for diagnostic tests, treatments, and supplies.
4. Write the physician's "order" on the Kardex exactly as it was entered in the client's clinical record.
5. Complete the communication process needed to implement medication "orders."
6. Place telephone calls as needed to complete the physician's "orders."
7. Recheck your completion of each step to assure accuracy and thoroughness.
8. "Sign off" your completion of transcribing the set of physician's "orders."

cating a STAT "order" to the involved staff member to assure timely follow-through is easier than trying to reverse the consequences of a delayed response to a STAT "order" for clinical laboratory studies because the staff member was unaware of the medical directive.

Basically, there are four types of errors. These are (1) omitting words or symbols in the entry; (2) misinterpretation of words or symbols used in the entry; (3) incorrect identification of the client; and (4) incorrect selection of the client's Kardex (LaFleur and Starr, 1986, pp. 250–251).

Due to the urgency of many clients' needs and the illegibility of the writer's penmanship, a nurse might misread a physician's "order." An order might be missed entirely in the transcription process, or part of an order might be left out. As a result, the client's medical plan might be incorrectly implemented, or left unchanged when important changes were indicated. Errors of these types commonly include omission of a laboratory study, drug, or parenteral fluids. The incorrect procedure or route of administration could be used or the medical intervention could be scheduled incorrectly. All of these errors could cause serious harm (Northrup, 1987, pp. 43). Errors of omission can be avoided by making special effort to read each word and symbol in the "order" and to consistently use symbols required by agency policy to indicate completion of various aspects of the transcription process. To avoid errors of omission it is important for client care managers to use the same symbols used by unit clerks in the transcription process.

Closely related to errors of omission are errors resulting from incorrect interpretation of a physician's "order." This type of transcription error occurs when words, common abbreviations, or symbols are incorrectly understood. For example, "QD" (every day) and "QID" (four times a day) often look very similar, as do "QD" (every day) and "OD" (right eye). If the context and content of the "order" are not evaluated, misinterpretations can readily occur. This is particularily true if the "order" is written hastily. To avoid incorrect interpretations of physician's "orders," the "order" must clearly make sense in terms of diagnosing or treating the client's active health concerns. To make sense of a physician's "order," the nurse must understand both the nature of the client's health problem and the anticipated consequences of the medical intervention. If it is a drug "order," for example, the nurse needs to know the drug's action; dosage range, route, and frequency; and appropriateness for the client's condition. If the "order" lacks clarity, the client care manager is obligated to contact the physician for additional information.

The client care manager might err in transcribing physician's "orders" incorrectly by picking up the wrong client's imprinter or addressograph plate. An addressograph is used to print client identification information on clinical record forms. As a result, other departments would implement the medical directives for the wrong clients, since they often do not review the actual physician's "orders." To avoid this type of error, those who transcribe "orders" need to identify clients by matching exactly the information on the client's clinical record with that on the addressograph or imprinter, rather than using the client's room number. These errors are likely to decrease when physicians enter their medical directives directly into computerized interdepartmental systems. These systems reduce the need for client addressograph plates, or separate client identification equipment.

Another common error in transcribing physician's "orders" occurs when the nurse selects the wrong client's Kardex and writes another client's physician's "orders" on it without matching it with the identification on the chart. This error can be avoided by carefully matching both the client's and attending physician's names on the Kardex with those on the clinical record before duplicating the "order." In addition, concentration is needed to assure that Kardex forms are returned to their proper location after use.

Overall, errors in the transcription process can be avoided by completing each of the recommended steps in proper sequence. Due to distractions and interruptions, the client care manager might need to make a special effort to avoid errors of omission, duplication, or misinterpretation of physician's "orders." Concentration is also needed to assure that clients are correctly identified on requisition forms and Kardexes before medical directives are transcribed.

COMMUNICATING CHANGES IN CLIENT CONDITIONS

Client care managers are expected to **communicate changes in a client's condition** to the attending physician, the interdisciplinary team, client, and family or significant others. With the increasing acuity level of clients in both acute and long-term care facilities, the likelihood is high that clients' conditions will change significantly. Often, a change of condition indicates that the client is physiologically unstable and that related nursing attention is urgently needed.

Information about a change in the client's condition can come from various sources, including nurses' observations, reports from other staff, and the client or the client's family. In response, the client care manager completes a nursing assessment of the client's current status. This involves collecting information about vital signs, a detailed description of the client's symptoms and discomforts, and responses to the medical plan in effect. Some examples of changes in a client's condition that require additional nursing observation are responses to medically prescribed therapies, such as analgesics; dietary modifications; changes in fluid intake; weight gain or loss; and the inability to maintain functional independence in activities of daily living. In addition to the client's concerns and perceptions, observations of interdisciplinary staff and family members are included in the nursing assessment. If the assessment leads to the conclusion that the client's physiological status or functional abilities have changed significantly, medical evaluation is needed.

The nurse has a responsibility to notify the physician of changes in the client's status in a timely manner. Depending on the urgency of the client's medical needs, if the physician does not respond within a reasonable time, the nurse should seek other sources of assistance as described by agency policy and organizational responsibilities. The client care manager informs the physician of the nursing assessment. Often the physician gives "orders" to remedy the client's problems. Transcribing these "orders" results in revisions of the client's medical and nursing plans of care.

Since the nurse is responsible for coordinating interdisciplinary efforts on the client's behalf, he or she is expected to inform the health team members of the changes in the medical plan. Frequently, these changes involve several other departments (e.g., dietary, pharmacy, laboratory, rehabilitation services, or pastoral care).

In addition, the client care manager is expected to contact and inform the designated family member or significant other about the change in the client's condition and in the plans of care. Generally, the family asks about the nature of the change and seeks information on why the "orders" were changed. The family or significant other generally wants to know what actions have been taken to provide the needed care (e.g., medical evaluation) and what revisions in the medical plan have been made. Both the client and the family benefit from factual information offered in a tactful, sensitive manner. They are entitled to such information, and involvement in the interaction usually helps them to take an active part in addressing the problems confronting them.

The changes in the client's condition, nursing assessment, and responses need to be documented in a timely manner (Allen, 1989, pp. 62–64; Feutz-Harter 1989, pp. 8–9). In addition to transcribing the physician's "orders," nursing progress notes need to include the following information:

1. Date and time entry was made
2. The nursing assessment
3. That physician was informed, and how (e.g., by telephone)
4. Actions taken and revisions made in the plan of care
5. The information given, and to whom (e.g., client, and name of family member)
6. Responses of the client and family and any special requests they may have

This type of detailed documentation, rather than vague references such as "physician informed of change of condition," helps nursing staff to provide the needed follow-up and to communicate with interdisciplinary staff when indicated. It also provides a complete legal record of care provided and client responses should a legal dispute arise.

■ SUMMARY

One type of dependent nursing functions performed by client care managers is the transcription of physician's "orders." Depending upon the agency's purpose and staffing, unit clerks may share some of the responsibilities associated with transcribing physician's "orders." The nursing activities associated with this function are often complex, requiring effective and efficient communication with many different members of the interdisciplinary team.

To be complete, the physician's "order" must clearly indicate what the medical plan is and must direct when and how it is to be carried out. Who carries out the directive depends upon the agency's purpose, services, and organization. To communicate efficiently, approved abbreviations and symbols that are interpreted consistently by all agency staff are used.

Physician's "orders" vary in type and form. The client care manager needs to comply with agency policies to assure that the client's medical needs are addressed in a timely manner. Before transcribing any physician's "order," the nurse needs to determine that it is consistent with the client's condition and safety and to seek clarification if the medical directive is unclear, ambiguous, or dubious. The client care manager needs to comply with agency policy before transcribing "orders" entered by a physician's assistant.

Principles for transcribing "orders" are strategies used to communicate efficiently and accurately. The transcription process is sequenced to assure that the "orders" are systematically communicated to those who are responsible for implementing them without error or inefficiency. The steps are organized so that interruptions and distractions will not result in omitting any components during the transcription process.

Client care managers are expected to communicate changes in client conditions. Subsequently they often transcribe physician's "orders" to make the needed revisions in the medical and nursing plans of care in a timely manner. In addition, the client care manager communicates these changes and revisions to the involved interdisciplinary team, client, and family or significant others. Detailed documentation of the client care manager's coordination of activities helps the nursing and interdisciplinary team provide the needed follow-up care.

▆▆▆▆ APPLICATION EXERCISES

a. You are admitting to a private room a client who has a wound with copious foul smelling drainage which may be infectious. Indicate whether you would: (1) obtain a culture; or (2) wait until you receive a physician's "order" to do so. Give reasons for your actions.

b. Your assigned client with a history of chronic obstructive pulmonary disease quickly becomes dyspneic, disoriented, and ashen. You are unable to contact the attending physician immediately by telephone to discuss the client's change in condition. Identify your next intervention. Give reasons for your decision.

c. A physician writes an "order" for chemotherapy using abbreviations that are not approved at your agency. Describe what you are expected to do prior to transcribing it, according to your agency's policy.

d. A client questions you why she is unable to continue taking medicines she took previous to admission. She is worried she will get sicker. Describe your nursing interventions to her nursing needs. Give reasons for your actions.

e. A client's condition has worsened necessitating medical evaluation. The physician believes that the client needs multiple diagnostic studies and transfer to another unit. Describe the nursing responsibilities associated with transcribing such physician's "orders" at your assigned agency.

REFERENCES

Allen, AMB: Telephone documentation, *Orthop Nurs* 8(2):62–64. (March-April, 1989).

American Nurses' Association. *Nursing: a social policy statement,* Kansas City, Mo, 1980 American Nurses' Association.

Cohen MR: Avoiding errors caused by drug suffixes, *Nurs* 21(2):48–49. (February, 1991).

Creighton H: *Law every nurse should know,* ed 4, Philadelphia, Pa, 1981, W.B. Saunders.

Creighton H: Nurse's failure to follow physician's orders, *Nurs Manage* 20(1):18–19. (January, 1989).

Cushing M: Who transcribed that order? *Am J Nurs* 86(10):1107–1108. (October, 1986).

Cushing M: Law and orders, *Am J Nurs* 90(5): 29–30, 32. (May, 1990).

Doctor's verbal orders and license revocation, *Regan Rep Nurs Law* 25(5):2. (October, 1986).

Feutz-Harter S: Documentation principles and

pitfalls, *J Nurs Adm* 19(12):7–9. (December, 1989).

Guarriello DL: When doctor's orders aren't the best medicine, *RN* 47(5):19–21. (May, 1984).

LaFleur MW, Starr W: Chapter 7: Transcription of doctor's orders. In *Health Unit Coordinating,* ed 2, Philadelphia, Pa, 1986, W.B. Saunders.

Langdon CLG: The legal burden of questionable orders" *Nurs Life* 4(5):22–25. (September-October, 1984).

Maher VF: Your legal guide to safe nursing practice. *Nurs* 19(11):34–41. (November, 1989).

Manthey M: "What are doctors' orders, anyway? *Nurs Manage* 20(1):26–27. (January, 1989).

Northrup CE: Don't overlook "routine" orders, *Nurs* 17(3):43, (March, 1987).

Nurse's Reference Library: Practices: legal risks, ethics, human relations, career management, Springhouse, Pa, 1984, Springhouse Corporation.

Rhodes AM: Carrying out physicians' orders, *Matern Child Nurs J* 15(3):193. (May/June, 1990).

Rocereto LR, Maleski CM: Following orders . . . and other obligations: 8 legal questions, *Nurs Life* 4(6):18–19. (November/December, 1984).

Tammelleo DA, Gill D: When following orders can cost you your license, *RN* 47(3):13–14. (July, 1984).

MANAGING OTHERS

chapter nine

USING PERSONAL STRENGTHS TO CREATIVELY MANAGE OTHERS

Completing this chapter should enable you to:

1. Describe the application of human development theories in identifying employee motivations and needs.
2. Describe important characteristics of an organization's culture.
3. Identify five phases of organizational development as stages of growth and change.
4. Describe types of power staff nurses can use to influence others.
5. Describe characteristics of effective leadership.
6. Discuss common leadership styles.
7. Discuss major functions of nursing leadership.
8. Describe the nursing leadership function of providing role models.
9. Describe the nursing leadership function of providing staff direction.
10. Describe the nursing leadership function of providing feedback, including criticism and praise.
11. Describe nursing methods used to evaluate the success of the work group.

KEY CONCEPTS:

human relations management
  human development theories
    continuities
    changes
characteristics of an organization's culture
phases of organizational development
evolution (growth)
revolution (change)
phases of organizational development
sources of influence
  power
    knowledge
    positional

      personal
leadership
leadership style
authoritarian or directive
democratic or participatory
laissez faire or nondirective
nursing leadership functions
  role modeling
  directing
  providing feedback
    criticism
    praise
  evaluating success

■■■■■ DEVELOPING A CLIENT CARE MANAGEMENT STYLE

As described in Chapter One, the terms "management" and "leadership" are used interchangeably in some nursing circles. Actually, the two terms have different meanings (Kotter, 1990, pp. 103–104). Nursing "management" refers to the judicious use of resources to achieve client goals. It includes responsibility for directing and controlling the process. Nursing "leadership," in comparison, refers to skills used to guide others in such a way that followers accept direction voluntarily, without relying on an individual's organizational authority. Entry-level staff nurses use leadership skills to benefit themselves and their clients. That is, entry-level staff nurses use leadership skills to maximize their effectiveness as client care managers, directly benefiting those receiving care, as well as indirectly improving their nursing practice. As client care managers, staff nurses can learn to build on personal strengths to increase their effectiveness in helping others, emphasizing attitudes and positive personal strengths rather than negative perspectives or vulnerabilities. Effective staff nurses manage others creatively by accenting their own talents, strengths, and interests and those of their co-workers to provide quality care to clients.

In today's evolving information era, health care environments confront staff with demands for complex changes deeply rooted in societal trends. The evolving cultures (patterns of interactions related to accepted values and behaviors) in these service-oriented work environments place considerable emphasis on human relations skills. Consequently, the client care manager's effectiveness depends largely upon the individual nurse's **human relations management** skills. In a recent study, Platz, Biordi, and Holm (1991, p. 15) reported that "human management skill was ranked as the most important criterion of effectiveness for chief nurse executives as well as middle-level nurse managers. With the increasing emphasis on decentralizing organizations and the efficient use of scarce human resources, entry-level staff nurses will be expected to use human management skills too (Manthey, 1990a, pp. 19–20). These skills relate to personal leadership characteristics. Consistent with the evolving emphasis on specified outcomes as integral to quality of care, client care managers will continue to be expected to develop scarce human resources (Blancett, 1990, pp. 4–5).

Applying Human Development Theories

To gain insight into client behavior, nurses learn to apply human motivation theories. For example, many nurses are familiar with Maslow's theory and other theories used to describe human development throughout the life span. In a similar manner, nurses apply these theories to learn about the motivations of the people with whom they work and to identify factors underlying an employee's behaviors and perceptions of work experiences. Since most members of the nursing work group are adults, nurses can apply **human development theories** that address the concerns of adulthood to understand co-workers' motivations. If the entry-level staff nurse understands a co-worker's motivations, he or she is likely to be able to identify that person's personal strengths, upon which meaningful relationships can be established.

A brief review of a developmental psychology textbook reveals many current human development theories. Basically, each theory describes predicted developmental **continuities** and **changes** typically occuring throughout adulthood. Such theories help the nurse to anticipate biological, psychological, and social continuities and changes that affect co-

Common Biological Continuities and Changes During Adulthood

Continuities	Changes
1. Genetic background.	1. Decreasing function related to disease or disuse.
2. Adaptation within limits of physiological reserves.	2. Decreased immune response to cellular deviation.
3. Increasing individual differences due to "wear and tear" of living.	3. Decreased endocrine response to maintain metabolic rate, reproduction.

workers. For example, adults are influenced by the biological continuities of their genetic inheritance, and also by biological changes associated with increasing chronological age. The box above lists common biological continuities and changes associated with adult human development. Some common changes include altered immune and endocrine responses and decreased reserves for adapting to physiological deficits.

The box below lists common psychological continuities and changes associated with adult human development. Some common psychological continuities include personality structure, intelligence, and cognition. Some common psychological changes include increased introspection and increased response time to stimuli.

The box on p. 121 lists common social continuities and changes experienced by adults. Common social continuities include persistent basic values and corresponding roles. For example, an individual whose basic values are consistent with self-esteem and respect for the rights of others is likely to continue to hold such values throughout adulthood. Similarly, an individual who gained great personal satisfaction from fulfilling the role of a parent is likely to continue to value that role for as long as it is feasible to do so. Common social changes include loss of roles, such as worker, spouse, or friend and decreased personal resources, such as body function, positive self-image, and income.

The common continuities and changes of adulthood need to be considered to gain in-

Common Psychological Continuities and Changes During Adulthood

Continuities	Changes
1. Continuation of personality structure.	1. Increased introspection.
2. Consistent or increased intelligence, especially verbal.	2. Increased response time to stimuli.
3. Continued patterns of perception or cognition.	3. Increased caution in the interest of accuracy.

Common Social Continuities and Changes During Adulthood

Continuities	Changes
1. Persisting basic values	1. Increased social losses, for example, of friends and family

2. Continuing basic roles within personal limits	2. Decreased personal resources
	   a. body function
	   b. positive self-image
	   c. income, economic resources

sight into the motivations of co-workers in an effort to maximize their individual productivity. The client care manager can use these insights to identify the co-worker's strengths and vulnerabilities. Such an approach might also increase the client care manager's sensitivity to the concerns and needs of individual members of the work group.

Becoming Acquainted with Important Characteristics of an Organization's Work Culture

The culture or ecology of the work environment strongly influences the behavior of members of a work group. The culture of a work group derives from its values, techniques, and particular ways of doing things, and from the basic beliefs and inherent assumptions, goals, practices, and concerns of its members (Jameton, 1990, pp. 443–445). The nature of the work environment makes social demands on each member of the nursing work group. The culture of the work environment usually involves organizational values, norms, and interpersonal strategies (del Bueno, 1986b, pp. 15–20). By gaining insight into the work group's values, norms, and expectations, client care managers develop sensitivity to other forces that motivate the behaviors of its members.

Individual employees have unique characteristics and motivations. In the same way, the **characteristics of organizational cultures** or patterns of interrelationships within work groups differ. Coeling (1990, pp. 26–30) described how entry-level nurses can use information about organizational cultures to adapt their behavior to various dimensions of the work environment. The culture of the nursing work group is rooted in its history and traditions. The group's values are reflected in deliberate or unintentional choices. For example, a culture might value physiological client needs over those that are primarily psychological or emotional in nature. The leadership style used by key members of the work group provides clues about how decisions are made by the group.

Patterns of helping each other or working together to complete assigned client care indicate the group's commitment to teamwork rather than individual competition and achievement. Entry-level staff nurses need to be sensitive to how feedback is given to the group, including the types of behaviors that openly receive positive recognition and those that are criticized. They need to notice how much emphasis is placed on following routines, policies, and procedures and how much on learning new methods and using flexibility and creativity. These patterns of behavior, or norms of the work group, are used to judge the acceptability of members' behaviors, including those of new graduates joining

---

Questions to Describe a Nursing Work Group Culture

Physical/psychological focus

Is it considered more important to first meet clients' physical needs or their psychosocial needs?

How important is it to be organized and efficient?

How important is it to understand the client's point of view and to respect the client's values?

Large/small power distance

Does the nurse manager have a more autocratic or democractic style?

Who can tell another staff nurse what to do?

Are some nurses more powerful than others? If so, what gives them their power?

Individualism/collectivism

Does an individual nurse or the whole group tend to decide what nursing care a client needs?

Do nurses tend to work alone to complete their assignments, or do they work together to finish the work of their shift?

How acceptable is it to compete with fellow nurses?

Criticism/approval

Do nurses tend to criticize each other directly or indirectly?

Does criticism tend to occur in public or private?

How and by whom is positive approval given?

Strong/weak uncertainty avoidance

Do the nurses tend to value and stay with past ways of doing things or to get excited about learning and applying new approaches?

How important is it to follow policies and procedures?

To what extent do nurses feel there is one right way to do things?

Coeling HV: Organizational culture: helping new graduates adjust, *Nurse Educ* 15(2):27, 1990.

the group. If entry-level nurses are unaware of or insensitive to work group culture, they are unlikely to change their behavior to meet prevailing expectations and less likely to remain with the work group. The box above includes a list, "Questions to Describe a Nursing Work Group Culture," compiled by Coeling (1990, p. 27). She recommends that entry-level staff nurses use these questions to become familiar with the organization's culture and to guide their adjustment to it. Effort expended to identify the characteristics of one's work group culture is likely to be very worthwhile.

Relating Organizational Development to Work Group Culture

Work environments of health care organizations vary widely. With the increasing interrelatedness of organizations and their corresponding competitiveness, much has been written about creating cultures that provide high-quality customer service (Curtin, 1990, pp. 7–8; Hicks and Silva, 1984; Kramer and Schmalenberg, 1991b, pp. 51–55; Manthey, 1990a, pp. 16–17; Peters and Waterman, 1982). These authors emphasize various methods of developing desired values and norms to increase employee productivity and effectiveness.

Analysis of the stages of development of an organization's culture provides insight into the work group culture. As described by Hannan and Freeman (1989, p. 68), when members within an organization agree on its norms, it becomes more resistant to change. However, the actions of individual members of the group can significantly influence the organization. Hannan and Freeman indicate that the actions of individual workers matter more to the subunits of an organization than to the organization as a whole, but they do matter (Hannan and Freeman, 1989, p. 40). As members of a subunit of the health care organization, namely the nursing department, entry-level staff nurses influence its culture. They can support desired changes without eroding the organization's strengths. Based on information about the development of the organization's culture, they can identify which aspects contribute to its success and need to be continued and which are sources of conflict and require revision.

Five important characteristics of an organization are its

1. Age
2. Size
3. Stages of evolution
4. Stages of revolution
5. Rate of growth within its respective industry (Greiner, 1972, pp. 38–39)

An organization's age influences its history and its patterns of response to management problems and principles. For example, the evolving emphasis on decentralization in health care organizations helps explain the ineffectiveness of many centralized systems that were less responsive to the increasing complexity of health care.

Closely related to the organization's age is its size. As the success of an organization leads to increasing demands for services, its size increases and the nature of the organization changes irreversibly. Increased size magnifies the organization's need for communication and coordination among workers.

Understanding **phases** of **organizational development** helps to gain insight into the agency's work culture. An organization's stages of **"evolution,"** or growth, are characterized by continued expansion without significant change in the organization's typical patterns of activities (Greiner, 1972, p. 40). Its stages of **"revolution,"** or change, on the other hand, are characterized by considerable turmoil and revision of management practices and patterns (Greiner, 1972, p. 40). Surviving organizations experience intermittent periods of evolution and revolution throughout their life cycles.

Health care organizations are also influenced by the rate of growth of the health care industry. Witness the popularity of "downsizing" as health care costs have escalated. Periods of evolution or relatively smooth expansion can be delayed if there is increased demand for services. Periods of revolution or marked changes in methods of operating are difficult to delay when demand for services significantly declines. Client care managers need to understand the historical background of the organizational culture where they work to better predict the likelihood that it will change markedly or continue without substantially altering the processes it uses to provide client care.

Phases of organizational development occur throughout an organization's life cycle. To survive, organizations pass through at least five major phases of growth (Greiner, 1972,

p. 37). Each phase is characterized by an evolutionary stage of growth and a revolutionary stage of crisis. These phases include

1. Growth through creativity: crisis of leadership
2. Growth through direction: crisis of autonomy
3. Growth through delegation: crisis of control
4. Growth through coordination: crisis of red tape
5. Growth through collaboration: crisis of ? (The focus of this crisis is difficult to predict but will be related to collaboration.)

These stages are depicted in Figure 9-1. By analyzing the historical features of health care organizations the client care manager can gain insight into the processes of change occurring within them. In addition, they can appreciate that solutions used during evolutionary stages of organizational development sow seeds for the problems that give rise to revolutionary stages. Change is the only constant in organizational development.

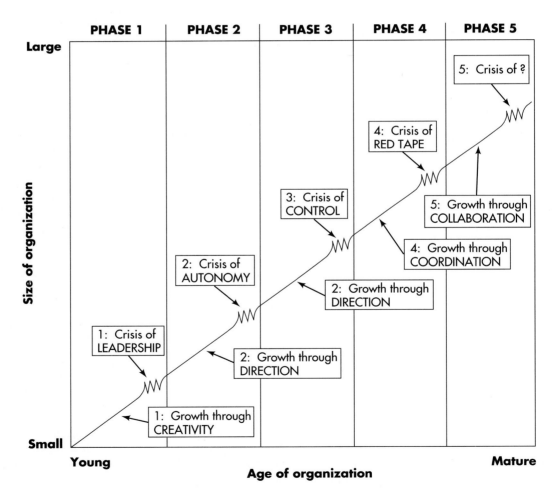

Fig. 9-1.   Phases of organizational development, including stages of evolution and revolution. (From Greiner L: Evolution and revolution as organizations grow, *Harvard Bus Rev*, July/August: 41, 1972.)

Developing a Personal Leadership Style

Staff nurses as client care managers use various **sources of influence** or **power,** to lead others. They use personal talents, strengths, and leadership skills to maximize scarce human resources to provide high-quality care. Using nursing leadership skills is an integral part of the client care management process. The actual leadership characteristics used and corresponding activites vary with the personal management style of the nurse, the setting, and the characteristics of client needs. Each nurse communicates personal power differently to influence others and to motivate them to provide the needed client care. For example, one nurse might use charisma to guide others. Another nurse might use self-confidence in nursing knowledge and skills to relate effectively to other members of the work group.

The nature of the work environment influences the type of leadership skills that enhance the client care manager's effectiveness. For example, the nursing leadership skills used to complete many concrete tasks in a busy surgical unit are likely to differ from those used to care for clients in a rehabilitation setting with fewer scheduled activities. In addition, due to differences in acute and long-term care staffing mixes, leadership characteristics vary with the composition of the work group, the pattern of service delivery, and the organization's priorities (Smith, 1987, pp. 513–514).

Power

To mobilize the resources required to complete client care activities within the nursing work environment, staff nurses use **power** from several sources. Though difficult to define specifically without reference to situational variables, power generally refers to the staff nurse's "ability to do [what is necessary] to achieve nursing objectives" (Gorman and Clark, 1986, p. 129). Basically, staff nurse power or ability to influence others in the work group stems from three major sources.

Knowledge   Knowledge is very influential. Due to his or her education in nursing, the client care manager has developed a source of power based on nursing **knowledge.** This knowledge enables the nurse to understand client situations and what needs to be done to meet clients' needs. Organizations that strive to provide quality health care and reward excellence in providing it are typically strongly influenced by professional knowledge. Consequently, nurses with greater knowledge typically gravitate to more influential positions within such health care environments. For example, clinical nurse specialists often exercise considerable power in mobilizing resources for clients they serve. Similarly, some patterns of nursing service delivery using differentiated practice rely on greater nursing knowledge as the key basis for differentiating levels of practice. The image of nurses as knowledgeable professionals is evolving, albeit all too slowly. That is, the perceived power of nurses as a function of their professional knowledge is creating an increasingly positive image of nurses among members of other disciplines, such as administrators, physicians, and the public, and among nurses themselves (Kramer and Schmalenberg, 1991a, pp. 52–54).

Positional power   The client care manager's position within the organization is another source of power. This source of power is often referred to as organizational authority or **positional** power. Within centralized organizational structures, persons occupying positions near the top have greater positional power than those providing direct care. Within decentralized organizations, client care managers are gaining the positional power to provide effective care directly, including legitimate clinical decision-making authority. del Bueno referred to this type of influence as political power (del Bueno, 1986a, pp. 125). To benefit from this gain in organizational power, the client care manager must consistently use it to provide needed nursing services in a timely manner according to agency and professional standards of practice.

Personal power   Another major source of influence is **personal power** related to an individual's charactersitics. These charactersitics include appearance, verbal and nonverbal communication skills, and personality strengths. The importance of personal appearance is often communicated to nursing students by dress codes, though this is not frequently stressed as a component of personal power available for influencing others. The individual's choice of clothing, including its fit, style, and cleanliness, influences the perceptions of co-workers. It also conveys messages about the nurse's sense of self-esteem and worth. Indeed, the client care manager's appearance is an example of the use of nonverbal communication skills to influence others. Other nonverbal communication skills include eye contact, body language, facial expressions, and use of touch and silence. Such techniques can be used to communicate interest and concern for others and enthusiasm for providing needed client services.

Another aspect of personal power is the individual nurse's verbal communication skills. Using proper terminology within the health care setting is a method of communicating competence. On the other hand, use of vulgar language, though it may be common in one's personal life, has great potential for offending clients, families, and co-workers. Consequently, this type of language is avoided to enhance one's personal power. In a similar manner and for the same reasons, written documentation incorporates proper terminology. Special attention to accurate spelling, punctuation, and legibility supports a positive image of one's competence. Further, the client care manager carefully selects words that accurately describe the nurse's plans and observations and actions taken to provide care.

The personality characteristics of client care managers are important sources of personal power. Some individuals exude enthusiasm for nursing and exhibit considerable charisma in relating with others. Other nurses are soft-spoken, quiet, and focus on meeting client needs by demonstrating exemplary active listening skills. What is important is not that differences exist, but that every client care manager possesses strengths that can be used to influence others (Knippen and Green, 1990, p. 7). Each individual has personal strengths. These personality characteristics can be used to encourage others to do the right things or to do things right for clients. Focusing on these individual strengths helps identify and develop leadership skills. In this way, scarce human resources can be mobilized.

Identifying Leadership Styles and Personal Strengths

Many scientists have attempted to define leadership and delineate the characteristics of people who are effective leaders. However, a universally acceptable definition has not been found. In the context of client care management skills, **leadership** refers to the nurse's ability to get co-workers to voluntarily behave, without coercion, in desired ways. That is, to do the right things in the right way. The nurse's personal use of power enables her or him to guide, persuade, or "lead" others to perform nursing duties and activites effectively and efficiently.

Leadership style refers to the individual's pattern of relating to others or how the leader "gets along" with members of the work group. The leadership skills used to manage client care vary from nurse to nurse. The individual leadership styles of client care managers reflect the skills used by each nurse to influence co-workers to do the right things correctly.

Three common leadership styles are authoritarian or directive, democratic or participatory, and laissez faire or nondirective. No one leadership style is best. Rather, the best leadership style is the one that most effectively influences others to do the right things correctly in a specific situation.

Authoritarian or directive leadership style.   An **authoritarian** or **directive leadership style** is one in which the leader attempts to influence others though the use of positional power or organizational authority. An authoritarian leader directs others by telling them what to do and when and how to do it. This approach is usually effective in emergency situations where the client depends upon others to do the right things correctly within severe time limits. Little or no time is available for teaching, trial and error, or trying to reach a consensus among co-workers. In such circumstances, the staff nurse is obligated to be directive.

Democratic or participative leadership style.   A client care manager using a **democratic** or **participatory leadership** style seeks and uses input in making decisions that affect others. A democratic leader using a participatory leadership style encourages others to take part in establishing the policies and procedures used by the group. To the extent possible, the leader strives to make decisions by reaching a consensus based on mutual agreement of the group members. This approach is often effective in developing work schedules and assignment plans in an effort to obtain the commitment of those involved.

Laissez faire or nondirective leadership style.   The **laissez faire** or **nondirective leadership style** is characterized by a deliberate effort not to interfere or to intervene as little as possible with the activities of the work group. Though frequently criticized, this approach allows members of the work group to be flexible, self-directed, and creative in fulfilling their work responsibilities. This approach can be quite effective if members of the work group are highly skilled and self-motivated to do the right things correctly for clients. If some members of the work group are inexperienced or accustomed to directive leadership styles, they are likely to express dissatisfaction with this style. When a nondirective leadership style is used, minimally skilled members of the work group may not address client needs efficiently, relying on trial-and-error methods in the absence of adequate direction. This method makes it very difficult for minimally skilled members to meet high-priority needs in a timely manner; they may not even recognize urgent client needs. Using this leadership style with workers who are inexperienced or minimally skilled could place clients at unreasonable risk.

Being a Follower

This discussion of leadership characteristics and styles may seem daunting to a beginning nurse. The entry-level nurse might humbly question whether leadership skills can be applied by someone who has little practical experience as a client care manager. To the extent feasible, the entry-level nurse needs to avoid "mind talk" that minimizes her or his potential for leadership and to resolve to begin by developing effective follower skills. Client care managers are expected to be effective followers in many traditional nursing organizations. Being an effective follower involves being able to think for oneself and take initiative in completing work (Kelley, 1988, pp. 142–148). The box on p. 128 describes common characteristics of effective followers.

The staff nurse who strives to be an effective follower encounters opportunities to demonstrate personal strengths, knowledge, and organizational know-how and to practice leadership. Gaining experience as an effective follower is likely to prepare the staff nurse

---

Characteristics of Effective Followers

1. Demonstrate superb self-management skills
   a. Can think for themselves and know their strengths and vulnerabilities
   b. Can work independently without close supervision
   c. See themselves as equals of the leaders they follow; are apt to openly disagree with leadership unapologetically and are less likely to be intimidated by organizational structure
   d. Recognize that leaders are following the lead of others
   e. Try to appreciate the goals and needs of the team and organization
2. Demonstrate commitment to the agency's mission and goals
   a. Support leaders who are focused on the agency's goals instead of their own
   b. Are loyal to organizational needs
3. Develop competence useful to the organization
   a. Hold higher standards than are required by the work culture
   b. Value and participate in professional development activities
   c. Take on extra work after they do excellent work in completing their core responsibilities
   d. Contribute to team work
   e. View co-workers as colleagues instead of competitors
   f. Often identify problems and take initiative in presenting solutions
4. Demonstrate courage, honesty, and credibility
   a. Establish a pattern of independent critical thinking
   b. Trust their own knowledge and judgment and consequently are trusted by others
   c. Stand up for what they believe in
   d. Are insightful and open in expressing their concerns to superiors
   e. Can keep leaders and colleagues honest and informed

Adapted from Kelley RE: In praise of followers, *Harvard Bus Rev* 66:142–148, 1988.

for future nursing leadership situations. The effective follower role is often a temporary position albeit a necessary one because every leader depends on followers. That is, the beginning staff nurse, by being an effective follower of nursing leaders, frequently encounter opportunities to practice leadership skills. The formal organization depends on effective followership at the staff nurse level, which also includes use of leadership skills in managing care for a group of clients.

Some nurse leaders have articulated the need for nursing students to prepare to be effective followers when beginning their careers (Guidera and Gilmore, 1988, p. 1017; Murphy, 1990, pp. 68–69). This suggestion does not detract from the value of staff nurses. Rather, it acknowledges the need for staff nurses to function as followers to support effective leaders working toward the common goal of excellence in quality care. Effective followers can succeed without a strong leader, and they can help a leader to succeed. Both leaders and followers need to promote client focused organizational cultures. Being effective followers may well be entry-level nurses' niche in the organization while they gain experience working with effective leaders. Indeed, effective followers readily exercise leadership qualities to help others get the right things done correctly for clients. Considerable savvy and expertise are needed to follow nursing leaders effectively and not dwell on negative features of the situation or sabotage the organization. Effective followers focus on common goals: they demonstrate commitment to providing quality care to clients and to sustaining nursing as a caring profession.

PERFORMING NURSING LEADERSHIP FUNCTIONS WHILE MANAGING CLIENT CARE

Common **nursing leadership functions** performed by client care managers make use of the nursing process and corresponding clinical decision-making skills. The client care manager determines what clients need during the assigned time period within the context of long-term goals, what resources are available to achieve these goals, and how individual client outcomes can be best achieved within the resource constraints of the situation. The nurse's leadership approach incorporates both short-term and long-term client goals. Basically, the leadership functions include

1. Influencing staff to commit to individual client goals
2. Providing role modeling as a method of providing care
3. Providing feedback through constructive criticism and honest praise
4. Determining the extent of staff success in enabling clients to meet individual goals.

Motivating Co-workers to Commit to Individual Client Goals

By using power derived from nursing knowledge, organizational position, and personal attributes, client care managers contribute to the culture of the health care environment and motivate groups to identify with the results of their work. The services provided need to be consistent with the agency's mission or purposes. The desired results are satisfied customers—clients who met personal goals, which often match those established by the agency's standards of care. Client care managers use leadership skills to organize and develop the people they work with while providing quality care for clients.

Entry-level staff nurses are expected to contribute to team building (Tenzer, 1986, pp. 195, 197, 199–200). In this role, they clarify priorities to help the work group focus their efforts to meet individual client care objectives. They encourage open communication, friendliness, and an atmosphere of having fun working together. They avoid punishing staff when conflicts arise, striving instead to resolve conflicts by retaining staff commitment to common goals of client care. They use effective verbal and nonverbal communication skills when relating to members of the work group.

To help a work group resolve common problems, the client care manager focuses on individual client goals and identifies barriers to acceptable solutions (Cook and Dias, 1984, pp. 16–17). Specific communication strategies are used. For example, the nurse deliberately tries to emphasize positive gains. This approach does not mean that negative staff behaviors or client setbacks are ignored, but that communication focuses on helping staff improve care rather than stopping undesired behaviors. Another communication strategy is to describe specific behaviors and suggest alternative approaches, rather than labeling the behavior or attack the person. For example, if a staff member does not adhere to a client's plan of care, the client care manager might point this out. He or she would then follow with a discussion of reasons for carrying out the plan, rather than telling the staff member that he or she is uncooperative or hard to work with. In addition, comments about staff performance are offered frequently, privately, and as soon as appropriate to reinforce the desired behaviors. Only in urgent client situations where danger is imminent does the nurse comment on inadequate staff performance.

The client care manager actively listens to expressed staff concerns and promotes open communication among group members. Nursing assessments of client needs and the interventions used to meet them within the limitations of available resources are central to communication activities. Client care managers focus on short-term client goals while remaining mindful of those in effect for the long term. They communicate by their actions that each staff member can contribute to meeting common goals and developing an enjoyable work environment.

Serving as a Role Model

A common characteristic of nurses who positively influence co-workers is an ability to serve as **role models.** Role models consistently demonstrate positive attitudes and behaviors, such as those described in the ANA's Code for Nurses. Their actions speak louder than words. Role models use their behaviors to teach others, realizing that what they do often communicates more clearly than what they say (del Bueno, 1989, p. 100). Consequently, what role models say needs to correspond to what they do and how they do it. Role models use nursing knowledge as the basis for their clinical decisions. They make a special effort to keep up to date with current practices and perform nursing procedures according to agency criteria and legal and ethical requirements. When they recognize limitations in their nursing knowledge or skills, they seek help from others. Role models present a positive image of themselves as individuals and as competent members of the profession.

As mentioned earlier, client care managers influence their work groups by both their verbal messages and nonverbal behaviors. By deliberately serving as examples, they communicate their expectations to co-workers. Both client care managers as leaders, and their followers, need feedback to determine their effectiveness. As leaders, client care managers soon "get the message" if their followers do not perform their work in desired ways. Without followers, client care managers are not leaders. Followers follow voluntarily, which explains why follower responses and feedback strongly influence leadership behavior. If a leader's influence does not lead to the desired responses, the leader should seek feedback from co-workers. Most nursing leaders actively seek feedback from their work groups to help them evaluate staff perceptions. Using the feedback enables them to continue to lead effectively.

Seeking and Providing Feedback

Client care managers complete communication processes by regularly informally **providing feedback** to the work group. The primary purpose of feedback is to help co-workers improve client care. Feedback is based upon observations of client responses and staff behaviors. Formal feedback is typically given at infrequent intervals to meet agency requirements for employee performance evaluation. Informal feedback provided in various ways helps co-workers meet client care objectives. For example, the nurse might communicate the feedback in face-to-face conversation or written messages or by encouraging co-workers to openly communicate directly with each other. Effective feedback is specific and descriptive rather than judgmental of the individual as a person. Feedback is generally more effective when it is given promptly after the behaviors are observed. It needs to be clearly stated in words the co-worker can readily understand. Too much feedback at one time can be overwhelming and threatening to the co-worker. The client care manager also avoids providing feedback that is likely to humiliate, demean, or embarrass co-workers. Effective feedback relates specifically to client care and the specific behaviors of co-workers.

Informal feedback is usually interpreted as either criticism or praise (Simpkin, 1991, pp. 4–5). The client care manager's pattern of providing feedback needs to include both. The type of feedback given depends upon the co-worker's behavior and its effects on client care. Generally, praise is given to reward desired behavior while criticism is provided to suggest alternatives believed to result in more desired behavior.

Using Nursing Process Skills to Help Co-workers Evaluate Their Effectiveness

As mentioned earlier, client care managers help co-workers clarify and comprehend individual client goals. Co-workers are reasonably expected to work toward helping clients meet these goals. Obviously, this leadership function requires that the client care manager direct staff or clearly communicate expectations of co-workers, as well as nursing plans and the strategies to carry them out. Throughout the workday, client care managers seek feedback from co-workers and assess client responses. This information is used to determine which goals clients met and which require further staff effort. Client care managers treat co-workers as important members of the group and share responsibility for the care provided. An integral client care management leadership function is to **evaluate** the **success** of the nursing work group. In this way, they share successes and rewards with co-workers when client outcomes are met. More specific nursing strategies used to supervise and evaluate the work of co-workers are presented in Chapter Eleven.

■ USING CRITICISM AND PRAISE TO STRENGTHEN COWORKERS' CAREGIVING BEHAVIORS

Client care managers are expected to contribute to a high level of morale among co-workers and to maintain co-workers' motivation to provide high-quality client care. How they accomplish these results depends upon their effective use of leadership skills. Client care managers need to creatively communicate perceptions of co-worker behaviors in a sensitive and tactful manner. The purpose of the communications is of paramount importance, whether the feedback is in the form of criticism or praise.

Providing Constructive Criticism

Client care managers are expected to provide constructive **criticism** to co-workers. Though many hesitate to constructively criticize the behaviors of co-workers, they can learn to do so with skill and thus contribute to effective team building. Before giving feedback about a co-worker's behavior, the manager needs to remember that its primary purpose is to help the individual provide better client care. If the feedback is given in such a way that it labels the behavior of the person, it is likely to be resented. If the criticism is obviously given in a spirit of helpfulness, it is more likely to be heard and accepted.

Prior to criticizing a co-worker's behavior, the client care manager should observes the individual's demeanor for signs of frustration and examines herself or himself for signs of hurry or upset. Any criticism given when either party is under stress is less likely to motivate the co-worker to make desired changes in behavior. Feedback given or received when either person is not ready is less likely to be interpreted accurately.

It is important to learn the facts surrounding the co-worker's behavior, which help identify situational factors contributing to the behavior. Factual information also helps to determine which factors were under the co-worker's control and which were not. Insight into the situation surrounding an inadequate performance can help the client care manager suggest reasonable and realistic alternative approaches. Drawing hasty conclusions about what happened or criticizing the co-worker's attitude should be avoided.

The client care manager considers alternative possible causes for a co-worker's inadequate work performance. As discussed earlier, the co-worker may be motivated by common human developmental needs as well as norms and values reinforced by the work group culture. The client care manager encourages the co-worker to describe his or her perceptions of the situation and makes suggestions as to possible improvements. Frequently, the individual brings up important points that the client care manager was unaware of. The approach also allows the individual to "save face" and maintain a sense of self-worth. Often the co-worker can point out negative aspects of the behavior in question and suggest appropriate changes.

A key component of providing constructive criticism to most co-workers is to use a friendly approach and actively listen (Luke, 990, p. 7). For example, the co-worker might simply be asked, "What happened?" The client care manager seeks clarification when the co-worker's statements or suggestions are unclear, at the same time conveying confidence in the co-worker's ability to make the needed changes. In addition, the client care manager needs to give reasons for the desired changes using behavioral terms. For example, instead of saying, "You frustrate people," the client care manager might say, "Have you tried giving clients plenty of time to follow your directions? Some people feel very frustrated when they're best efforts aren't fast enough." This assures that the co-worker's behavior is not a consequence of a lack of information about staff expectations.

To avoid giving criticism that results in embarrassing, demeaning, or threatening the co-worker, the client care manager carefully decides when and where to give it. As mentioned, both parties need to be calm enough to hear and accurately comprehend what is communicated. Anxiety or anger diminishes the likelihood of such comprehension. Unless a client's safety is at immediate risk, criticism of the co-worker's behavior needs to be offered in private. This reduces both the potential for embarrassment and the likelihood that the criticism will be interpreted as a form of punishment. Often the criticism is stated after opening with a genuine compliment or description of the co-worker's typical performance, to preserve the individual's feelings of competence and self-confidence (Pollock, 1971, pp. 47–48). Such an approach often prepares the co-worker to listen carefully to the constructive criticism.

The purpose of constructive criticism is to prevent the recurrence of particular behaviors, to strengthen what the co-worker is doing appropriately, and to promote the desired changes for the proper reasons—because the desired behavior is the right thing to do for clients, not merely because one wants to avoid punishment. The box on p. 133 lists key considerations for giving constructive criticism and features to avoid to effectively provide this type of feedback.

Giving Praise to Build Co-worker Strengths

It is a curious phenomenon that **praise,** which is a very powerful reward and fun to give, is infrequently offered. Praise is a strong motivator because it addresses the common human need for recognition and approval (Luke, 1991, p. 3). The purpose of giving praise is to reward desired work performance. Client care managers are encouraged to use several strategies when praising co-workers to build on their strengths. Every member of the work group has strengths worthy of honest recognition.

Often, client care managers hesitate to praise a co-worker's performance because they believe it is common to the work group and want to avoid the appearance of favoritism. Generally, everyone who deserves praise should receive it. Perhaps the praise could be

Providing Constructive Criticism

1. Remember that the primary purpose of constructive criticism is to improve client care.
2. Select a time that corresponds to the needs of both the giver and the receiver.
3. Learn about the circumstances surrounding the co-worker's behavior.
4. Distinguish situational factors under the co-worker's control from those that are not.
5. Suggest reasonable alternative behaviors.
6. Actively listen to the co-worker's suggestions for change.
7. Use a friendly approach to communicate confidence in the co-worker's abilities.
8. Explain reasons for the suggested changes in behavior.

given in a group setting, where it is more likely to be fairly distributed. On the other hand, an individual co-worker's work might be recognized in private or in the group, depending upon the nature of the performance and its value within the organizational culture. In any event, praise needs to be given frequently to assure that good work is never taken for granted.

Praise, like criticism, is necessarily based in fact. Frequently, a manager's attention to

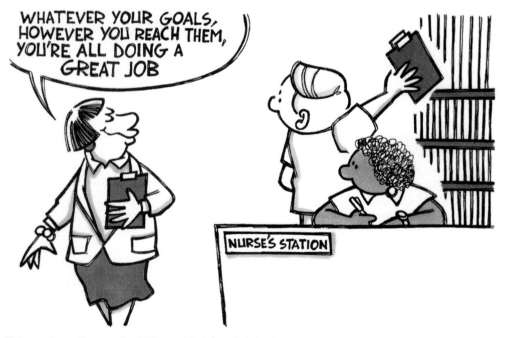

False praise or flattery should be avoided since it is insincere.

details of complex client care situations and staff responses to them provides numerous opportunities for honest praise. Staff members are likely to be aware of their unique talents and strengths and use them routinely. Though seemingly commonplace, creative responses to client needs should be recognized to assure their repetition. If use of unique talents and strengths is not rewarded, it is less likely to be used, to the detriment of clients.

False praise or flattery should be avoided since it is insincere. In addition, it is often given to gain something rather than to reward desired behaviors. Flattery is likely to offend coworkers, rather than motivate them to continue to do good work.

Praise is a very effective leadership tool when offered honestly and in such a manner that it increases workers' self-esteem. It can be a powerful reward, and it is far less costly than wage or salary increases. It has rarely, if ever, been overused in heatlh care environments, where cost effectiveness is often the preoccupation. Praise is a communication skill that can frequently be used to strengthen creative use of individual talents.

Recently, the importance of rewarding special achievement as a method of helping positive work cultures evolve has been recognized (Trofino, 1987, pp. 11–12). Methods of communicating approval throughout the work organization are needed to reward the numerous effective responses made to meet client needs. Many new challenges depend on creativity as well as effective clinical decision making on behalf of quality client care. Wouldn't it be fun to work in a setting where praise is given by and to co-workers as frequently as it is given to nursing staff by clients and families they serve?

SUMMARY

Effective staff nurses manage others creatively by emphasizing their own talents, strengths, and interests and those of their co-workers. To help manage this process they can apply human development theories to gain insight into the motivations and behaviors of co-workers. These theories help to identify common continuities and changes that occur during adulthood.

The organizational culture also influences staff behavior. Sensitivity to the norms, values, and expectations of the work group culture helps the entry-level staff nurse make the adjustments needed to succeed as a client care manager. Understanding the background development of the organization helps the staff nurse predict future growth and changes.

Entry-level staff nurses can use personal strengths, positional authority, and nursing knowledge as sources of power within the work environment to help the team provide needed nursing care for the assigned group of clients. They also need to adapt their leadership styles to fit the nursing situation. Often, staff nurses assume the role of effective followers to practice leadership skills and to support the organization and its leaders.

Common staff nurse leadership functions include motivating co-workers to make a commitment to individual client goals, serving as a role model, seeking and providing feedback, and contributing to team building. Staff are encouraged to give praise and constructive criticism honestly, in a timely and tactful manner. Praise is an inexpensive tool that staff nurses can give to reward effective staff efforts and desired behaviors.

APPLICATION EXERCISES

a. Interview a co-worker. Identify the individual's stage of human development by reviewing her or his biological, psychological, and social continuities and changes over the last ten years.

b. Describe the nursing work group culture by answering the questions suggested by Coeling.

c. Identify the predominant leadership style you most frequently use to influence your nursing peers. Describe your sources of power.

d. A co-worker's comments to a client about another colleague (in your presence) casts doubt on the colleague's competence. State what you would you do, where and how.

e. The morale of your nursing work group is slipping somewhat. Members express feeling overworked, underpaid, and unappreciated. Describe what you would do to help without increasing financial costs.

REFERENCES

Blancett SS: Human development renaissance, *J Nurs Adm* 20(7/8):4–5, (July/August, 1990).

Coeling HV: Organizational culture: helping new graduates adjust, *Nurse Educ* 15(2):26–30. (March/April, 1990).

Cooke PC, Dias D: Teambuilding: getting it all together, *Nurs Manage* 15(2):16–17. (May, 1984).

Curtin LL: Creating a culture of competence, *Nurs Manage* 21(9):7–8. (September, 1990).

del Bueno D: Power and politics in organizations, *Nurs Outlook* 34(3):124–128. (May/June, 1986a).

del Bueno DJ: Organizational culture: how important is it? *J Nurs Adm* 16(10):15–20. (October, 1986b).

del Bueno D: Our actions drown out our words, *RN* 32(8) August:100, 1989.

Ehrat KS: Leadership in transition, *J Nurs Adm* 20(10):6–7. (October, 1990).

Gorman S, Clark N: Power and effective nursing practice, Nurs Outlook 34(3):129–134. (May/June, 1986).

Greiner LE: Evolution and revolution as organizations grow, *Harvard Bus Rev* 50(4):37–46. (July-August, 1972).

Guidera MK, Gilmore C: In defense of followership, *Am J Nurs* 88(7):1017. (July, 1988).

Hannan MT, Freeman J: *Organizational ecology,* Cambridge, Mass, 1989, Harvard University Press.

Hick CR, Silva MA: *Creating excellence: managing corporate culture, strategy, and change in the new age,* New York, 1984, New American Library.

Jameton A: Culture, morality, and ethics, *Crit Care Nurs Clin North Am* 2(3):443–451. (September, 1990).

Kelly RE: In praise of followers, *Harvard Bus Rev* 66:142–148. (November-December, 1988).

Knippen JT, Green TB: Reinforcing the right behavior, *Supervis Manage* 35(4) April: 7, 1990.

Kotter JP: What leaders really do, *Harvard Bus Rev* 68:103–111. (May-June, 1990).

Kramer M, Schmalenberg C: Job satisfaction and retention: insights for the '90s, *Nurs 91* (3):50–55. (March, 1991a).

Kramer M, Schmalenberg C: Job satisfaction and retention: insights for the '90s, Part 2, *Nurs 91* (4):51–55. (April, 1991b).

Luke RA: How to give corrective feedback to employees, *Supervis Manage* 35(3) March: 7, 1990.

Luke RA: Meaningful praise makes a difference, *Supervis Manage* 36(2) February: 3, 1991.

Manthey M: Nursing: an ecological perspective, *Nurs Manage* 21(8):16–17. (August, 1990).

Manthey M: Three simple rules, *Nurs Manage* 21(12):19–20. (December, 1990).

Murphy D: Followers for a new era, *Nurs Manage* 21(7):68–69. (July, 1990).

Patz JM, Biordi DL, Holm K: Middle nurse manager effectiveness, *J Nurs Adm* 21(1):15–24 (January, 1991).

Peters TJ, Waterman RH: *In search of excellence,* New York, 1982, Warner.

Pollock T: *Managing others creatively,* New York, 1971, Hawthorn Books.

Simpkin GD: Getting your staff to do what you want, *Supervis Manage* January: 4–5, 1991.

Smith MM: Getting ahead in the corporate culture, *Am J Nurs* 87(4): 514–515 (April, 1987).

Tenzer I: Team building, *AORN J* 43(1):195, 197, 199–200. (January, 1986).

Trofino J: Shaping the environment for professional nursing practice, *Nurs Adm Q* 11(4):11–12. (Summer 1987).

chapter ten

COORDINATING AN INTERDISCIPLINARY TEAM

Completing this chapter will enable you to:

1. Describe the interdisciplinary team as an organizational resource.
2. Describe principles used to promote effective working relationships within the interdisciplinary team.
3. Describe barriers to interdisciplinary team effectiveness.
4. Describe the duties of the client care manager in coordinating the efforts of the interdisciplinary team.
5. Describe principles of coordinating the priorities of the interdisciplinary health team.

interdependencies

interdisciplinary team

cooperation

collaboration

organizational provisions

   common language

   mission statement

   structured time and place

interdisciplinary team goals

client priorities

role conflict

value nursing contributions

work culture of interdisciplinary team

principles for promoting effective working relationships

barriers

interdisciplinary team priorities

THE INTERDISCIPLINARY TEAM AS AN ORGANIZATIONAL RESOURCE

With the increasing emphasis on managing information in the evolving health care arena, nurses are becoming more interdependent with other members of the health team. **Interdependencies** require members of different disciplines to rely on each other to meet individual client needs effectively and efficiently. Nurses are learning that "We can't know it all and we can't do it all" (Carroll, 1987, p. 43). This realization reflects the need for health care organizations to support the work of **interdisciplinary teams.** Such teams are composed of members of several disciplines providing services to individual clients. This chapter describes staff nurse participation on interdisciplinary health teams within the context of the client care manager's role as a coordinator of such group efforts.

Client care managers coordinate nursing staff efforts to satisfy clients' nursing needs. Because of their pivotal position within the health care organization, they also coordinate the efforts of members of the interdisciplinary health team. This coordinating function of client care managers requires staff nurses to understand the priority needs of individual clients, the agency resources available to meet them, and the process the organization uses to meet them effectively and efficiently. Client care managers must also understand why client's priority needs change throughout the treatment process. For example, early in a client's hospitalization, respiratory therapy might be needed to satisfy needs for adequate ventilation and to prevent complications. Later, physical therapy might be the highest priority to maximize mobility. Still later, discharge planning activities might involve a variety of disciplines to enable the client to live at home with a chronic health problem. Background knowledge of this type enables client care managers to anticipate evolving client care activities and helps them organize the interdisciplinary team's efforts to complete them.

Coordinating the diverse efforts of the interdisciplinary team requires skills in human relations and group work. Not only do individual client needs change from day to day, but the composition of the interdisciplinary team is often in a state of flux as well. The culture of the health care team strongly influences what members expect of each other, who makes clinical decisions, how clinical decisions are made, and how treatment programs are carried out. Obviously, each culture reflects what the health team members perceive as their overall purpose and goals and how they are rewarded for success in their endeavors. Coordinating interdisciplinary efforts provides staff nurses with numerous opportunities to influence the work culture and the quality of care clients receive on a daily basis.

Effective health teams are very valuable resources. Without them, the agency typically cannot efficiently provide quality care. Client care managers play a key role in their success. Persistently trying to organize seeming chaos into goal-directed activities on behalf of clients is an arduous, demanding nursing function. Many client care managers learn to perform coordinating duties more effectively as they gain experience as a member of the work group. They also learn about the interpersonal dynamics involved in team building.

Identifying the Interdisciplinary Team as an Organizational Resource

Many health care organizations, though not all, divide the work of client care along functional or departmental lines. Consequently, each discipline is formally organized as a unit or department with its own policies and procedures. These should be consistent with the agency's overall philosophy, purposes, policies, and procedures. Each member of the interdisciplinary team has a primary identification with and commitment to a specific discipline and its knowledge, values, and skills. Each discipline's routines, which reflect its contributions to client care, guide its members in carrying out their functions and duties. The disciplinary routines of staff nurses entail complying with therapy schedules, providing feedback, and answering requests for specific follow-through on treatment programs.

Cooperation and **collaboration** are key to interdisciplinary team work. Staff nurses enable clients to adhere to varying schedules and respond to requests to maximize client benefits from services received. As individual client needs change in response to treatment, interdisciplinary team members need to communicate and collaborate with each other to

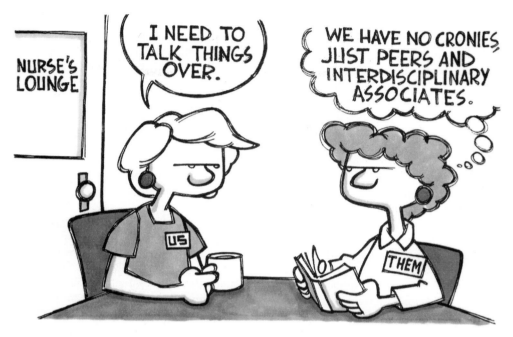

The more complex the organization, the more likely interdisciplinary conflict is to occur.

assure that priority needs are addressed. If communication and collaboration with the interdisciplinary team are inadequate, conflict occurs and the quality of client care suffers. The larger and more complex the organization's work force, the more likely interdisciplinary conflict is to occur (Guy, 1986, pp. 111–121) unless deliberate efforts are made to avoid it.

Due to the interdependencies of various professions, many health care organizations make several different types of **organizational provisions** to enable their interdisciplinary teams to address evolving client needs in an efficient and effective manner. Most disciplines use unique knowledge bases and language to support their work. Consequently, to work together, the interdisciplinary team needs a **common language.** At times, the same word or abbreviation has different meanings in different disciplines. For example, mg means "milligrams" to RNs, MDs, and pharmacists, while it might mean "muscle groups" to physical, occupational, and recreational therapists. If confusion of this sort is not clarified, errors or conflict can result.

In addition, effective interdisciplinary teams need a commonly understood overall goal or mission to guide them in setting priorities and identifying roles and responsibilities to clients within a specific setting. The **mission statement,** which defines the organization's unique purpose, reflects the group's overall goals. It guides team effort toward accomplishing their most important purpose. Team commitment to the mission also helps members to identify with each other and as a meaningful group within the agency (Weiss, 1990, p. 5). As a group, members share the team's success and accept responsibility for its lack of success. The group identifies areas where it can improve its performance as a whole. The members are more likely to reach client care goals as a team than they would be as individuals.

The organization's mission, as understood by members of the interdisciplinary team, guides the team's effort. To do so, the mission needs to promote a positive culture of working together. That is, as the group works together, norms or mutual expectations need to evolve that support an atmosphere in which interdisciplinary team members mutually respect each other and the team as a whole. Such an atmosphere promotes open communication among members, including free expression of opinions and active listening. Interdisciplinary team members need to be encouraged to consult, collaborate, and evaluate team efforts without fear of retaliation. Unless a specific effort is made to develop positive working relationships, they are likely to be replaced by less effective interpersonal relationships. In a work atmosphere that promotes team building, members are more likely to trust and believe in each other and in what each discipline can contribute to the team's efforts in meeting individual client needs. As such, interdisciplinary teams offer staff nurses opportunities to practice their leadership skills.

Another important requirement of an effective interdisciplinary team is a **structured meeting time and place.** Health care organizations need to provide meeting times and places for their interdisciplinary teams to communicate and collaborate (Moulder, Staal, and Grant, 1988, p. 339). These regularly scheduled and structured conferences are in addition to the day-to-day episodic interactions that occur while members of the interdisciplinary team provide care. Providing for meetings encourages the team to discuss concerns and individual treatment responses to promote efficiency in addressing changes in client needs in a consistent and timely manner. Frequently, organizational support also includes developing staffing patterns that allow interdisciplinary team members to work together

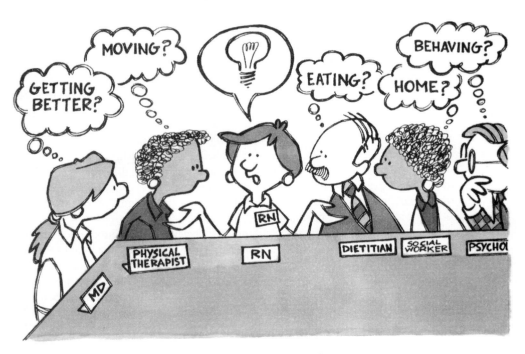

Effective communication is very important to the interdisciplinary team.

long enough to clarify roles and expectations and to become familiar with the common routines of the involved disciplines.

Another common provision made by health care organizations committed to effective interdisciplinary teams involves allocating resources so that team members can share information. This enhances personal effectiveness in ways that would be difficult through individual effort alone. Sharing of knowledge of skills among team members often increases the value and credibility of the team. Sometimes, sharing expertise might entail continuing education programs and in-service orientation programs. By collaborating with each other, members of the team promote each other's success and the view that the team is an organizational resource. A work environment or culture that rewards open communication and sharing of individual knowledge and skills also promotes creativity in addressing individual client needs.

Health care organizations use valuable staff time and human resources to support interdisciplinary teams. It costs the agency money to provide time for team members to meet, confer, share, plan, and evalute the extent of their success. Effective interdisciplinary teams and team-building efforts reflect the organization's priorities in providing client care. As such, they are valuable organizational resources.

Comparing the Agency's Mission with Interdisciplinary Team Goals

A health care agency's goals are likely to be stated in broad, general terms in a mission statement, as described earlier in this chapter. **Interdisciplinary team goals,** on the other hand, reflect the special needs of the clients they serve and the knowledge and skills needed to meet them. Interdisciplinary team goals concern specific individual client needs and activities.

The goals of the interdisciplinary team must be consistent with the agency's purposes and goals. If they are not, conflict is likely to result, and the team might not reach its goals due to lack of organizational support in the form of time, staffing, equipment, or supplies. To avoid unnecessary conflict, the health care agency needs to communicate changes in its mission in a timely manner. Subsequently, the interdisciplinary team can incorporate these changes into their goals and activities to avoid conflict and frustration.

Valuing the Contributions of Each Discipline

Due to the complexity of modern health care, every client is likely to use the resources of an interdisciplinary team. Health problems that require care in an institutional setting are likely to require care from several disciplines. The composition of the interdisciplinary team corresponds to the type and complexity of services needed. For example, a client requiring primarily diagnostic services is likely to interact with a different group of professionals than a client who is receiving rehabilitation for a chronic health problem or one receiving supportive care for a terminal illness.

Client priorities also shape the contributions made by various disciplines. No single discipline or member of the health team always provides first-priority care for all clients. Rather, the desired outcomes mutually agreed upon by the individual client, family, and staff are used to identify priorities and organize the team's efforts. Priorities determine how the client spends time in the health care setting and how each discipline contributes to the client's well-being. Obviously, the interplay of all these variables can cause confusion and **role conflicts** (incompatible or inconsistent expectations between interdisciplinary team members).

To avoid role conflict as evidenced by gaps or overlap in services provided, each member of the interdisciplinary team needs to understand what is expected of him or her and what can reasonably be expected of members of other disciplines. These expectations are usually determined by the primary characteristics of the client's situation, which include type of setting, nature of client needs, individual member's perceptions of the potential contributions of his or her discipline, and how these perceptions are communicated to other members of the interdisciplinary team. In specialized settings, such as those focusing on psychiatric or rehabilitation services, different disciplines are available than in general hospitals or typical long-term care settings, where interdisciplinary teams are more traditional. Typical acute care settings usually provide more extensive diagnostic services than long-term care settings. In addition, communication among members of the interdisciplinary team is complicated by the fact that it occurs in various ways—face-to-face, by telephone, through automated information systems, or by written request forms.

Who does what depends on the combination of disciplines in an interdisciplinary team and the client's needs. The individual member of a specific discipline may determine what is appropriate. For example, some physical therapists assist clients with exercises to strengthen upper extremities. Others might refer such clients to other disciplines, such as occupational therapy. Some activity therapists might become centrally involved in developing spiritual programs, while others might assume a supportive role in such programs.

Since it is staff nurses who frequently spend the most time with clients on a twenty-four hour basis, they usually are expected to coordinate interdisciplinary team efforts. To do this, they use knowledge of the client's needs and goals, of the composition of the interdisciplinary team, and of the special skills and talents of members of the work group.

Staff nurses need to **value their nursing contributions** to the interdisciplinary team as well as efforts made by other disciplines. Many nursing students learn about the common contributions of various health disciplines early in their careers. Less frequently they gain experience as a member of an interdisciplinary team that would help to gain insight into the dynamics of such group work. Later, as entry-level staff nurses managing client care, they learn about special skills and contributions of individual members of the interdisciplinary team. With a cooperative spirit, they need to openly communicate and collaborate with other team members in an effort to meet specific, more complex client needs. By following through on identified special needs of clients, and communicating concerns to other disciplines, effective teams are built. Members learn to value each other's contributions while improving the quality of care clients receive.

PROMOTING EFFECTIVE WORKING RELATIONSHIPS ON THE INTERDISCIPLINARY TEAM

Client care managers are expected to promote effective working relationships on the interdisciplinary team. Persistent effort is needed to develop and sustain such relationships. As coordinator of interdisciplinary efforts, the client care manager has numerous opportunities to practice leadership skills aimed at contributing to team building.

As mentioned earlier, each member of the interdisciplinary team needs a clear idea of the group's overall purpose to give meaning to their work. This principle emphasizes the importance of the group's goals and need for a language commonly understood by its members. Client care managers must not assume that everyone knows why the group exists and what it is expected of its members. To do so is to invite conflict. By actively listening to the interactions of team members, the client care manager can identify differences in individual perceptions of the group's overall goals. Such differences need to be clarified to avoid conflict within the group. As discussed in Chapter 9, Coeling (1990, pp. 26–30) described five major categories of information that new graduates might use to analyze their work group cultures to help them adjust their practice to the norms and expectations of a specific nursing setting. The box below gives a similar list of group characteristics that nurses might use to analyze the **work culture of the interdisciplinary team.** Analyzing these factors will also help new graduates adjust their personal behaviors to the interdisciplinary team.

Each member of the interdisciplinary team needs to feel that he or she contributes to helping the group meet its goals. This need may seem obvious, but it can be difficult to achieve. Historically, nurses have struggled for professional autonomy, perhaps at the risk

---

Questions to Ask to Understand the Work Culture of the Interdisciplinary Team

Team emphasis: physiological or mental and emotional client needs

Does the team consider it more important to address a client's physiological or mental and emotional needs first?
How important is it to the team to be organized and efficient?
Does the team focus on the client's point of view and respect the client's values?

Team dynamics: use of power by individual members

Does the group's coordinator use a more autocratic or democratic leadership style?
Who can tell members what to do?
Are some members more influential than others? If so, what is the source of their influence?

Team spirit: collaboration or rivalry

Does a member or the whole group tend to decide what the interdisciplinary plan is for individual clients?
Do members tend to work alone to carry out their respective interventions?
How acceptable is it to compete with other members?

Team building: rewards and discipline

Do members tend to criticize each other directly or indirectly?
Do members receive constructive criticism publicly or privately?
How are team efforts reinforced? By whom?

Team fashions: tradition or creative change

Do members tend to value and stick to doing things in customary ways or get excited about learning and applying new approaches?
How important is it to follow policies and procedures?
To what extent do members feel there is one right way to do things?

Modified from Coeling H: Organizaitonal culture: helping new graduates adjust, *Nurse Educ* 15(2):27, 1990.

of decreased collaboration with others, especially physicians. More recently, consistent with existing interdependencies, nurses are appropriately emphasizing cooperation and collaboration as goals for interacting with interdisciplinary team members (Marsden, 1990, pp. 422–424). Rather than competing with each other, interdisciplinary members need to determine priorities of care with client and families, and then plan how best to address them as a team. Though sometimes difficult to measure, the discipline's contribution to a client's care affects the plan's success meeting desired outcomes. A discipline's authority to make decisions is not synonymous with the value of its contribution to client well-being. Rather, the group emphasizes the contributions of participating disciplines to efficiently carry out an effective care plan.

The interdisciplinary team needs relevant, accurate, consistent, and constructive feedback about its success in meeting client goals. As mentioned in Chapter Nine, feedback helps the work group judge its effectiveness and identify areas needing further development. This feedback consists of factual information relating to the specific goals of individual clients. To be most effective, feedback needs to be timely and to be given in such a manner that it is readily understood by all team members. Through its form and style, it rewards positive behaviors while helping the group to avoid unproductive effort. Team members rarely tire of hearing about their successes when they are described accurately and sincerely.

The interdisciplinary team is strengthened when positive behaviors are recognized—that is, when desired efforts toward the group's goals are rewarded. Rather than commenting, "You did a good job," one might say, "Your careful monitoring of M.T.'s discomfort helped her to avoid a serious reaction to the antibiotic." This is not to imply that group activities are not aimed at improving team performance (Weisberg, Grandin, and Pack, 1989, p. 87), but that it is important to regularly acknowledge specific team efforts that promote the group's success. More generally, open communication and expression of opinions free the group's creativity to identify healthy conflict within the group and identify new solutions. Using this creativity, the group may be able to solve old problems within the system that were interpreted earlier as individual performance problems.

Developing mutual respect and effective collaboration among interdisciplinary team members is a very complex process. Each discipline's unique knowledge base evolves in response to changing client needs, and the discipline's members are likely to be the most knowledgeable about these changes. Entry-level staff nurses need to acquaint themselves with interdisciplinary team members as individuals. They need to appreciate others' special interests in responding to various client needs. Members of the team often need to be encouraged to seek help regularly from each other. Sharing special knowledge and skills promotes mutual respect, trust, and appreciation of the value of each other's contributions, which increases the value of the team's expertise. Such an approach also permits individual members to recognize limitations without risking a client's well-being. With the information explosion and the variety of interests pursued by individual members of interdisciplinary teams, sharing knowledge and skills needs to become an established norm in the work cultures of health care organizations, instead of being perceived as ego trips. The new knowledge and skill are likely to benefit clients and increase individual team member confidence and morale.

The opposite of seeking help is offering it. Most disciplines are willing to offer constructive help to each other. This sharing is likely to persist when team members trust each other and expect colleagues to receive help, without taking offense, when the goal is to improve the quality of client care. In such a work environment, offering help is likely to pro-

Principles for Promoting Effective Working Relationships on Interdisciplinary Teams

1. Each member has a clear idea of the group's overall purpose, which gives meaning to the team's work.
2. Each member feels that he or she makes valued contributions to help the team meet its goals.
3. The team receives relevant, accurate, timely, and constructive feedback about its success in meeting its goals.
4. Team effort is rewarded, that is, desired behaviors are reinforced.
5. Members are encouraged to seek help regularly.
6. Members are encouraged to offer help willingly.

mote self-esteem and appreciation of the contributions of other disciplines. Of course, sensitivity and tact are needed, as in all communications used to promote effective working relationships. The box above summarizes **principles for promoting effective working relationships** on interdisciplinary teams. The box below summarizes some "tried-and-true" approaches conducive to positive working relationships.

Overall, strategies for working effectively with an interdisciplinary group require staff nurses to demonstrate the value of nursing knowledge and skills by using them with confidence (Coker and Schrieber, 1990, pp. 46–48). This encourages other members of the health team to respect nursing contributions as well. In addition, by seeking to clarify the roles and expectations of various other members of the health team, staff nurses can learn

Core Communications for Team Building

The SIX most important words:
"I APPRECIATE YOUR TRYING TO HELP"

The FIVE most important words:
"YOU DID A NICE JOB"

The FOUR most important words:
"WHAT IS YOUR RECOMMENDATION?"

The THREE most important words:
"IF YOU PREFER"

The TWO most important words:
"THANK YOU"

THE MOST IMPORTANT WORD:
"WE"

about the special knowledge and skills used in other disciplines to care for clients. By reinforcing positive behaviors such as seeking and offering help, each member of the interdisciplinary team can maximize the effective use of available interdisciplinary knowledge and skills on behalf of clients.

BARRIERS TO INTERDISCIPLINARY TEAM EFFECTIVENESS

Given the complexities of client care and the variety of disciplines, work cultures, and individual personalities involved, it is not surprising that the interdisciplinary team is sometimes unsuccessful. Considerable potential for conflict exists. Eliminating interdisciplinary teams is not an option; the interdependencies of the various disciplines involved in providing health care are likely to continue or increase in the future. Every discipline shares responsibility for enhancing interdisciplinary cooperation for the benefit of clients. Thus, the skills needed to resolve interpersonal conflict, as described in Chapter Six, are very useful for team members.

The ability to identify common **barriers** to interdisciplinary team effectiveness helps the client care manager improve the team's effectiveness. Since an interdisciplinary team is an expensive agency resource, its effectiveness merits thoughtful nurturing. Sometimes a health care agency bears the expense of an interdisciplinary team without adequately evaluating the benefits clients derive from it. The health care agency and individual members of the group share responsibility for the team's success. While coordinating the team's efforts and acting as client advocates, client care managers are often aware of missed opportunities. By being aware of barriers to the teams' effectiveness, the staff nurse is in a good position to nurture the group's success.

In the hectic, stress-filled health care work environment, clients often feel extremely vulnerable. Health care workers try to do the best they can with the resources they have. In such an environment, the care actually received by clients is fragmented and lacks focus even though the health team is highly motivated and skilled. Often, if the health team has not worked together for long, the group senses the need for common goals. Unless the group has sufficient time and a place to meet and share concerns, it suffers from a lack of direction. Unless the agency's mission and overall interdisciplinary team goals are clear, its members often continue pursuing their respective disciplines' goals for clients. Each discipline is intent upon providing the best care possible, but without an overall perspective from the client's point of view. As a result, priorities of care are often not identified. Clarification of the agency's mission or values can help to identify barriers of this sort.

Each discipline is likely to observe the client in a slightly different situation. Different disciplines' approaches and treatment methods lead to different perceptions of the client's suitability and responses to treatment (Hodes and Crombrugghe, 1990, pp. 73–75). To the client, these varying expectations may appear to be in conflict, when in fact they may merely represent the different interpretations of health team members. Sometimes, past experiences influence the values and attitudes of individual members of the health care team toward specific client situations. For example, a client experiencing difficulty controlling bowel elimination, might be prematurely omitted from scheduled speech therapy sessions away from the nursing unit to avoid embarrassing "accidents." At the same time, other disciplines might have made special effort to adjust their interventions to enable the client to attend, given that speech therapy is a high priority. The client is likely to experience frustration and difficulty in expressing it to the team. The team needs to communicate with each other, including the client to avoid being distracted from its priorities. Consequently,

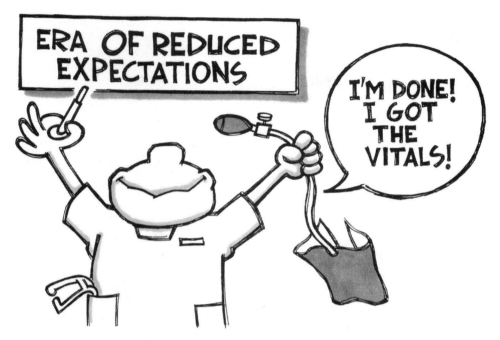

In the hectic, stress-filled health care work environment, the care received by clients is often fragmented, even though the health care team is highly motivated and skilled.

a special effort is needed to clarify goals, approaches, expectations, and values to enable the health team to meet individual health care needs in a timely manner. When conflicts arise, it is critical to analyze the situation, rather than attempt to fix blame on specific team members.

As the technology evolves to permit the rapid transmission of information, health care workers will be confronted with the challenge of keeping up with current knowledge in their discipline. The need for a common language is likely to increase to meet these information needs. The specific detailed information required to address a client's situation is often available only through automated systems (Swenson-Feldman and Brugge-Wiger, 1985, pp. 44–46). Staff nurses are expected to use automated systems to document care so that members of all disciplines have access to current information regarding client needs. Special effort is needed to communicate current information in a common language so that it is accessible to all disciplines.

An effective health team knows who is expected to carry out each part of the care plan for every client. Without a current written plan of care, avoiding overlaps and gaps in care is difficult and evaluating the effectiveness of the team's contributions and the plan in general is nearly impossible. To prevent overlaps and gaps, each member of the interdisciplinary team must know what the plan is and what is expected of team members from each discipline. As technology evolves and knowledge bases expand, continued effort is needed to clarify the various roles of each discipline on the health team. Identification of individual client priority needs helps each discipline to anticipate what contribution it might make toward enabling the client to meet desired outcomes.

Marked differences in personality can interfere with interdisciplinary team effectiveness, but this type of barrier may be less common than is often thought. Before attributing the cause of the team's ineffectiveness to "personality conflicts," it is sound practice to first ensure that other types of barriers are not at fault. As the team focuses on individual client goals and establishes effective communication processes to meet them, the norms of the work culture are likely to help members focus on major issues and concerns that interfere with the group's work instead of on individual idiosyncracies.

If the individual idiosyncracies of members of the team continue to result in interpersonal conflict, they need to be resolved using the suggestions discussed in Chapter Six. No one is expected to change his or her personality. Rather, each member involved in the conflict is expected to try to change behaviors in an effort to provide quality client care in a responsible manner.

PRIORITIES OF THE INTERDISCIPLINARY HEALTH TEAM

As the cost of health care escalates and the acuity of client health conditions rises, care during illness becomes more complex. The interdependencies of the health team also increase. Clients depend on their care givers to respond to their urgent needs in an effective and timely manner. In addition, because of the scarcity of human resources, a high value is placed on staff time and its efficient use to meet individual client needs. The client's well-being, if not survival, depends on early identification of urgent needs and their management as top staff priorities.

Client care managers are expected to help the **interdisciplinary team** address **priority** client needs. To begin, the team needs to focus its efforts on individual client goals and assessed health problems. To assure that the client receives services as planned, the client care manager needs to differentiate nursing priorities from those identified by the interdisciplinary team to meet client goals. For example, nursing staff might place high priority on client comfort, while the interdisciplinary team might focus their efforts on increasing the client's physical mobility, endurance and strength. To support the client's lack of attendance at other high priority therapies, to avoid discomfort in such situations is not in the client's best interest. Often, due to the complexity of the care needed, much nursing time and effort are consumed addressing nursing care. However, the staff nurse also needs to address interdisciplinary interdependencies to assure that the client receives the right care at the right time.

To avoid omitting important aspects of quality care, the client care manager needs to participate in interdisciplinary activities to help organize activities on the basis of *client* needs and priorities, rather than those of a specific discipline (Summers et al, 1988, pp. 665–670). Further, desired client outcomes need to be described in terms of both long- and short-term goals to avoid costly complications or inefficiency. Defining both long- and short-term goals provides important time frames to help staff plan for changes in individual client treatment programs and to evaluate patterns of responses to treatment. These goals help the team to plan continuing care and communicate as needed concerning available community resources in a timely way.

Given the hectic pace of health care, special effort is needed to identify specific plans and guidelines to measure the progress of individual clients. Such planning helps the team to reduce inefficiencies and to avoid neglecting life-threatening priorities of client care. To address this organizational need of interdisciplinary teams, meeting times and places are structured to enable the group to communicate concerning individual client goals at regular intervals and to revise plans in a timely manner.

◼◼◼ COORDINATING EFFORTS OF THE INTERDISCIPLINARY TEAM

Client care managers are expected to coordinate the efforts of the interdisciplinary team. This entails knowing individual client care priorities and communicating them to the appropriate members of the interdisciplinary team in a timely manner. Coordinating, however, does not include any decision-making authority for other disciplines or on behalf of the client (Gadow, 1989, p. 541; Shaffer and Preziosi, 1988, p. 603). Rather, the nurse acts as a client advocate, helping to articulate concerns and communicate them to the interdisciplinary team. The staff nurse, by following several guidelines, can perform coordination duties efficiently and effectively.

First, to assure that priority needs are met, the interdisciplinary team needs to remain client-centered. The team focus guides the focus of nursing. This focus of efforts is, first, and foremost, on client needs; accordingly, staff scheduling, socialization, agency efficiency, and economizing are no more than second in importance.

As changes in client needs occur, they are communicated to affected members of the interdisciplinary team. Feedback helps the team to evaluate client responses to their plan and care.

Second, as coordinator of the interdisciplinary team, the client care manager shares responsibility for enabling the client to meet desired outcomes of care. In this capacity, the client care manager frequently explains to clients, families, and staff why routine actions have been taken in the client's behalf. This accountability is shared with other members of the team. If a client has questions about the specific knowledge, skills, or methods used by members of another discipline to provide complex interventions, the nurse usually asks that member of the team to answer them. The nurse might also ask a team member to explain a complex treatment to assure that the client has accurate information. Such situations might arise when a client receives complex diagnostic preparations, drugs, dietary interventions, or specific exercises.

Third, the client care manager supports the team effort to carry out the plan. This support includes providing information and reinforcing explanations of the approaches used by other members of the team. Sometimes, to promote effective use of time, the nurse might assemble needed equipment and supplies. Obviously, each member of the team shares responsibility for performing all procedures and treatments safely. Consequently, each member of the team makes his or her needs for special equipment known to the agency staff expected to obtain them. In addition, the nurse frequently helps clients to prepare for scheduled procedures and treatment sessions so that members of other disciplines can provide them efficiently. Such preparation often includes providing comfort measures in anticipation of the treatment, enabling the client to wear special attire, or scheduling activities to maximize the benefits the client derives from the procedures.

Fourth, the client care manager shares responsibility for developing the interdisciplinary plan of care and communicating it to involved team members. To succeed, the client care manager needs to clearly understand what the plan is and be able to clearly describe it to others, using a common language. This responsibility includes promptly entering nursing information into the clinical record used by other disciplines to enable them to carry out the details of individual treatment plans. This information must be accurate, legible, and accessible when others need it to complete their activities in a timely manner. For example, changes in dietary plans associated with diagnostic studies are communicated to the nutrition department to assure that the client receives adequate nourishment at appropriate times—for example, when the client no longer needs to remain NPO upon successful completion of a procedure.

Fifth, the client care manager communicates changes in the goals or interventions of interdisciplinary care plans to affected team members. Other disciplines are often efficiently brought up to date on such changes when the team regularly schedules a time and place for this activity. Communication forms are often used to transmit routine information, but it can be transmitted electronically if the agency's information system is sufficiently automated. If scheduled sessions with the client need to be changed or discontinued on short notice, this should be communicated as soon as possible to enable members of other disciplines to revise their work plans and use available time effectively. A common example is the need to inform the physical therapy staff when a client is unable to attend a scheduled therapy session due to discomfort or activity intolerance.

The nursing staff shares responsibility for carrying out the interdisciplinary plan with other members of the health team. In addition, the client care manager participates in evaluating the team's success in enabling individual clients to achieve desired outcomes. To evaluate client progress, the client care manager needs to know what the interdisciplinary plan is, who is doing what to carry it out, and what time frame for outcomes is anticipated. Frequently, the time frame corresponds to the client's insurance coverage program requirements. Such information is invaluable to the client care manager in coordinating interdisciplinary efforts and helps in planning for the client's continuing care for as long as it is needed. Client care managers often use information about the client's health insurance benefits to plan and evaluate outcomes of care and if ncessary to refer the client to other less costly services available in the community.

COORDINATING PRIORITIES OF THE INTERDISCIPLINARY TEAM

Each discipline represented on the team believes it can help achieve outcomes desired by the client and family. Each team member approaches the client's situation from the perspective of his or her own discipline. Accordingly, each discipline has specific goals for each client, which need to be consistent with the team's overall goals for these individuals. Individual client goals and priority needs guide the team's efforts, rather than addressing a simple plurality of goals of several disciplines. Working toward common goals for individual clients requires cooperation and collaboration among team members. Without open communication, neither cooperation or collaboration is likely to occur. Nurses, like members of other disciplines represented on the interdisciplinary team, need to make a specific effort to assure that client needs and goals are clearly understood and written references for them are readily accessible.

Client care managers need to make specific efforts to establish nursing goals with individual clients that are consistent with overall goals. These goals guide nursing staff activities and help the client care manager to coordinate the interdisciplinary team's efforts. Usually, the long-term goals established depend on the client's length of stay at the agency. The time period involved will vary, depending upon the type of agency and the client's individual needs. Shorter-term goals refer to gradations of client accomplishments required to succeed overall.

To increase effectiveness and efficiency, information about the client's responses and condition needs to be communicated to the interdisciplinary team at regular intervals. Unless a structured process for this communication is established, the client's care is likely to be fragmented and deviate from the plan. In addition, opportunities to reinforce the client's progress can be missed, making it more difficult to sustain the client's motivation and team morale.

Feedback about the client's progress and the team's success are critical in monitoring progress toward overall goals. Gaps and overlaps in team efforts often surface; frequently, they result from lack of information that exists but is not readily accessible. Team members need to concentrate their efforts on meeting client goals, and avoid blaming one another. If conflicts arise, differences in goals and perceptions need to be identified and clarified. The team's plan is revised to meet priority client needs, in a spirit of collaboration and cooperation rather than competition among disciplines.

SUMMARY

The information era has increased the interdependencies of members of the health team. Client care managers are expected to coordinate the efforts of the interdisciplinary team to improve quality and reduce fragmentation of care on behalf of clients. They use skills in human relations and group work to succeed, emphasizing cooperation and collaboration.

Interdisciplinary teams are a valuable organizational resource. They need a common language, mission, and a structured time and place to discuss common concerns, client priorities, and corresponding treatment plans. Each member of the team is committed to the values of a specific discipline, and his or her contribution reflects that discipline's unique knowledge and skills. In addition to valuing their own discipline, members learn to value the contributions of other disciplines to meet priority client needs.

Client care managers use their leadership skills to contribute to team building. They communicate their concerns and skills through what they say and do. Specific effort is needed to strengthen desired patterns of behavior and to provide feedback to the team about client responses to treatment programs. In the interest of providing quality care, team members are encouraged to seek help from others and to offer it as well. By identifying barriers to interdisciplinary team effectiveness, client care managers can avoid destructive conflict. They can use communication skills to resolve conflict to enable the group to focus on client needs and goals.

Client care managers use their nursing knowledge to identify priorities for the interdisciplinary team. They actively communicate plans of care to the interdisciplinary team and provide timely information when client conditions and plans change. By referring to individual client short- and long-term goals, they help the team evaluate a plan's effectiveness and make arrangements for the client's continued care as long as it is needed. They provide feedback to help the team identify successes and areas needing further development. The team is encouraged to collaborate and cooperate as colleagues, rather than compete.

APPLICATION EXERCISES

a. Give three examples of interdisciplinary team member behaviors reflecting cooperation and collaboration that promoted the recovery of clients for whom you have provided care. Describe your nursing contributions in these situations.

b. Make a list of five terms that you believe have the same meaning for all members of the interdisciplinary team. Verify the meaning of each of these terms with at least three different interdisciplinary team members.

c. Get acquainted with the work culture of the interdisciplinary team by systematically answering the questions suggested in this chapter. Identify any surprises.

d. Note communication patterns among interdisciplinary team members while participating in a conference. Make a list of the ways that positive relationships among interdisciplinary team members were promoted. Describe two circumstances caused by communication barriers.

e. Compare your nursing priorities with those of the interdisciplinary team for one of your assigned clients.

REFERENCES

Carroll PF: Turf wars: time for a truce? *Nurs 87* 17(12):43. (December, 1987).

Coeling HV: Organizational culture: helping new graduates adjust, *Nurse Educ* 15(2):26–30. (March/April, 1990).

Coker EB, Screiber R: "The nurse's role in a team conference, *Nurs Manage* 21:(3):46–48. (March, 1990).

Gadow S: Clinical subjectivity, *Nurs Clin North Am* 24(6):535–541, 1989.

Guy ME: Interdisciplinary conflict and organizational complexity, *Hosp Health Serv Admin* January/February: 31(3):111–121, 1986.

Hodes JR, Crombrugghe PV: Nurse-physician relationships: difference of perspective is one reason for continued nurse/physician conflict, *Nurs Manage* 21(7):73–75, July, 1990.

Marsden C, Ethics of the "doctor-nurse game," *Heart Lung* 19(4):442–424. (July, 1990).

Moulder PA, Staal AM, Grant M: Making the interdisciplinary team approach work, *Rehabil Nurs* 13(6):338–339. (November-December, 1988).

Shaffer FA, Preziosi P: Nursing: the hospital's competitive edge, *Nurs Clin North Am* 23(3):597–612. (September, 1988).

Summers PM, Nadermann N, Turnis RM, Lynn P, Rechlin R, Hentges J, Roche, A: Quality management: program design—an interdisciplinary approach, *Nurs Clin North Am* 23(3):665–670. (September, 1988).

Swenson-Feldman E, Brugge-Wiger P: Promotion of interdisciplinary practice through an automated information system, 7 (4):–47. (July, 1985).

Weisberg J, Grandin JA, Pack M: The wheel of care, *Geriatr Nurs*, March/April: 10(2):86–87, 1989.

Weiss DH: Total teamwork: how to build an effective team, *Supervis Manage* 35(8):5. (August, 1990).

chapter eleven

SUPERVISING AND EVALUATING THE WORK OF OTHERS

OBJECTIVES

Completing this chapter will enable you to:

1. Describe how client satisfaction influences an agency's definition of quality care.
2. Describe indications, characteristics, and goals of client advocacy.
3. Explain the functions of supervision.
4. Describe the characteristics of effective supervision.
5. Explain the principles of evaluating client care provided by others.
6. Describe the essential characteristics of the supervisory relationship between the client care manager and supervisees.

KEY CONCEPTS

consumerism
quality care
  perspectives
    client
    staff
    agency
  components
    structure
    process
    outcomes
client advocate
  autonomy

paternalism
beneficence
maleficence
supervision
  functions
    characteristics of effective supervision
evaluation of client care done by others
  standards for quality care
  criteria
responsibility for action or nonaction of subordinates

SATISFYING CUSTOMERS AS A FOCUS OF CLIENT CARE MANAGEMENT

Entry-level staff nurses supervise and evaluate the work of others with whom they share responsibility for providing care to clients. To fulfill the responsibilities of this component of the staff nurse's role, nursing services must focus on satisfying client needs. To effectively supervise the work of others aimed at meeting client needs requires that the entry-level staff nurse, as client care manager, must become a client advocate from time to time. While supervising the work of the nursing work group and coordinating health care teams, the staff nurse continuously evaluates the effectiveness of client services they provide. Satisfying customers, both clients and staff, is the focus of the staff nurse's efforts.

THE RISING TIDE OF CONSUMERISM

Consumerism, a social movement that aims to protect clients or recipients from inferior or dangerous services, has arrived in the health care industry. Client satisfaction is a prerequisite for a health agency's success. The staff nurse reponsible for meeting clients' needs is also expected to promote clients' satisfaction with services received. This responsibility complicates the supervisory process because it requires that the perspectives of both clients and staff be respected.

With the evolution of the information era, clients expect to choose how they will use their time, resources, and talents. This includes expecting to participate in making the decisions that affect how their individual health care needs are managed. As Toffler predicted (1980, pp. 265–288), modern technology develops more options for individuals in many aspects of daily living, including health care. Increased availability of health care information helps consumers obtain up-to-date information, think independently, and be assertive about their needs. As a result, some providers of health care perceive that clients are more demanding than they seemed to be a decade or more earlier (Sinclair, 1990, p. 63).

As health care consumers, clients today have greater access to current information. Many clients learn about available health care services, technology, and equipment from the mass media. They expect detailed attention to be paid to their individual needs. Concurrently, due to present health care financing mechanisms related to primary economic trends, clients personally pay a greater proportion of the costs of their health care. These trends influence health care strategies. Many health care providers compete to maintain or increase the number of clients they serve. Health care organizations have responded by offering a greater variety of programs and services, in addition to those traditionally provided. Most providers believe that satisfied clients are more likely to return to them for needed health care. Realizing that satisfied clients expect to actively participate in their care, providers involve them in decision-making. Satisfaction with the quality of health care received is closely related to whether the client received the care that he or she perceived as necessary. Indeed, client satisfaction is becoming an accepted and established measure of quality care (Nelson et al, 1989, p. 185).

To help evaluate their services and measure client satisfaction, many health care organizations request feedback from their clients after discharge. Though the reliability of this approach should be questioned, this method has identified some important facets of client satisfaction that have been confirmed by more systematic study. For example, client perceptions of the amount of time spent waiting for services has been delineated as one key factor related to their satisfaction with health services received (Hildman and Ferguson, 1990, pp. 26–29). The findings of such studies are used to plan specific organizational efforts to increase promptness in providing services. Ultimately, focusing upon client satisfaction with services received is a common method of improving the quality of care. In this way, the rising tide of consumerism in mainstream society is having profound effects upon the quality of health care.

DEFINING QUALITY OF CARE

Quality care, services that consistently produce desired results, is a universal concern in health care organizations. Due to their different vested interests, clients and providers perceive quality of care from different **perspectives. Clients** define quality care from their perspective: "They [providers] looked like they knew what they were doing"; "They explained things to me"; "I got better." The value of incorporating client perspectives into definitions of quality care is slowly being recognized (Lehmann, 1989, p. 227; Nelson et al, 1989, pp. 185–186). Health care providers or **staff** define quality care from a different perspective, considering such factors as the acuity of the client's illness; availability of resources (staffing, equipment, and time required to address client needs); and standards of care provided in comparison to standards of practice they believe are essential for quality care. From the **agency's** perspective, important issues include providing the resources needed by anticipated target populations, developing processes for delivering services, and creating explicit, established standards of care.

When considering critical characteristics of quality care, it is necessary to remember that both quality and evaluation always involve an element of subjectivity. Quality is evaluated in the eyes of the beholder. Evaluation always involves an element of subjectivity (del Bueno, 1990, p. 4). Evaluation involves ranking the importance of various benefits, or

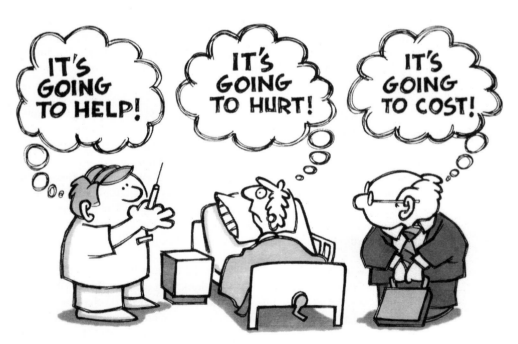

Due to their different priorities, clients, staff, and agencies perceive the quality of care differently.

placing "value" on various aspects of quality care. Although different components of quality care are measured and corresponding data collected and interpreted, evaluation of care ultimately involves a subjective judgment by the evaluator.

While supervising the work of others, staff nurses need to distinguish client perceptions, which are often based on personal experience, from those of staff, which are usually based upon professional standards of practice and institutionally established standards of care (Patterson, 1988, pp. 628–629). Client care managers share responsibility for assuring that every staff member understands the agency's definition of quality care. Sharing a common definition helps staff to develop the system and language required to guide direct-service staff. Commitment to the agency's definition of quality care is so important that many health care organizations consume considerable resources to make it explicit and explain its ramifications to staff. The staff uses this definition and related goals and standards as the basis for developing a system and process for providing quality care.

Basically, quality health care consists of three basic **components:** structure, process, and outcome (Wright, 1984, p. 458).

Structure

The **structure** of quality care is how the agency organizes its resources to match the specific needs of the client population it serves. Structure is reflected in staffing patterns and equipment and other agency resources made available to care for clients. For example, the structure of quality care for acutely ill pediatric clients differs from that needed by chronically ill middle-aged adults. The structure for pediatric clients would involve other key decision makers, while middle-aged clients are likely to make decisions about their own care. The basic parts of the service program are likely to differ in terms of staffing, equipment, and use of other agency services and resources. If the agency provides care only for pediatric clients, its purpose and mission and the methods used to address them will differ from those of an agency whose client population includes persons of varying ages throughout the lifespan. The structure needs to program flexibility into its responses to the wide variety of health problems presented by its client population.

Process

Closely related to the structure is the **process** used to provide quality care. The process depends on the nature of the client's needs and how the staff uses resources to address them. For example, an acutely ill client is likely to need more diagnostic services, whereas a chronically ill person is likely to require more monitoring, counseling, and support. The emphasis in the process of providing quality care is likely to change from admission to discharge. The process of providing quality care is not synonymous with the nursing process, though the nursing process is used to promote quality care. The process of quality care encompasses broader agency activities. Nurses apply the nursing process to meet nursing practice standards while also complying with the agency's standards to provide quality care.

The process of quality care varies with the client's health problems and responses to treatment. The client's perception of interactions with care providers affect her or his satisfaction with the services received. After the client has been discharged, many health organizations collect data about consumer satisfaction with various tasks of care and types of services received. Those data are used to identify which patterns of staff activities promote client satisfaction and which merit further examination. Obviously, this type of retrospective study does not help clients directly, and some dissatisfied clients are unlikely to describe their perceptions in writing. Relying on this method of evaluation alone is unlikely to promote accuracy or reliability.

Recently, emphasis has been placed on decentralizing nursing service organizations. The need to focus organizational resources at the direct-service level to plan the process of providing quality care is being realized more frequently (Albrecht, 1990). Where this is occurring, staff nurses are likely to gain organizational influence to develop systems of care that are responsive to individual client needs. The evolving systems of care are more likely to be sensitive to the needs of both the client and the staff actually providing the quality care.

Outcomes

Recently, **outcomes,** or results, indicative of quality care are receiving more attention. These outcomes include client and staff perceptions and cost effectiveness (Hoesing and Kirk, 1990, p. 11; Nelson et al, 1989, p. 185; Welch, 1989, p. 469). In the past, quality care was often equated with ideal rather than realistic care. Consequently, the actual results of services provided and the costs of quality care were neglected. With increased concern about the costs of health services and increased proportions of expenses being directly paid by private individuals, client satisfaction and costs can no longer be ignored. Many health care agencies use management information and decision support systems to delineate the costs and benefits of various strategies and desired outcomes within the context of available resources (Coleman, 1989, p. 383; Lehmann, 1989, p. 223). By focusing on outcomes that clients desire, health care providers are developing customer-driven services. Health care providers have given lip service, but without action, to client-centered care for many years. The evolving methods of financing health care and the rising tide of consumerism and its associated competitiveness are stimulating continued focus on consumer interests and client-driven systems of quality care.

The Meaning of Quality Care

The benefits of developing a commonly understood language to discuss the components of quality care and what quality means to various members of the health care team are slowly being recognized (Frankl, 1990, pp. 52–65). However, the need for a common language and agreement by the nursing team about the meaning of quality care is not decreased because it is so difficult. Developing a common understanding of quality care requires staff at every level of the organization to comprehend the agency's mission and priorities and the processes used to address them. Staff nurses need to comprehend the structure, process, and outcomes of quality care established by the health care agency. Once they comprehend the primary purpose of the agency, the staff providing care directly to clients should understand the critical need to "do it right the first time" and avoid "rework" to promote efficiency and cost-effectiveness. Providing quality care requires that effective supervision be readily available to assure that staff providing direct services reliably and accurately identify client needs and have the necessary resources to address them.

Quality care issues do not revolve around differentiating the realistic from the ideal. Rather, quality care usually focuses on what clients perceive their needs to be (Nelson et al, 1989, pp. 185–186) and how the agency uses resources to meet them in a cost-effective manner (Hoesing and Kirk, 1990, pp. 10–15). Without satisfied clients, there is less need for health care agencies, including nursing services, and consequently, less need to employ nurses! The issues of quality care are complex and unlikely to disappear in the forseeable future.

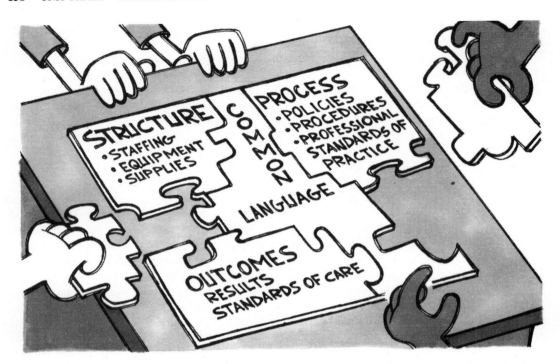

Developing a common understanding of quality care requires staff at every level of the organization to understand the agency's mission and priorities and the processes used to meet them.

Due to the persistence of the quality care issue, the need for nurses to act as client advocates is likely to continue. Staff nurses use knowledge of the needs of both the clients and the health care agencies, to provide care and oversee and coordinate services provided by others (Pagana, 1987, p. 51). Comprehension of the agency's definition of quality care usually strengthens the nurse's commitment to take independent nursing action to respond to client needs in a timely manner (Pinch, 1985, p. 39). Staff nurses, as advocates, use their assertiveness skills to communicate client needs to other team members as often as necessary until they are addressed within the agency's predetermined parameters of quality care.

ACTING AS A CLIENT ADVOCATE

Acting as a client advocate is not easy, smooth, or without risks, but it is critically necessary. **Client advocates** actively support client rights (as legally required) and make a special effort to defend client participation in decisions affecting them (Johnstone, 1989, pp. 31–34). Advocacy includes taking actions to secure the client's **autonomy,** or independence, in exercising their rights. Client advocacy is needed in many types of situations. Clients are entitled to understand their rights as consumers of health care and to receive support in making decisions consistent with their individual goals, values, and lifestyles. (The box at right lists client rights in acute care settings. The next box on p. 160 describes client rights that nurses are obliged to protect in any setting.) The primary purpose of client advocacy is to provide the client with information about her or his needs and available options. When a client makes an informed decision, he or she can reasonably expect that the

AHA's Patient's Bill of Rights

1. The patient has the right to considerate and respectful care.
2. The patient has the right to obtain from his physician complete current information concerning his diagnosis, treatment, and prognosis in terms the patient can be reasonably expected to understand. When it is not medically advisable to give such information to the patient, the information should be made available to an appropriate person in his behalf. He has the right to know, by name, the physician responsible for coordinating his care.
3. The patient has the right to receive from his physician information necessary to give informed consent prior to the start of any procedure and/or treatment. Except in emergencies, such information for informed consent should include but not necessarily be limited to the specific procedure and/or treatment, the medically significant risks involved, and the probable duration of incapacitation. Where medically significant alternatives for care or treatment exist, or when the patient requests information concerning medical alternatives, the patient has the right to such information. The patient also has the right to know the name of the person responsible for the procedures and/or treatment.
4. The patient has the right to refuse treatment to the extent permitted by law and to be informed of the medical consequences of his action.
5. The patient has the right to every consideration of his privacy concerning his own medical care program. Case discussion, consultation, examination, and treatment are confidential and should be conducted discreetly. Those not directly involved in his care must have the permission of the patient to be present.
6. The patient has the right to expect that all communications and records pertaining to his care should be treated as confidential.
7. The patient has the right to expect that within its capacity a hospital must make reasonable response to the request of a patient for services. The hospital must provide evaluation, service, and/or referral as indicated by the urgency of the case. When medically permissible, a patient may be transferred to another facility only after he has received complete information and explanation concerning the needs for and alternatives to such a transfer. The institution to which the patient is to be transferred must first have accepted the patient for transfer.
8. The patient has the right to obtain information as to any relationship of his hospital to other health care and educational institutions insofar as his care is concerned. The patient has the right to obtain information as to the existence of any professional relationships among individuals, by name, who are treating him.
9. The patient has the right to be advised if the hospital proposes to engage in or perform human experimentation affecting his care or treatment. The patient has the right to refuse to participate in such research projects.
10. The patient has the right to expect reasonable continuity of care. He has the right to know in advance what appointment times and physicians are available and where. The patient has the right to expect that the hospital will provide a mechanism whereby he is informed by his physician or a delegate of the physician of the patient's continuing health care requirements following discharge.
11. The patient has the right to examine and receive an explanation of his bill regardless of source of payment.
12. The patient has the right to know what hospital rules and regulations apply to his conduct as a patient.

From American Hospital Association: *Policy: a patient's bill of rights,* Chicago, Ill, 1975, The Association.

Nursing's Role in Patient's Rights

According to the NLN statement, nurses have a responsibility to uphold patients' rights:

☐ To health care that is accessible and meets professional standards, regardless of the setting.

☐ To courteous and individualized health care that is equitable, humane, and given without discrimination as to race, color, creed, sex, national origin, source of payment, or ethical or political beliefs.

☐ To information about their diagnosis, prognosis, and treatment—including alternatives to care and risks involved—in terms they and their families can readily understand, so that they can give their informed consent.

☐ To informed participation in all decisions concerning their health care.

☐ To information about the qualifications, names, and titles of personnel responsible for providing their health care.

☐ To refuse observation by those not directly involved in their care.

☐ To privacy during interview, examination, and treatment.

☐ To privacy in communicating and visiting with persons of their choice.

☐ To refuse treatment, medications, or participation in research and experimentation, without punitive action being taken against them.

☐ To coordination and continuity of health care.

☐ To appropriate instruction or education from health care personnel so that they can achieve an optimal level of wellness and an understanding of their basic health needs.

☐ To confidentiality of all records (except as otherwise provided for by law or third-party payer contracts) and all communications, written or oral, between patients and health care providers.

☐ To access all health records pertaining to them, to challenge and correct their records for accuracy, and to transfer all such records in the case of continuing care.

☐ To information on the charges for services, including the right to challenge these.

☐ To be fully informed as to all their rights in all health care settings.

From National League for Nursing: *Nursing's role in patient's rights.* New York, 1977, National League for Nursing.

care providers will support these decisions in ways that enable clients to carry out the related plans of care.

An advocate helps clients obtain the information needed to exercise their rights. This information includes knowledge about the nature of individual health problems and alternatives that might be used to manage or treat them. This information, which is often provided by various members of the interdisciplinary team, enables the client to decide upon the treatment options that best match her or his goals, values, and lifestyle. Sometimes clients have difficulty understanding explanations due to language barriers. Sometimes time constraints, the process of care, and the nature of the services provided inhibit the transmission of information to the client (for example a client who is critically ill and anxious might not comprehend hurried technical explanations). Or certain procedures might be embarrassing or unacceptable due to a client's cultural or spiritual beliefs. However, these circumstances to not negate the client's right to understand available treatment options and to make informed decisions about the plan of care.

Client care managers need to understand the rights of health care consumers. In addition, they need to understand that **paternalism, beneficence,** and **maleficence** inhibit client autonomy. Paternalistic care providers act in a "fatherly" way, as if they know better than the client what is to be done. Beneficent providers do what they think is in the client's best interest, not what the client thinks is best. The maleficent provider determines the care plan on the basis of avoiding harm or risk to the client, but again, the decision is not made by the client. The correct role for an advocate is to help clients obtain the information needed to make *their own* informed decisions about their care.

Another facet of advocacy in modern, fast-paced health care environments requires that the client care manager communicate client responses to care in a timely manner. Services should match client needs, not agency routines or procedures. This assures that both legal requirements and the client's long-term interests are served and that shorter-term, less cost-effective methods are not used. If the complexity of client needs conflicts with the staff's ability to respond to them or the agency's need to contain costs, the situation is prime for client advocacy. Such situations require that the client care manager communicate the client's needs to the direct service staff and other involved interdisciplinary team members. Often, these efforts also require collaboration with staff from other agencies to analyze the client's situation and identify solutions that satisfactorily address the individual's needs. As mentioned in Chapter Six, conflict resolution involves risk. To overlook or neglect client rights to avoid such risks or to take a path of convenience or expedience can jeopardize the longer term interests of both the client and the agency.

EFFECTIVELY SUPERVISING THE WORK OF OTHERS

Supervision is actively monitoring or overseeing the activities of others. To supervise the work of others as a client care manager means to "oversee" client care activites. The function of supervision is often communicated to the work group by the organizational chart, position descriptions, or patterns of nursing service delivery. Having supervisory responsibilities often implies that the client care manager has a broader perspective on what needs to be done and different ("better" implied) methods of doing it based on nursing commitment, credentials, and authority. The primary **functions** of supervision include providing the desired perspective and work environment that supports agency goals and monitoring the extent to which these goals are met. Effective supervision helps the staff in several important ways. **Characteristics of effective supervision** are the types of activities the client care manager performs to coach, monitor, and judge the effectiveness of work performed by the health care team.

First, to supervise others, the client care manager takes an active part in maintaining suitable working conditions. Specific attention is given to the culture of the work group. Supervisees are encouraged to communicate concerns and questions to assure that staff responsibilities can be met. The client care manager understands the language of the organizational culture and seeks to clarify misconceptions and agency goals. By reinforcing performance expectations, satisfactory effort can more readily be recognized and rewarded.

Second, the client care manager is expected to clearly understand the needs of assigned clients and what agency resources are needed to meet them. To create a supportive environment to meet client needs involves supervisory responsibility to provide adequate

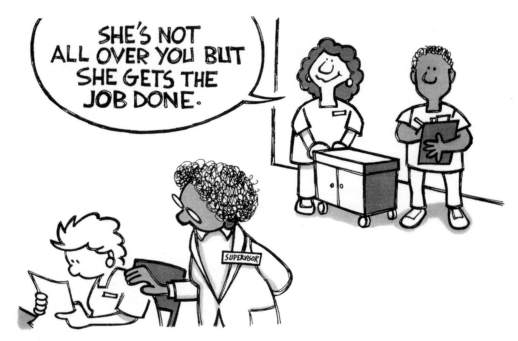

Characteristics of effective supervision are illustrated by the types of activities the client care manager performs to coach, monitor, and judge the effectiveness of work performed by the health care team.

equipment (Killian, 1990, pp. 34–35), supplies, and staffing. Supervisees are asked to report malfunctioning equipment, insufficient supplies, or help required to provide quality care safely. Often, to respond to the requests of co-workers, the client care manager needs to know how to operate equipment according to its manufacturer's specifications and how to troubleshoot when malfunctions are reported. To promote cost-effectiveness, the client care manager observes how co-workers use equipment and supplies and acts as a resource person to enable staff to learn to adapt client care to specific situations. Again, the client care manager focuses on client needs within the context of agency guidelines and oversees the use of its resources in providing care.

A client care manager is likely to encounter certain common situations when supervising the work of others. For example, a co-worker might procrastinate instead of completing activities efficiently, and so have to complete key tasks late in the day or after the end of the work day. Conferring with this co-worker earlier in the shift, the client care manager can inquire about the progress of various client care activities and suggest changes in the co-worker's work organization or time management. For example, the manager might offer to help the co-worker in ambulating clients earlier in the shift to assure that client goals are met. Or the client care manager might reinforce the expectation that the co-worker will ask for help from others, and plan with them according to mutually acceptable schedules, rather than wait until it is convenient for everyone later in the shift, which often does not happen.

Client care managers are also likely to encounter the feeling that there is inadequate staff to meet the variety of needs of the group of assigned clients. The client care manager needs to take the time and effort to actively listen to the expressed concerns and to determine what type of help is actually needed by the group. Can client care activities be adapted to better suit the work schedules? Can the staff be taught different techniques for meeting client needs, such as sequencing activities to maximize exercise, comfort, and rest? Are additional staff members needed to provide safe and effective quality care in accordance with agency standards? Co-workers expect reasonable responses to their expressed concerns; if their concerns are minimized or ignored, they often learn not to communicate them, or find different methods of responding to what they perceive as frustrating or unworkable circumstances.

Third, client care managers are often expected to orient, train, and guide co-workers according to their individual learning styles and needs, consistent with their backgrounds, experience, and assigned client needs. Sometimes, this supervisory responsibility involves selecting co-workers who are comfortable acting as desired role models. Orientation activities can be planned for the supervisee and another co-worker working together so that the new employee can demonstrate skills while assisting the role model. The co-worker acting as a role model is thereby recognized for positive performance and encouraged to share her or his knowledge and skills with others. The client care manager needs to make a special effort to assure that the planned learning activities enable the new employee to develop and demonstrate needed skills. The expectations of all people involved in learning activities need to be made explicit so that they can be met rather than guessed at.

Fourth, while supervising the work of others, client care managers try to stimulate a desire for self-improvement in supervisees. As mentioned in Chapter Nine, client care managers are more effective if they use leadership skills. While overseeing the work of others and interacting with them, client care managers are expected to criticize and praise co-workers to help them improve their work performance. Depending upon the client care manager's leadership characteristics and communication skills, open, direct, tactful messages can often be used to stimulate a co-worker's desire for self-improvement. As a role model, the client care manager can teach supervisees about the need for life-long learning by conveying self-confidence, enthusiasm, and commitment to acquire new knowledge and skills on a daily basis.

Fifth, client care managers guide supervisees in the use of talents and development of special skills. Within the limits of a co-worker's position description and performance expectations, the client care manager teaches supervisees how to use unique talents and skills that enhance the quality of care. For example, some co-workers have the unique communication skills needed to convey empathy and concern to clients. Often they use active listening techniques that skillfully enable clients to reflect upon their circumstances in a very helpful manner. Recognizing and reinforcing the use of such skills enhances the quality of client care. Much can be gained by the supervisee when the supervisor recognizes and reinforces special capabilities.

Sixth, while overseeing the work activities of supervisees, the client care manager has a superb opportunity to act as a role model and demonstrate desired attitudes, skills, interests, and work habits. The manager can provide an example of the desired attitudes and behaviors involved in providing quality care on a daily basis. This teaching method is very powerful; it is also very demanding. As an imperfect human being and a lifelong learner, the client care manager functioning as a role model is in a very vulnerable position. However, sharing unique talents and skills with others in a sensitive manner reinforces the agency's goals and enhances the quality of care.

The box on p. 164 lists common characteristics of effective supervision.

Common Characteristics of Effective Supervision of Client Care

- ☐ The client care manager actively provides suitable working conditions, including adequate staffing, equipment, and supplies.
- ☐ The client care manager clearly understands the needs of assigned clients and what agency resources are required to meet them.
- ☐ The client care manager orients, trains, and guides co-workers according to their individual learning styles and needs, consistent with their backgrounds, experience, and assignments.
- ☐ The client care manager tries to stimulate desire for self-improvement in supervisees.
- ☐ The client care manager encourages supervisees to use unique talents and develop special skills.
- ☐ The client care manager demonstrates desired attitudes, skills, interests, and work habits.

Providing effective supervision for co-workers is very challenging. However, if co-workers do not perceive that their supervision increases their effectiveness or efficiency, the resulting quality of care is not improved. This unfortunate consequence can occur if the client care manager rewards or reinforces behaviors by emphasizing incorrect performance or inadequate effort while overseeing the work of others. Attempting to change co-workers' behavior in health care settings by coercion is usually ineffective. Rather, the client care manager needs to emphasize desired efforts to enable supervisees to improve their performance. Client care managers who provide effective supervision usually use a wide variety of teaching skills. These skills are based upon knowledge about human motivation, communication, interpersonal relationships, and principles used to change behavior. They are similar to the knowledge and skills used to teach clients.

As a teacher of supervisees, the client care manager is sensitive to the motivations of individuals and the influence of the culture on the work environment. By remembering the agency's mission, goals, and definition of quality care, the client care manager strives to help co-workers to develop and apply knowledge and skills used to care for assigned clients.

EVALUATING CLIENT CARE PERFORMED BY OTHERS

Beginning staff nurses participate in judging the quality of work done by their peers and subordinates. They are expected to evaluate peers' and subordinates' effectiveness in helping clients satisfy health care needs. This type of evaluation is different from formal employee evaluations in that it is done primarily to judge the success of an individual client's treatment program instead of the effectiveness of an employee's work performance. It is possible that entry-level staff nurses might be asked to provide feedback about the work performance of a nursing team member. However, this section focuses on evaluating success in helping a client to meet health care goals.

Client care managers share responsibility for the effectiveness of care performed by others under their supervision and direction. As described earlier, to effectively supervise the work of others, the client care manager needs to know the clients' needs and what services and available resources are required to meet them. This nursing knowledge and skills cover proper use of equipment, supplies, and procedures. The client care manager needs to clearly understand the agency's definition of quality care, its identified criteria for desired outcomes, its structure, and standards of care used to guide staff.

Evaluation of client care done by others requires knowledge of the agency's standards for quality care. The client care manager uses these standards to assess the adequacy of services provided and client outcomes. To evaluate the work of others, one must consider the client's entire situation in context, rather than examining various client characteristics (del Bueno, 1990, p. 6). The resulting judgment about the quality of care the client received is then likely to be more reliable, accurate, and enlightening. Nursing students often question the rationale for requiring them to develop skills needed to provide care to a variety of clients. Without such varied experience, however, they are likely to encounter difficulty when trying to determine the needs of a diverse group of assigned clients, as is required when one supervises the work of others. It is very difficult, if not impossible, to evaluate how effectively clients' needs have been met if the client care manager does not know what these needs are. Similarly, it is difficult to evaluate how effective other staff members are in meeting client needs, if the client care manager does not know the desired client outcomes and what is needed to achieve them. Evaluating the client care performed by others requires that the client care manager assess what clients need, determine the desired care outcomes within the context of the agency's standards of care, and determine the process for providing for them.

The client care manager evaluates the work of others throughout the workday. After assuring that the supervisees have the knowledge and skills required to complete their work assignments, the client care manager confers with them to obtain feedback and monitor progress. While meeting with supervisees, the client care manager makes a special effort to reinforce their strengths and minimize their weaknesses.

In most situations, emphasizing strengths has greater priority than minimizing weaknesses. Obviously, supervisees need the skills required to provide care safely. If a supervisee does not possess adequate skills, then the client care manager needs to assure that he or she acquires them. Having enabled supervisees to acquire the needed skills, the client care manager focuses on maximizing the supervisee's strengths and talents.

When conferring with supervisees, it is always important to meet in a private area where open, direct communications can occur. Discussing client needs and care within earshot of clients, families, or visitors invites difficulty. Co-workers know that clients can misinterpret terminology or contexts, and they feel inhibited about engaging in open, forthright discussions in the client care areas. It is tempting to discuss concerns at the bedside while observing other aspects of the client's condition, but the client care manager needs to respect co-workers' privacy. Such respect requires that detailed questioning and discussion occur in private so that the communication can be open, direct and truthful. Depending on the nature of the discussion, subsequent revisions in the care plans may result to assure that the client receives quality care suited to her or his needs. Effective and efficient communication cannot be assured if it takes place in the presence of clients, family members, visitors, or other staff.

Though the agency establishes standards of care to guide staff, they are only guidelines. Each **standard for quality care** is a component of quality care as defined by the agency. Each standard is operationalized by **criteria,** clinical indicators that reflect the staff's current practices, a knowledge of relevant literature, and the opinions of clinical experts. The criteria depict elements of process and outcomes of quality care as they relate to specific client conditions and anticipated responses to treatment (Lehmann, 1989, p. 223). Staff use these criteria to quantify or measure their effectiveness in achieving quality care and identifying areas that need further examination to improve services. A common set of criteria for a specific standard describes the client's

1. Knowledge of the health condition and its treatment
2. Skills needed to manage the situation
3. Knowledge of medications
4. Ability to adapt self-care behaviors
5. Current health or physiological state (Wright, 1984, p. 463)

Information about the extent to which these criteria are met helps staff to judge the effectiveness of the structure, process, and outcomes of care.

Standards of quality care and corresponding criteria are used to judge the work performance of staff. When overseeing the work of others, the client care manager needs to be flexible in determining acceptable variances in the work performance of supervisees. Evaluation of work performance includes considering the context of clients' circumstances and comparing agency standards for quality care. For example, the manager might consider whether client characteristics are atypical and contribute to the client's short- and long-term responses to treatment. Sometimes a client has a rare combination of diseases or symptoms that are difficult to treat, or the client experiences idiosyncratic responses to treatment. The client might not readily understand the nature of the health problems, or lack a support system. Client care managers accept responsibility for monitoring the efforts of supervisees to provide quality care as defined by the agency.

Client care managers apply several principles to provide effective supervision. The goals of effective supervision include maintaining or improving the quality of care provided and developing direct service staff capabilities. Managers often teach and coach co-workers (Davidhizar, 1990, pp. 42–44). In addition to role modeling positive and supportive attitudes, they actively help maintain the morale needed to sustain team efforts.

Client care managers are expected to judge the work performance of co-workers throughout the workday, on a daily basis. The basic frames of reference for such evaluation are the pertinent standards of care and the specific employee's job description. The job description provides background information about the minimal requirements expected of a given category of employee. It typically includes descriptions of organizational responsibilities, quantity of work, knowledge, attitudes, and skills. This information is used to establish common expectations between the client care manager and the supervisee.

While monitoring client responses to care provided by others, the client care manager provides specific feedback about the co-worker's work as it influences the quality of client care. Methods of controlling or reducing costs without compromising the effectiveness of care require constant attention. The manager provides concrete directions to the supervisee before, during, and after provision of care.

Constructive criticism is designed to maintain or improve the quality of care. Rather than offering general or vague comments, the client care manager, as an effective supervisor, describes behaviors or activities in concrete, observable terms. For example, instead of labeling the supervisee's behavior by saying, "Your clients are complaining about waiting. Can you organize your work better?" the client care manager might say to the supervisee, "Two of your clients didn't like waiting to get your help with personal cares this morning. You usually use your time wisely. What might you do differently to reduce their waiting?"

Specific suggestions are offered, based on the individual co-worker's strengths, motivations, talents, and skills.

As preparation for evaluating the work of others, the client care manager should understand the organizational culture, particularly how staff are rewarded for providing quality care (Casebeer, 1990, p. 42). When conferring with supervisees, the client care manager encourages them to evaluate their own work (DeSimone, 1984, p. 16). Information gleaned from self-evaluation efforts helps the supervisor to gain insight into the individual's perceptions, attitudes, and goals. Indeed, the experience might very well help the co-worker to review old goals and set new ones (Anderson and Davis, 1987, p. 48).

After minimal requirements are met, the focus of the evaluation needs to shift to accentuating the positive aspects of the co-worker's accomplishments and reinforcing desired behaviors. Comparing the client care manager's evaluation with that of the supervisee sets up a learning situation. By negotiating differences, meaningful goals can be identified. Client care managers can learn a great deal from involving co-workers in solving client care problems (Schmieding, 1990, pp. 58–60), though this approach is not used as frequently as it could be.

By guiding the supervisee to take an active part in solving client care problems, the client care manager can help supervisees' self-confidence grow from seeing their ideas put into action. Combining active listening with an invitation to discuss ideas often helps the client care manager to focus on the needs of both the co-worker and client. When summarizing the discussion, alternative methods and goals can readily be described in measurable terms.

To reinforce suggestions resulting from the evaluation of an individual's work, the client care manager needs to follow up on the supervisee's response to the agreed-upon plan (DeSimone, 1984, p. 17). Withholding corrective actions until scheduled performance reviews should be avoided. Rather, constructive comments should be offered as soon as possible, in a tactful, open, direct manner. Achievements need to be recognized and positive feedback given. To maximize learning from the work experience, discuss what worked and what didn't. Unsuccessful efforts also require recognition and revision depending upon client's responses (Davidhizar, 1990, p. 44). Lack of such feedback diminishes the effects of the client care manager's efforts.

Seeking feedback from the client, family members, and support system is consistent with the advocacy component of the client care manager role. Such feedback is also useful for defining quality care. A critical analysis of feedback is used to evaluate the client's total situation. Promoting meaningful communication patterns between direct service staff and their clients helps to evolve badly needed customer-driven health care systems.

ACCEPTING RESPONSIBILITY FOR THE ACTIONS OF SUBORDINATES

Effective client care managers accept **responsibility for the action and nonaction of subordinates.** When the client care manager provides effective supervision, certain conditions evolve and persist. Both client care managers and their supervisees clarify expectations of each other. Each member of the work group learns to assume responsibility for assigned client care and expects to answer for what he or she does. These conditions are based upon the assumption that the supervisor is a

1. Resource person for both clients and staff
2. Teacher of both clients and staff

3. Loyal employee (Curtin, 1990, p. 7)
4. Accountable member of the nursing profession answerable for the actions he or she takes (Johnstone, 1989, pp. 32–33; Luquire, 1988, p. 61).

Before the supervisor accepts this responsibility, the subordinates must possess four essential characteristics:

1. Subordinates must know what care the client needs
2. Subordinates must possess the required skills, equipment, and supplies needed to provide assigned client care services (Allen, 1990, pp. 14–15)
3. Subordinates must know the goals of individual clients
4. Feedback about client responses must be communicated to the work group to provide for continuity of care.

Each of these requirements demands attention from the client care manager. Inattention to these characteristics may result in liability for the actions of other health team members and one's own actions as a participant in the client's care (Rhodes, 1986, p. 315).

SUMMARY

Client care managers accept responsibility for supervising and evaluating the work of others with whom they share responsibility for providing care to assigned clients. Within the context of the agency's definition of quality care, the focus of supervisory efforts includes satisfying customers and supporting and developing staff.

In the recent past, client satisfaction has become an essential ingredient in quality care. Clients obtain considerable information needed to promote and maintain health from the mass media so they are becoming more sophisticated consumers. Due to the rising influence of client perceptions of the quality of health care they receive and changing mechanisms for financing spiraling costs, more customer-driven systems are likely to evolve. To provide quality care, client and staff perceptions and cost-effectiveness criteria are incorporated in the agency's structure, process, and desired outcomes. To remain competitive, health care agencies need to use valid and reliable methods to evaluate their success in providing quality care and they need to use this information to improve quality.

While fulfilling their supervisory responsibilities, client care managers are expected to protect client rights. The goals of advocacy activities include enabling clients to obtain information needed to exercise their rights and protect their autonomy in making decisions affecting individual plans of care. Advocacy activities often require the staff nurse to communicate client needs and concerns in a timely manner and to accept the risks involved in conflict resolution.

To effectively oversee the work of others providing client care, staff nurses accept responsibility for maintaining a safe working environment in which staffing, equipment, and supplies are adequate. They support the agency's definition of quality care by comparing actual outcomes and services with established standards. They participate in the orientation, training, and incidental teaching of staff to assure that needed care is provided safely, effectively, and efficiently. Another feature of effective supervision is the ability to stimulate co-workers to strive for continuous self-improvement by participating in self-evaluations of their performance. Closely related to these co-worker efforts are the supervisor's recognition and reinforcement of special talents, knowledge, and skills. The client care manager also acts as a role model while providing care to teach desired attitudes and skills.

The client care manager evaluates client care performed by others. To promote accuracy and reliability in judging effectiveness, the client's entire situation needs to be considered in context. Feedback from clients, families, and support systems is used to achieve quality care. This approach requires that the staff nurse know each client's needs and what resources are required to meet them. Standards of care are used as guidelines. Specific feedback is given in a place and a manner that reflects respect for both clients and staff and promotes effective communication. To gain from the evaluation, the client care manager must follow up with involved staff to assure that indicated changes occur and desired behaviors are rewarded.

For a supervisory relationship between the client care manager and supervisees to be effective, supervisees must know what client services are needed, how to provide them using agency resources, how to communicate feedback about client responses, and the extent to which individual client health care goals were met. When these conditions exist, the staff nurse can readily accept responsibility for the actions and nonactions of subordinates in providing quality care.

APPLICATION EXERCISES

   a. Many clients, as consumers of health care, pay for a portion of the costs of nursing services provided. Identify the specific phases of the nursing and management processes that provide opportunities for promoting client satisfaction.

   b. Describe specific components of quality care at your assigned agency in terms of the agency's structure, process, and outcomes.

   c. Give three examples of client advocacy that you witnessed while completing your clinical work assignments during the last week.

   d. Observe the behaviors of a nurse supervising the practice of staff nurses. List the principles of effective supervision you believe were applied that were reflected in the supervisor's behavior.

   e. A "float" LPN is assigned to your nursing work group. State what you can do as a staff nurse to demonstrate your acceptance of responsibility for her actions.

REFERENCES

Albrecht K: *Service Within,* Homewood, Ill, 1990, Dow Jones—Irwin.

Allen AMB: Changing liability of the nurse over the past decade, *Orthop Nurs* 9(2):13–15. (March/April, 1990).

Anderson PA, Davis SE: Nursing peer review: a developmental process, *Nurs Manage* 18(1):46–48. (January, 1987).

Casebeer L: Personnel decisions: "wheeling" toward better performance, *Nurs Manage* 21(8):42–44. (August, 1990).

Coleman RL: The use of decision analysis in quality assessment, *QRB* 15(1):383–391. (December, 1989).

Curtin LL: Old loyalties in the new organization, *Nurs Manage* 21(3):7–8. (March, 1990).

Davidhizar R: The manager as coach, *Adv Clin Care* 5(3):42–44. (May–June, 1990).

del Bueno DJ: Evaluation: myths, mystiques, and obsessions, *J Nurs Adm* 20(11):4–7. (November, 1990).

DeSimone A: How evaluations can improve performance, *RN* 47(7):15–16. (July, 1984).

Frankl KAJ: The language and meaning of quality, *Nurs Adm Q* 14(3):52–65. (Spring, 1990).

Hildman TB, Ferguson GH: Prompt service: a factor in patient satisfaction, *Nurs Manage* 21(12):26–29. (December, 1990).

Hoesing H, Kirk R: Common sense quality management, *J Nurs Adm* 20(10):10–15. (October, 1990).

Johnstone MJ: Professional ethics and patients' rights: past realities, future imperatives, *Nurs Forum* 24(3):29–34, 1989.

Killian WH: Equipment mishaps may result

in lawsuits, *Am Nurse* 22(6):34–35. (June, 1990).

Lehmann R: Forum on clinical indicator development: a discussion of the use and development of indicators. *QRB* 15(7):223–227, 1989.

Luquire R, Six common causes of nursing liability, *Nurs 88* 18(11):61–62. (November, 1988).

Nelson EC, Hays RD, Larson C, Batalden PB: The patient judgment system: reliability and validity, *QRB* 15(6):185–191. (June, 1989).

Nelson ML: Advocacy in nursing: how has it evolved and what are its implications for practice? *Nurs Outlook* 36(3):136–141. (May/June, 1988).

Pagana KD: Let's stop calling ourselves "Patient Advocates," *Nurs 87* 17(2):51. (February, 1987).

Patterson CH: Standards of patient care: the joint commission focus on nursing quality assurance, *Nurs Clin of North Am* 23(3):625–638. (September, 1988).

Pinch W: "Patient advocacy, ethical dilemmas and decision making: the importance of autonomy, *Imprint* 32(4):36–39. (November, 1985).

Rhodes AM: Liability for the actions of others, *MCN* 11(5):315. (September/October, 1986).

Schmieding NJ: Do head nurses include staff nurses in problem-solving? *Nurs Manage* 21(3):58–60. (March, 1990).

Sinclair VG: Potential effects of decision support systems on the role of the nurse, *Comput Nurs* 8(2):60–65. (April, 1990).

Toffler A: *The third wave,* New York, 1980, Bantam Books.

Welch CC: Entering a new era of quality care, *ANNA* 16(7):469–471. (December, 1989).

Wright D: An introduction to the evaluation of nursing care: a review of the literature, *J Adv Nurs* 9(5):457–467. (September, 1984).

chapter twelve

ASSIGING AND DELEGATING CLIENT CARE ACTIVITIES

OBJECTIVES

Completing this chapter should enable you to:

1. Differentiate between assigning and delegating client care.
2. Describe principles of client care assignment.
3. Compare responsibility, authority, and accountability.
4. Define liability.
5. Contrast the two types of negligence.
6. Describe the relationship of accountability to client care assignment.
7. Discuss key concepts underlying effective delegation.
8. Describe principles of delegation.
9. Describe principles to be considered before delegating client care activities to less skilled staff.
10. Describe the relationship of delegation to accountability for client care.

KEY CONCEPTS

assigning client care
delegating client care
principles for assigning client care
responsibility
authority
accountability
malpractice

negligence
   omission
   commission
liability
principles for delegating the work of
   client care managers

DIRECTING THE WORK OF OTHERS

Entry-level nurses in the client care manager role direct the work of others. This function usually entails assigning and delegating client care activities. How client care is assigned often depends upon the agency's organization and patterns of nursing service delivery and staffing. Careful consideration is given to individual employee qualifications and capabilities. Proper delegation requires similar considerations. To appropriately fulfill these management responsibilities, the staff nurse needs to understand the nature of these functions and common strategies used to perform them.

ASSIGNING VS. DELEGATING CLIENT CARE ACTIVITIES

Entry-level staff nurses are frequently expected to both assign and delegate client care activities in an attempt to provide quality care with available resources. They usually have opportunities to observe more experienced staff nurses assign and delegate client care activities (in accordance with the agency's organization, context, and work group characteristics) before they are expected to perform these functions themselves.

Assigning client care differs from delegating it. **Assigning client care** relates to the client care manager's function of allocating the work required to care for a group of clients to available staffing. To assign care, the manager must know what each client's needs are and what knowledge, skills, equipment, and supplies are required to meet them. Staff are paid to complete assignments in accordance with their credentials and position descriptions and, when feasible, individual talents and preferences. When completed, assignments include a matching list of staff, clients, and other activities describing the work to be done during a specified shift. The list designates specific staff responsibilities in meeting client needs and related nursing activities. **Delegating client care** refers to the client care manager's function related to leadership, management of resources, and staff development. Delegation involves asking someone else to perform a task that is one of your responsibilities (Nurse's Reference Library, 1984, p. 640) or work that you are being paid to do. Delegated client care is often not written, but done to make wise use of time and available staff resources. It emphasizes individual staff strengths and preferences. In practice, however, these very complex concepts are not mutually exclusive. The box below depicts components of assigning client care according to client needs. Care assignments are based on

Assigning Client Care

Work to be Done Based on Client Needs	Staff Assignment Considerations

Health condition:
  unstable
  unpredictable
  infectious
  complex
	Employee's scope of practice:
	  legal requirements
	  legal restrictions
	  employee's position description

Environmental factors:
  location of client to needed utilities
  number and frequency of time-consuming
    tasks
  interdisciplinary treatment schedules
	Agency's division of work:
	  formal organization
	  policies

Other needed agency resources:
  equipment
  supplies
  physical plant
  coordination of other therapies
	Employee's characteristics:
	  need for inservice education to use safely
	    and cost effectively
	  skills and special talents
	  credentials, personality
	  related experiences
	  attitudes

client needs and what the employee is expected to do with the agency's resources to meet them. Clients with unstable or unpredictable conditions require more complex assessment and monitoring than those with stable conditions. Clients requiring special infection control measures typically also require more time. Clients with complex needs for diagnostic or treatment procedures are likely to require more time and often more skilled care.

Many environmental factors can affect the nature of a work assignment. Generally, caring for clients located in the same area of the nursing unit requires less energy and time than caring for clients in rooms some distance apart. Clients with time-consuming needs, such as frequent monitoring of vital signs or collection of specimens, also require more effort. Clients with established treatment schedules involving other disciplines such as physical, occupational, speech, or group therapies, need special effort so that nursing care will be completed within limited time periods. Another factor that affects the amount of work to be done to meet a client's needs is the types of agency resources available. For example, if equipment is shared by all, staff must coordinate the use of it, which takes time and effort. The availability of supplies and the process for obtaining them can also affect how long it takes staff to complete assignments. The client care manager shares responsibility for making commonly used supplies readily available, and also those that are used less frequently, such as wound debridement trays used in assisting other disciplines in providing client care. The nature of the physical plant, such as the availability of toilets and sinks in private rooms or the lack of them in multibed wards, can also place additional demands on staff. The use of other therapies in the client's overall treatment plan may increase demands on nursing staff, who must assure that the client is prepared and available to participate as scheduled.

Agency functions also affect how the work involved in providing client care is divided. For example, critical care units expect to provide more highly skilled staff in lower ratios to patients than do long-term care agencies that provide convalescent or maintenance care. When **assigning client care,** the staff nurse designates which staff members are to care for specific individuals. This is usually based on responsibilities delineated in their position descriptions, legal scopes of practice, and educational backgrounds. An assignment implies an employee's responsibility to perform activities consistent with his or her position description, in accordance with legally accepted practices (Nurse's Reference Library, 1984, p. 643). The employee is expected to accept work assignments that meet criteria outlined as conditions of employment in her or his job description. Each employee assumes primary responsibility for completing the client care activities included in daily work assignments.

In addition, the individual characteristics of nursing staff members need to be considered when making assignments. Clients with certain personality characteristics, such as anxiety or low self-esteem, are often managed more effectively when matched with staff members who are talented in responding appropriately to such characteristics. Sometimes staff have special interests in common with clients, and matching them can add a special touch in care. Conversely, staff vulnerabilities need to be considered when clients require special approaches or procedures contrary to a nursing team member's disposition. A demanding client who expects follow-through on every detail is unlikely to fare well with a staff member who readily acknowledges that he or she "can't stand sweating the small stuff."

In comparison, a client care manager *delegates* various activities to promote efficiency and cost-effectiveness. Both clinical and nonclinical tasks can be delegated. For example, tasks needed to provide "bedside" care as well as those integral to marketing, public relations, or organizational health, might be delegated to various members of the work group.

Delegation can free time and promote staff development and effective time management. In contrast with assigning client care, **delegating client care** entails a manager's asking a co-worker to perform tasks or activities that are part of the manager's assignment, not part of the co-worker's assignment (Nurse's Reference Library, 1984, p. 640). Proper delegation of client care activities requires that the client care manager consider the employee's position description, the employee's legal scope of practice, and the complexity of individual client needs. The delegated activity is not part of the employee's work assignment, rather an addition to it. Note that the nature of the client care needed as well as the individual staff member's credentials, scope of practice, and individual characteristics need to be considered. In addition, the co-worker must voluntarily accept the delegated work and be motivated to learn about it.

The client care manager uses authority differently to direct staff when assigning care and delegating it. For example, a client care manager might *assign* a licensed practical nurse (LPN) to provide personal hygiene and dressing changes for a group of clients under her or his supervision and complete the corresponding documentation. This *assignment* is likely to be consistent with the LPN's position description and legal scope of practice. It would not be an appropriate assignment for a nursing assistant (NA) because of the need to understand principles of asepsis (needed to safely change dressings), which are usually not included in NA's legal scope of practice. The client care manager could also *delegate* to an RN the responsibility of monitoring the vital signs of a client during the client care manager's lunch break. This delegation is contingent upon acceptance by the RN, who must agree to complete the client care activity, in addition to completing her or his current assignment. If the RN has the needed knowledge, skills, and experience to provide the interim care safely, the delegation process can proceed. If not, the client care manager must assure that the RN has the needed knowledge, information, directions, and instruction before delegating the client's care. The client care manager accepts ultimate primary responsibility for the consequences of delegated tasks.

ASSIGNING CLIENT CARE

Generally, the entry-level staff nurse gains experience supervising the work of others before being asked to assign client care activities. Experience in overseeing the work of others helps produce insights into the complexities of client care and the diversity of persons (and corresponding qualifications, skills, and talents) providing it. Some **principles for assigning client care** can be followed to assure that the group's work is properly allocated so that all needs are satisfactorily met.

Assess Clients' Needs

First, the client care manager assesses the needs of all clients whose care will be assigned. This preliminary assessment might be done in several ways, including the collection of information directly from the client and from family, clinical record, classification system, or change-of-shift report. These assessments enable the nurse to determine, in a general way, what types of needs the group of clients have, what is planned to meet them, how complex the care is, and approximately how much time is needed to complete it. On the basis of this information, the client care manager sets priorities for her or his assigned group of clients. For example, clients who are responding unpredictably, who are threatened by serious complications, who have infectious conditions, who require complex nursing procedures or time-consuming care, or who are experiencing high levels of anxiety receive special consideration. When assigning care, the client care manager attempts to maximize the available staff knowledge, skills, and time to address each client's care safely and satisfactorily. Physiologically unstable clients require more expertise and time to assure that their needs are safely met. Nurses caring for clients who need extensive infection control measures require additional knowledge, skill, and time to assure the safety of the clients and others in the immediate environment. Special needs influence which staff are assigned to care for which clients. To promote effective infection control strategies, a staff member is generally not assigned more than two clients requiring such care during any shift. This strategy of assigning only two such clients requires the staff member to plan effective use of time and supplies as well.

Consider Staff Number and Type

Second, the client care manager usually knows the number and classifications of staff available to provide the needed care, either before or immediately after receiving the change-of-shift report. Agency policies, rooted in state laws that define and delimit scopes of practice, require that work assignments be consistent with the responsibilities, tasks, and activities included in corresponding staff position descriptions. The position descriptions for client care managers, as entry-level RNs, generally require that they accept responsibility for using the nursing process to determine client needs and establish, implement, and evaluate care plans to meet them. In addition, they often delineate dependent and interdependent functions on the client's behalf. For example, RNs are expected to communicate effectively with the interdisciplinary team and coordinate efforts made to enable clients and families to gain and maintain independence in self-care. In addition, after adequate preparation, client care managers perform a wide variety of nursing procedures using established guidelines provided by the agency or manufacturers of the equipment and supplies. As nursing establishes itself as a profession, RNs will be expected to assume greater responsibility for the scope of their practice, including accountability for those working directly under their supervision and direction.

In comparison, LPNs and NAs are dependent on other professionals to assess client conditions, analyze the information gathered, and establish safe and effective plans to respond to the identified needs. Various classifications of subordinate nursing staff rely on RNs to provide guidance and direction in responding to individual client needs. Consistent with their legal scopes of practice, each staff member is answerable for actions or nonactions taken to meet client needs. Accordingly, they share liability for any harm or injury they cause clients in the performance of their duties.

Generally, LPNs are prepared to implement established plans of care and to provide feedback about clients who are expected to respond predictably. They can usually be expected to perform procedures according to protocol, but are not prepared to evaluate client responses to various treatments, particularly those that indicate unstable physiological conditions requiring immediate attention. They are prepared to perform various infection-control procedures, apply principles of asepsis (sterile techniques required in various procedures designed to prevent or control infectious processes), and conduct established routines. Again, LPNs typically are not adequately prepared to assess, analyze, or evaluate client responses, though they are proficient in implementing established plans of care for physiologically stable clients and those with predictable conditions.

NAs, when assigned client care, have the narrowest scope of nursing practice, which corresponds to their educational background. Typically, they are prepared to provide routine personal hygiene measures, especially those related to the clients' activities of daily living. These activities include bathing, dressing, transferring, ambulating, repositioning, toileting, and feeding clients. In addition, they can record routine intake and output and other basic nursing routines that require them to perform specific hand-washing procedures and comply with universal precautions. However, NAs are not prepared to apply principles of asepsis. They can be expected to perform basic nursing procedures for which they have been prepared, and they are answerble for such actions.

When assigning client care, the client care manager determines who of the available staff is best able to provide each client's care. Remember that the agency is likely to use a classification system, policies, and position descriptions to match estimated client needs with available staff. These factors strongly influence what staff expect their work assignments to be. It is important to establish high performance expectations and work together to meet them (Schaffer, 1991; p. 146). It is up to the imagination and creativity of the client care manager to use specific detailed information about individual staff capabilities to maximize client care. For example, some staff are more efficient due to skills gained from experiences working with others in complex situations. Other staff members might be inexperienced, but be very good listeners for clients with less complex physical needs but greater emotional needs, such as the undergoing extensive diagnostic procedures.

In any event, the client care manager *must* assign care primarily on the basis of client needs and demonstrated staff competence to address them. Without such a foundation, it is not safe to assume that the client will receive safe and satisfactory care. If there is any question about the adequacy of the staff member's qualifications to provide the needed care, the situation must be clarified before assigning care. To enable staff to proceed safely, the client care manager asks questions, discusses mutual expectations, provides instruction when a staff member is unfamiliar with a specific approach or procedure, gives specific directions for adaptations, and plans with each member to ensure proper follow-through. The assignment is acceptable only when each staff member understands it and is adequately prepared to carry it out.

Demonstrate Trust in Co-workers' Abilities

Third, each co-worker is respected or treated as an individual with specific needs, who contributes to the group's effort and is recognized for contributing. Unless there is a specific reason not to do so, the client care manager expects each staff member to perform all functions and tasks delineated in her or his position description. Trust, though difficult to manage, is critical (Manthey, 1990, p. 28). Each staff member should be trusted to follow through on a client care assignment. To not trust a co-worker, without justification, diminishes the person's sense of self-worth and decreases the individual's value to the organization. All client care activities are important! By assigning staff in a way that challenges them to use their strengths and maximizes their contributions to quality care, the client care manager promotes the agency's efficiency and effectiveness.

Promote Continuity of Care

Fourth, to the extent possible, client care is assigned consistently to the same staff to promote continuity of care. That is, most clients benefit from receiving care from staff who have in-depth knowledge and experience. Although clients generally don't mind answering occasional questions when they really need to be asked, clients appreciate not being asked to answer the same questions repeatedly. Consistency in working relationships between staff and clients improves efficiency and effectiveness.

Avoid Disrupting the Logical Work Flow

Fifth, the client care manager helps staff organize work by assigning activities in similar locations and in combinations that are compatible with interdisciplinary treatment program schedules. Try as they might, each staff member can only be in one place at a time. If they are expected to be in two places simultaneously to complete care according to the team's schedule, work flow is likely to be disrupted. These disruptions, in addition to frustrating clients, often negatively affect nursing staff, other team members, and departments.

Describe Assignments in Detail

Sixth, after assuring that staff are adequately prepared to complete client care assignments, the staff nurse describes the desired care in concrete or measurable terms. Detailed information is usually available on individual plans of care or defined in nursing procedure manuals. If it is not, it is important that clarification be made. For example, it is not adequate to say, "Mr. J needs regular intermittent catheterizations"; rather, the staff member needs to know the frequency of the intermittent catherizations, and what amount of residual urine is to be reported immediately for further evaluation. This helps both the employee and the staff nurse evaluate the outcomes of care. To confirm that the assignee accurately comprehends the assignment, the staff nurse seeks feedback throughout the work day. Sharing mutual expectations about work provides a sound foundation for evaluation later. Specific information about the care provided and feedback about the client's responses to it provide clues to areas of continuing concern as well.

Assign ALL Aspects of Care

Seventh, though it almost goes without saying, responsibility for *all* of each client's care is explicitly assigned (Schaffer, 1991, pp. 147–148), including both concrete tasks *and* all functions involved in assessing, planning, and evaluating care. To ensure that customer-driven services are consistent with common nursing goals, the client care manager needs to avoid assigning *only* procedural aspects of client care. For example, frequently, only the nursing tasks (for example, monitoring vital signs, dressing changes, personal hygiene measures) involved in a client's care are considered when assigning it. It also takes knowledge. Assigning everything promotes caring attitudes and development of corresponding systems to divide the work involved in the desired client care.

To promote accountability for all of a client's care, only one person is explicitly assigned to each component of it. Expectations are clearly communicated in terms that enable staff to readily determine if the desired results were successfully achieved. Through an orientation that is unique to nursing, this method emphasizes the totality of the client's care. However, some organizations might vary assignment methods, and strive to retain focus on the client's totality as a person through its formal organization of the interdisciplinary team.

An assignment method might involve two types of responsibilities: (1) those that must be completed during each shift, and (2) those that occur over extended or indefinite periods of time. For example, in common primary nursing arrangements, a "primary nurse" is designated in combination with a staff nurse who is assigned care each shift. The "primary nurse" assumes responsibility for managing the client's response and evaluates the need to make changes in the plan based on emerging urgent needs that require immediate attention. In a modified team or functional nursing pattern of nursing service delivery, on the other hand, several persons might be assigned to manage a client's overall plan of care. In addition, on a daily basis, each client care manager might also be assigned another group of clients for an extended time period. These assignments would involve monitoring client responses and striving to assure continuity of care for a group of clients in addition to those assigned on a shift-by-shift basis.

By reviewing completed client care assignment sheets, a staff nurse should be able to identify who is assigned to complete each aspect of the client's care. The responsibility for completing client care assignments rests primarily with those employed to carry them out. But a manager can never totally delegate this responsibility to other staff; ultimately, the client care manager shares responsibility for the quality of care provided. An assignment method might involve two types of responsibilities: those that must be completed during each shift, and those that occur over extended or indefinite periods of time. For example, in common primary nursing arrangements, a "primary nurse" is designated in combination with a staff nurse who is assigned care each shift. In a modified team or functional nursing pattern of nursing delivery, on the other hand, several persons might be assigned. In addition, each client care manager might also be assigned another group of clients for an extended time period. These assignments would invove monitoring client responses to plan care and striving to assure continuity of care for a group of clients in addition to those assigned on a shift-by-shift basis.

By reviewing completed client care assignment sheets, a staff nurse should be able to identify who is assigned to complete each aspect of the client's care. The responsibility for completing client care assignments rests primarily with those employed to carry them out. But a manager can never totally delegate this responsibility to other staff; ultimately, the manager shares responsibility for the quality of care provided.

Consider Changes in Clients' Conditions

Eighth, to assure that clients receive needed care, the staff nurse considers the time and complexity of the designated activities, initially and throughout the workday. Client's conditions change, requiring reassessment of needs and perhaps different knowledge and skills to meet them. Sometimes, these changes in client conditions are anticipated and incorporated in the initial assignment. Typically, staff with greater knowledge and skills are assigned to care for less physiologically stable clients. At other times, a client's condition changes unexpectedly. Such clients require care monitoring and skilled responses by the client care manager, including changes in work assignments, to ensure that client needs are being adequately monitored, assessed, and addressed.

Consider Changes in Clients' Plans of Care

Ninth, changes in client conditions or plans to treat them can mean that staff need more help or instruction. Equipment, supplies, or treatment modalities may be prescribed that staff are unfamiliar with or that are beyond their scope of practice. If the nature of the client care remains within the assigned staff member's scope of practice, the client care manager needs to provide the additional help or instruction. Generally, the staff nurse initially learns about changes in clients' plan of care when transcribing physician's "orders." It is critical that the client care manager communicate these changes accurately and in a timely manner to assigned staff in the client's behalf. If the changes in the client's plan of

---

Guidelines for Assigning Client Care

1. Determine the amount of nursing care time required, and the complexity of the activities allocated.
2. Identify who, of the available staff, is best qualified to provide the client's care, considering attitudes, skills, demeanor, and efficiency.
3. Consider each staff member as an individual with a unique combination of needs, skills, and talents.
4. Strive to maximize continuity of care and reduce fragmentation.
5. Combine assignments to increase efficiency; consider treatment schedules and geographic locations of clients.
6. Describe the assignment in measurable terms; be specific about expected results.
7. Designate one person or an absolute minimum number of staff to be responsible for each client's care.
8. Plan to provide additional help, direction, or instruction as necessary to match the needs of individual staff members.
9. Communicate assignments clearly, preferably in writing.
10. Assign responsibility for holistic care; avoid assigning only nursing procedures.

---

care exceed the assigned staff member's scope of practice, the client care manager must reassign the client's care and make the provisions needed to provide it. The box above lists guidelines for assigning client care.

▮ LEGAL ASPECTS OF ASSIGNING CLIENT CARE

Thus far, this discussion of the function of assigning client care has emphasized the need to focus on assessed or identified client needs as an essential foundation for meeting this staff nurse responsibility (Feutz, 1988, p. 10). If the staff nurse does not know what care clients need, he or she cannot provide for the corresponding knowledge, skills, attitudes, and talents. The agency's resources, policies, procedures, or position descriptions cannot alone be used to designate which staff member can reasonably provide care; the clients' needs must also be considered. The agency depends on staff nurses to collect the information on clients' needs and to determine what needs to be done to meet them during the work shift.

As mentioned in Chapter Three, staff nurses are expected to provide accurate information about client needs demanded by the agency's classification system to help it provide adequate staffing. In addition, they are expected to assign available staff correctly to match client needs. The agency assumes responsibility for providing adequate staffing, in terms of both numbers and qualifications (Calfee, 1987, p. 26). If available staffing is inadequate, staff nurses are expected to communicate their concerns to their supervisors immediately to assure safe and adequate care (Creighton, 1986b, p. 14). Identifying the problem of inadequate staffing does not permit the staff nurse to decrease the standard of care below that required by law (Rabinow, 1985, p. 29). Clients are legally entitled to minimal standards of care whether or not the agency is adequately staffed. Client care managers share responsibility for ensuring that such standards of care are provided. These standards for safe practice are based on scopes of nursing practice as defined by state licensing agencies. In a court of law, these standards might be compared to actions that would be taken by a peer, or reasonable and prudent nurse, in similar circumstances.

The staff nurse, as client care manager, assumes **responsibility** for nursing judgments, decisions, and actions (Creighton, 1986a, p. 24). That is, the nurse expects to answer for situations that are under her or his control. In circumstances where control is shared, responsibility is shared also. In previous years, when the nurse acted as an agent of the health care organization, the agency was held accountable under the *respondeat superior* doctrine. That is, the agency, as "master," was assumed to exercise control over the nurse's actions and was accountable for the consequences of the nurse's judgments, decisions, and actions. As nursing gains recognition as a profession, individual nurses are likely to be perceived as being *personally* answerable for their judgments, decisions, and actions.

The staff nurse has the **authority** to judge the nature of client needs and the adequacy of staffing and to take action as necessary to obtain staffing. In other words, based on nursing knowledge and skills, the nurse has the personal power to determine client needs and the organizational power to obtain adequate staffing. The nurse also decides whether the qualifications of the available staff match the complexity of client needs. Qualified staff can promptly recognize and manage changes in clients' conditions (Feutz, 1988, p. 9). Obviously, the more complex the client's needs, the more knowledge and skill are needed to assess and manage them. Inexperienced, float, or "pool" (subcontracted by temporary staffing agencies) staff usually need supervision and often additional direction, if clients with complex needs are to receive safe care. If minimal standards of care are not provided and client safety is at risk, the nurse must take immediate action to alleviate the situation.

Accountability refers to being answerable for results. The staff nurse is accountable for the consequences of decisions made and actions taken in meeting the responsibilities of client care. The staff nurse's primary accountability is to clients, as stipulated in the standards of practice established by the profession. These standards are used as a foundation for judging the correctness and adequacy of care. To not adhere to accepted standards of practice and thereby place the client at risk or cause harm is **malpractice,** or professional misconduct. Nurses use malpractice insurance to manage the risk of being accused by clients of causing them serious harm or injuries. This method of managing risks is used to reduce the financial burden of resolving such accusations (Bernzweig, 1990, pp. 379–380). The individual nurse's need for malpractice insurance will be discussed in more detail in the Epilogue.

Secondarily, the nurse is also answerable to the agency and is expected to comply with its policies, procedures, and guidelines. Accordingly, to be accountable when assigning care, the staff nurse must know the agency's guidelines for determining the employee qualifications needed to respond adequately to various types of client needs. Again, the agency depends upon input from staff nurses about assessed needs and the adequacy of staffing. When staff nurses identify the problem of inadequate staffing, they are expected to immediately communicate specific information about the nature of the clients' needs and available staffing to their immediate supervisors. As mentioned in Chapter Four, attempting to complete an impossible assignment and consequently endangering clients is irresponsible.

Liability is legal accountability for client risks, danger, and injury caused by the nurse's malpractice or negligent acts.

Negligence involves either acts of **commission,** doing something that harms the client or acts of **omission,** not doing something that should have been done to prevent client harm or injury.

When the staff nurse assigns client care, the agency expects that nursing knowledge, skills, and standards will be the basis for designating what work each staff member is requested to do. The client care manager is authorized to allocate resources consistent with client and agency goals. Improperly assigning client care increases the nurse's risk of liability resulting from her or his own actions or the actions of others (Rhodes, 1986, p. 315). If the nurse acts responsibly, in accordance with agency policies and professional standards, the agency, as employer, can be held liable for the consequences of inadequate staffing. To the extent that the nurse is a participant in negligent acts believed to cause harm to clients, he or she shares liability. Proper assignment of client care is a big step in providing safe care, and it concurrently eliminates the nurse's liability in this matter.

ACCEPTING ACCOUNTABILITY FOR ASSIGNED CLIENT CARE

As mentioned earlier, assigning client care entails designating individual staff members to provide it, within guidelines provided by the agency's formal organization, policies, procedures, position descriptions, and systems of care. When staff nurses assign client care according to the agency's guidelines, they accept responsibility for performing this function. They also accept supervisory responsibility for client care. However, staff accept primary responsibility for completing their assignments and expect to answer for their actions. Assigned staff are accountable for completing the work allocated to them within the allotted time period, and for the consequences of their work. They accept responsibility for completing the assigned client care activities in a safe, efficient, satisfactory manner.

DELEGATING CLIENT CARE

Client care managers typically have many opportunities to delegate some of their assigned duties and tasks. The primary purpose of delegating client care is to shift some responsibility to another staff member to increase one's own effectiveness and efficiency and improve the skills, effectiveness, and efficiency of those accepting the delegation (Sondak, 1991, p. 5; Hanston, 1991, p. 126). Responsibility for duties and tasks can never be totally delegated, however.

Delegating differs significantly from assigning client care. However, several characteristics of proper delegation are similar to those involved in client care assignment. Assigning client care is a required function. It is regularly done to properly allocate the work that staff are employed to do. Delegating work is optional, or done by choice. Client care managers can delegate only those client care activities that are part of their own work assignments, not those already assigned to others. Client care assigned to others can be reassigned, but not delegated. RNs have the most inclusive legal scope of practice of the various classifications of nursing staff, which permits them to assign or delegate a range of activities to RNs, LPNs, and NAs.

Many staff nurses have great difficulty delegating work effectively to available staff (Lane, 1990, p. 46). Often, whether any client care is delegated depends on the norms of a specific work culture. Predominant staff perceptions of the purposes of delegation often condition client care managers (Lawrie, 1990, p. 1). Some cultures encourage delegation while others do not; norms of the work environment, often unspoken, can work to reinforce or punish those who delegate work. For example, a culture's prevailing attitude may be

"We all work together until we're all done" or "Everyone is expected to do a fair share around here." Client care managers in such a culture might hesitate to delegate any client care activities assigned to them, fearing that they might appear incompetent, disorganized, or lazy.

A different work culture might encourage client care managers to delegate in the interests of cost effectiveness. However, managers might hesitate to grant their delegatees decision-making authority consistent with the responsibility needed to follow through efficiently. In such a case the delegation defeats its purpose because the delegatee spends considerable time and effort relaying information instead of using the delegated authority to make decisions needed to complete activities smoothly and efficiently. Fear of liability for the actions of others is often given as a reason for not delegating (Salmond, 1990, p. 41).

Some nurses might hesitate to delegate client care activities because doing so frees up time for them to do activities that are more complicated or with which they are less familiar. Others believe that since they can perform an activity proficiently, nothing is to be gained by delegating it to other available staff. In fact, other staff often welcome the challenge of learning new skills or increasing their proficiency in performing them. Some client care managers avoid delegating care for fear of "dumping" extra work on staff. These explanations are invalid in most situations.

Whether or not client care is delegated is a personal decision of the staff nurse, and not a scheduled or clearly defined requirement of the position. To develop skills used in delegating care to increase one's own effectiveness and efficiency and those of co-workers, client care managers need to constantly seek opportunities to delegate.

Depending on the nature of the client care activities and qualifications of available staff, many characteristics of the process of delegation are similar to those used to assign

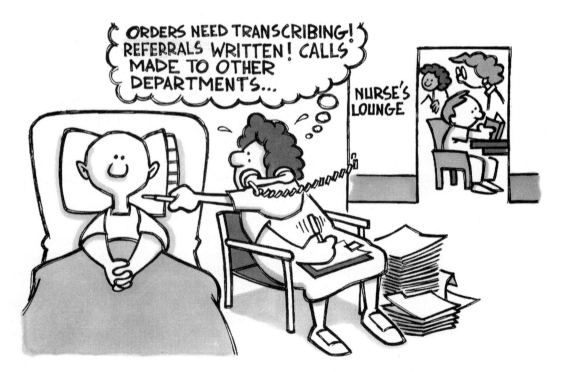

By not delegating effectively, the client care manager takes on extra work.

client care. When assigning client care, the manager needs to know the strengths and weaknesses of the staff to whom the work is allocated. When delegating care, it is also important that the delegator know her or his own personal strengths, likes, dislikes, and vulnerabilities. This helps the nurse to delegate to improve care quality and staff capabilities, not to seek personal gain or avoid activities that are personally distasteful.

There are several **principles for delegating work of assigned client care managers.** The box below lists requirements for properly delegating work to others. The client care manager needs to know what is involved in the activities that are being delegated, within the context of her or his own position description and that of the delegatee. The tasks to be delegated need to be consistent with these position guidelines. In other words, is this work similar in type and complexity to that routinely expected of this type of staff member? If the answer is yes, this work could be delegated. In addition, the delegated tasks need to be consistent with the individual's capabilities, interests, and skills since the delegatee needs to voluntarily accept the additional work, rather than be required to do it. Receiving the delegatee's approval ensures that he or she accepts responsibility for completing the specific tasks and accepts accountability for the consequences of actions taken.

To effectively delegate client care, the client care manager needs to communicate expectations clearly and completely. The delegatee should be able to describe what results are expected and what types of client responses or variations need to be reported to the client care manager. Sometimes, due to lack of open communications, the client care is not delegated because "it takes less time to do it myself." However, skills needed to delegate effectively are developed through practice, and typically, efficiency also increases with practice. Before delegating client care, the desired results need to be clear in the manager's own mind and that of the person who will strive to achieve them. The desired results need to be described in concrete, descriptive terms, so that client outcomes and characteristics can be readily used to determine whether the delegatee was successful. Open discussions

---

Requirements for Delegating Duties and Tasks

1. Determine the extent and complexity of client needs or the nature of the work to be delegated.
2. Identify the employee to whom tasks or duties are to be delegated.
3. Determine that the work is consistent with the employee's position description and normal duties.
4. Clearly communicate expectations and desired results using concrete, measurable terms; convey both trust and sufficient authority.
5. Obtain the employee's voluntary acceptance of the work request.
6. Keep communication lines open while providing needed direction, instruction, and supervision.
7. Compare actual results with desired goals; give constructive feedback and praise to reward the employee's efforts.
8. Constantly work toward increased productive use of time and resources and efficiency required to provide cost-effective quality care.
9. Practice, practice, practice!

help the delegatee to express concerns and questions and agree on mutual expectations of the delegation.

Preparing to Delegate Client Care

The client care manager needs to address several criteria to successfully delegate client care. Usually, the manager has gained some experience working with the delegatee before actually delegating various activities to her or him. These experiences help the client care manager become familiar with the other staff member's attitudes, knowledge, and skills. They also give the client care manager a chance to evaluate the staff member's skills. Prior to delegating any client care, the client care manager needs to determine that the staff member has the capacity to complete it.

The client care manager needs to ensure that the types of client care delegated are consistent with the agency's policies. That is, the type of work being delegated must be consistent with that normally performed by the delegatee's employee classification. A unit clerk can be asked to requisition supplies, while nursing staff can perform various procedures involved in client care. If delegated work is not consistent with agency policy and position descriptions, the employee is less likely to have repeated opportunities to practice new skills to perform them efficiently. The care needs to be delegated to the type of employee who is likely to perform it correctly or who might reasonably be expected to perform this type of work in the future.

The client care manager needs to trust the delegatee to complete the delegated work according to established standards or mutual expectations. A positive working relationship reduces any reservation the client care manager might have about granting the subordinate the authority needed to complete the tasks. If the client care manager expresses confidence in the delegatee's capacity to complete the tasks, he or she is also likely to believe in her or his abilities. A trusting relationship also promotes open and effective communication, so clear instructions and directions can be given. This increases the chances that the delegatee will readily accept accountability for the consequences of her or his actions.

For the delegatee to make decisions to obtain desired client outcomes, the delegator needs to grant sufficient authority. In other words, the person performing the client care activities needs authorization to modify activities to achieve desired results. Requiring the individual to repeatedly confer with the delegator before making necessary decisions is frustrating and inefficient. If the delegatee's decision-making authority is limited, the limits need to be clarified at the time the tasks are delegated, not throughout the process of completing them. It is critical that the co-worker receive recognition and praise for safely and satisfactorily completing delegated care. The manager seeks feedback both to help the co-worker and to sharpen delegation skills. With practice, delegation can become an extremely valuable tool for managing time and building effective working relationships. Ultimately, everyone benefits—clients, staff, and the agency.

Remember that one purpose of delegation is to help the co-worker learn and practice new skills. To be successful, the experience needs to be positive without unnecessarily risking the client's safety. If the delegatee makes a mistake, the staff nurse, as delegator, needs to explain the error and teach the person how to perform the activity correctly. If too much supervision, humiliation, or frustration is involved in completing the delegated tasks, the delegatee is likely to avoid accepting responsibility for other delegated tasks, and the client care manager is unlikely to use available time and resources more efficiently over the long haul. The client care manager needs to practice delegating activities to improve the quality of care, time management, and development of scarce human resources.

Though there are risks involved, if reasonable precautions are taken, delegating client care leads to satisfying work experiences.

Accepting Accountability for Delegated Tasks

The client care manager accepts primary responsibility for the consequences of delegation and shares legal accountability for them. These consequences can relate to one's own actions in delegating and also to the actions or nonactions taken by the delegatee. If client safety is risked and the individual suffers injury or harm, the client care manager may be liable. When undesired results occur, questions are asked concerning who was responsible for the client's care and why and how the activities were delegated. When reviewing the delegation process, the apppropriateness of the delegation and the qualifications of the staff to whom the care was delegated are considered. Remember, when the delegatee practices within an assigned role, he or she is responsible for the consequences. The staff nurse is responsible only when the nurse clearly delegates a task that lies within the professional practice role (Lane, 1990, p. 46).

Authority, responsibility, and accountability for delegation rest primarily in the staff nurse's decision-making role. That is, the staff nurse has administrative control over the actual delivery of care and is responsible for "protecting and promoting the common good" (Sullivan and Brown, 1989, p. 563). The client care manager determines the nature of the client's needs as well as the co-workers's capacity to meet them. By including all the components of proper delegation, the client care manager becomes an active participant in the delivery of care with the co-worker (Reis, 1991, p. 12). Consequently, the client care manager shares liability for the actions or nonactions of the co-worker. These legal parameters apply in situations where the client care manager has delegated care to others or has accepted delegation from others. When delegation is performed properly, no injury or harm occurs and everyone benefits; only when it is performed improperly does the potential for liability exist. Proper delegation is a skill well worth refining.

◼ SUMMARY

Staff nurses are expected to assign and delegate client care to available staff while managing care. Assigning client care involves allocating the work to be done and designating who is to do it. To complete this function, work is allocated according to assessed client needs and guided by agency policies, organizational structure, position descriptions, and legal scopes of practice. Care assigned to others can be reassigned but not delegated. In contrast, care assigned to the client care manager can be delegated. Both client care and nonclinical work can be delegated. Proper delegation of tasks is based on the complexity of the work and the staff member's legal scope of practice, assigned role, attitudes, knowledge, and skills. The delegatee must voluntarily accept the work request.

When making assignments, the client care manager needs to understand the types of client needs each classification of staff member is prepared to meet and the legal limits established for her or his scope of practice. The RN assumes responsibility for assessing client needs and judging the adequacy of available staffing to meet them. Client care is assigned consistent with legal guidelines; consequently, each staff member is responsible for her or his own actions and nonactions taken to complete them. Special consideration is given to clients with unpredictable, physiologically unstable, infectious, or other complex conditions; the RN is expected to make special provisions to ensure that minimal standards of safe care are provided. These standards reflect compliance with established standards of practice, and no exception is made for inadequate staffing. Client care is assigned on the basis of assessed needs and the staff's competence to provide it.

Client care assignments consider continuity of care, geographic location of clients, scheduled treatment programs and related nursing staff demands, and individual staff interests, skills, and talents. To the extent possible, client care is assigned to one person, to reduce fragmentation and need for coordination. Staff need respect, recognition, and trust to sustain effective working relationships. Assignments include all aspects of client care to promote a holistic approach integral to nursing care, focusing on the tasks of care is avoided.

Staff assume primary responsibility for completing the work assigned to them. Consequently, they accept liability for the consequences of their actions. The client care manager shares responsibility with the agency for obtaining staffing adequate to provide minimal standards of safe care. Accordingly, the client care manager is accountable for decisions made and actions or nonactions taken to assure safe care or avoid harm or injury to clients. The client care manager is legally liable for malpractice or negligent acts that result in client injury or harm.

Client care managers delegate various aspects of their work to increase their productivity and to increase the quality of care by developing the skills of other staff. Many nurses are hesitant to delegate. Sometimes this reluctance results from characteristics of the work culture or personal fears, but if proper guidelines are followed and preparations made, delegation can improve the quality of care. The staff nurse is responsible for assessing client needs and matching them to the staff member's nursing skills, attitudes, and qualifications; in addition, expectations and instructions need to be clearly communicated to delegatee. The delegatee voluntarily accepts the delegated work. The client care manager supervises the staff member's performance and provides feedback to help achieve the desired results. The client care manager grants the delegatee the authority needed to complete the work smoothly; the work relationship is built on trust and confidence in the individual's abilities. If mistakes occur, the staff member receives corrective feedback to enable her or him to perform the activities safely in the future. The staff member needs praise and recognition for accepting and successfully completing delegated care activities.

Client care managers assume primary responsibility for the consequences of delegated work. This responsibility relates to their decision-making role in determining client needs and how to meet them. When client care is properly delegated, no injury or harm is likely to occur. Management skills used to properly delegate client care are well worth nurturing to increase the client care manager's effectiveness and productivity. Use of these skills is instrumental in helping others increase their productivity as well.

■■■■■ APPLICATION EXERCISES

    a. Your nursing work group consists of another staff nurse, two LPNs, and two NAs. Identify those activities that you can assign to each category of nursing staff.

    b. Your group of twenty clients includes some with stable conditions and others who are not physiologically stable. Describe guidelines you would use to assign client care to available staff.

    c. Contrast nursing authority with accountability for meeting client needs.

    d. Describe which activities and functions a staff nurse can delegate to members of the nursing work group. Give reasons for your answer.

    e. Describe approaches you would use to promote positive experiences for your delegatees.

REFERENCES

Bernzweig EP: *The nurse's liability for malpractice,* ed 5, St. Louis, Mo, 1990, C.V. Mosby.

Calfee BE: Understaffing, *NursingLife* 7(6):25–29. (November/December, 1987).

Creighton H: Understaffing—Part I, *Nurs Manage* 17(4):24,27–28. (April, 1986a).

Creighton H: Understaffing—Part II, *Nurs Manage* 17(5):14,16. (May, 1986b).

Feutz SA: Nursing work assignments: rights and responsibilities," *J Nurs Adm* 18(4):9–11. (April, 1988).

Hanston RI: Delegation: learning when and how to let go, *Nurs 91* 21(4):126, 128, 131, 133. (April, 1991).

Lane AJ: Nurse extenders: refocusing on the art of delegation, *J Nurs Adm* 20(5):40,46. (May, 1990).

Lawrie J: Turning around attitudes about delegation, *Supervis Manage* 35(12):1–2. (December, 1990).

Manthey M: Trust: essential for delegation, *Nurs Manage* 21(11):28–29. (November, 1990).

Nurse's Reference Library: *Practices,* Springhouse, Pa, 1984, Springhouse.

Rabinow Jean: Inadequate staffing? Don't take chances with risky solutions, *NursingLife* 5(4):28–30. (July/August, 1985).

Reis DG: Appropriate delegation of activities, *Nurs Manage* 22(1):12. (January, 1991).

Rhodes AM: Liability for the actions of others, *MCN* 11(5):315. (September/October, 1986).

Salmond SW: Clinical support workers: a help or a hindrance to the shortage crisis? *Orthop Nurs* 9(5):39–46. (September/October, 1990).

Schaffer RH: Demand better results—and get them, *Harvard Bus Rev* 69(2):142–149. (March/April, 1991).

Sondak A: Delegation: getting to the heart, or gut, of the matter, *Supervis Manage* 36(3):5. (March, 1991).

Sullivan PA, Brown T: Unlicensed persons in patient care settings: administrative, policy, and ethical issues, *Nurs Clin North Am* 24(2):557–569. (1989).

chapter thirteen

CONDUCTING CLIENT CARE CONFERENCES AS A MANAGEMENT TOOL

OBJECTIVES

Completing this chapter should enable you to:

1. State the purposes of client care conferences.
2. Distinguish client care conferences designed to manage care from those designed to teach others.
3. Describe the process used to prepare for a client care conference.
4. Describe the process of conducting a client care conference.
5. Describe strategies to increase the effectiveness and efficiency of client care conferences.
6. Describe various methods of evaluating the effectiveness of client care conferences.

KEY CONCEPTS

conducting a client care conference as a
   management tool
process of conducting a management
   conference
   identify clients who could benefit

prepare and plan
purpose
conduct the meeting
evaluate effectiveness
structure

CLIENT CARE CONFERENCES

Entry-level staff nurses are expected to manage client care using a variety of management skills in many different organizational contexts. They are expected to direct, supervise, and coordinate the efforts of interdisciplinary teams to enable clients to meet their health needs in a cost-effective manner. A client might not make anticipated progress for many reasons, a common one being that some of the many people involved in the client's treatment are not following the same plan of care. To address this problem, the nurse can **conduct a client care conference as a management tool** to improve the quality of the client's care. When used selectively and skillfully, this technique is very effective in identifying current client needs and matching staff approaches to meet them. The nurse conducting the conference believes that the client's care will be improved enough to justify the expense of the meeting.

In the past, many nurses did not develop the skills needed to participate or conduct conferences, especially those involving interdisciplinary team members [where roles might overlap] (Coker and Schrieber, 1990, p. 46). As a consequence, many nurses have trouble valuing the contributions nurses can make to work effectively with other members of the team.

Nursing students are usually familiar with the types of conferences conducted for teaching purposes. A clinical conference (sometimes referred to as a "preconference" or "postconference") held for teaching purposes usually has as its primary purpose to teach others, including fellow students and staff. The "ground rules" for conducting the meeting reflect its teaching purposes; such conferences include specific categories of information and discussion and are scheduled according to the needs and goals of the learners. They are evaluated in terms of their effectiveness in addressing the learners' needs (Skurski, 1985, pp. 166–168).

Another common type of clinical conference is that which is regularly scheduled for the interdisciplinary team to help coordinate routine activities and update plans of care. Nursing students often participate in these conferences while working with psychiatric or chronically ill clients. The work group regularly schedules time to meet to systematically review treatment plans for each client. These conferences increase the effectiveness and efficiency of interdisciplinary teams by providing regular opportunities for members to express their concerns, share observations, and plan or revise client care plans. These interdisciplinary team conferences are an integral part of coordinating efforts on the client's behalf.

Change-of-shift reports are another type of clinical conference used to manage care, though they are not the type of conference that staff nurses use at their discretion to manage client care. Rather, these conferences are regularly scheduled sessions that give staff nurses an opportunity to discuss client needs, concerns, and progress to promote continuity of care.

Clinical conferences designed to help staff manage a client's care better with available resources are the focus of this chapter. This type of management conference is designed, planned, and implemented at the staff nurse's discretion to improve the quality of care received by clients at serious risk. Conducting a management conference, like proper delegation, requires distinct nursing skills. Nurses who use these skills regularly refine them with practice, to the benefit of clients.

Management conferences consume agency resources, primarily scarce staff time. Staff time is expended to better manage the care of clients at high risk for potential complications, or do not make expected progress to services provided due to the complexity of individual circumstances. Because management conferences use staff time, they are costly, but failing to recognize clients who could benefit from such conferences is even more costly in terms of ineffective expenditure of staff time, equipment, supplies, and facilities to achieve desired client outcomes.

Management conferences are used to help staff recognize complex client problems and their possible causes, as well as to identify and evaluate proposed solutions that are acceptable to both client and staff. That is, the client benefits from the care plan adjustment and staff gain insight into the individual's situation. Having participated in formulating the plan, staff increase their commitment to carry it out. Staff nurses conduct management conferences to build staff commitment to individualized plans of care, to facilitate desired staff approaches, and to coordinate the various disciplines involved.

The **process of conducting a management conference** involves four phases:

1. Identifying clients who could benefit
2. Preparation
3. Implementation
4. Evaluation and follow-up

Successfully conducting such a conference requires the client care manager to attend to various considerations in each phase.

CLIENTS WHO COULD BENEFIT FROM A CONFERENCE

Client care managers accept responsibility for **identifying clients who could benefit** directly from being the subject of a management conference. Characteristics that increase a client's risk of responding ineffectively to treatment vary. Common characteristics that indicate serious risks include

1. Language or communication barriers
2. Extremes in chronological age
3. Complexity of disease processes
4. Staff unfamiliarity with treatment approaches
5. Unusual client coping styles
6. Lack of meaningful or supportive relationships

As entry-level staff nurses gain experience, they become familiar with common patterns of client response to various health conditions and to typical treatment processes from admissions to discharge. Nursing students who choose to develop skills needed to conduct management conferences might turn to their resource persons such as clinical instructors or experienced staff nurses to help them identify clients who could benefit from such a conference.

As they gain experience, staff nurses learn to differentiate common individual variations from characteristics that indicate that a client is at serious risk for potential complications or is unable to make desired progress to meet care goals. A client might, for example be confronted with language or cultural barriers that complicate her or his ability to understand the purposes of various diagnostic procedures or treatments. This might delay informed consent and active participation based on comprehension of desired behaviors. Or a client experiencing a multiplicity of diseases and complications might perceive treatment goals differently from health care providers. As a result, there may be conflict instead of a mutually agreed-upon program of treatment. Sometimes, clients are assumed to understand disease processes affecting them without receiving adequate instruction and are unable to carry out the self-care procedures required to manage safely at home. Clients may feel overwhelmed by the many demands placed upon them by family and staff, and be unable to use coping mechanisms that were effective in the past in enabling them to adjust.

Rather than setting discharge dates without regard for the client's need to meet prospective payment requirements, staff can make timely interventions on the client's behalf. This can help to establish workable plans that are acceptable to both clients and their families and staff. The client care manager is in a very good position to identify clients at special risk, such as those confronted by complex situations not adequately addressed by agency routines or those who are not achieving desired client outcomes within the anticipated time frames. Accordingly, the client care manager can mobilize agency resources in the client's behalf. Conducting a management conference can lead to more effective use of available resources.

In some health care organizations, any member of the health care team can suggest that a client care conference be held (Jaeger, 1988, p. 62). This approach encourages staff to openly communicate their concerns about client care. However, the client care manager often determines when a management conference is needed to benefit a specific client (Ceccio, 1986, p. 42). The best time to identify such clients is when the client care manager evaluates an individual's progress in meeting the desired outcomes of a current plan. Does the current plan address the client's actual problems and needs? If the answer is no, the nurse needs to consider what changes in the client's condition, treatment, or response may indicate serious risks or complications. Does the client's response relate to lack of information or skills or inadequate preparation for discharge? If the answer is yes, a management conference could be an effective strategy for taking action. A management conference can be a very efficient approach to developing a workable plan to guide those caring for the client.

Generally, a potential candidate for a management conference is a client with complex needs who has been admitted within the last 24 hours and needs a care plan developed, has developed new problems or needs, or has long-term needs that should be re-evaluated. By deliberately concentrating on identifying clients who could benefit and by providing opportunities to practice communication skills, management conferences can be a viable, cost-effective strategy to coordinate team effort (Reed, 1987, p. 66).

PREPARING TO CONDUCT A MANAGEMENT CONFERENCE

Client care managers **prepare for and plan** management conferences. When a client is identified as being at serious risk or as not making anticipated progress, the nurse begins to formulate the specific purpose of the management conference. The box below lists some common purposes of management conferences. The client care manager continuously evaluates client success in meeting desired outcomes and reacts when clients are identified who could benefit from a management conference.

The **purpose** or specific objective for holding a meeting must be clearly stated.

Common Purposes of Management Conferences

1. To obtain input about the client's responses to treatment
2. To gain insight into the causes of the client's behavior and responses
3. To identify current priorities of client needs
4. To identify and evaluate proposed plans for addressing client needs
5. To build staff commitment for implementing desired approaches to client needs
6. To revise client care plans in a timely manner
7. To promote interdisciplinary team communication needed to coordinate care
8. To resolve differences in perceptions of client responses needed to guide treatment plans
9. To formulate discharge plans that address complex client needs
10. To promote efficiency and success in satisfying client needs in a cost-effective manner

Frequently, more than one purpose for a management conference can be readily identified. The purpose must be identified, verbally or in writing, prior to preparing to conduct the meeting. The purpose guides identification of nursing staff and interdisciplinary team members needed to participate in the conference.

Consider a pediatric client suspected of being a victim of child abuse, who is experiencing discomfort related to multiple abdominal and skeletal injuries, and exhibiting delayed emotional and social development. This situation would require careful attention to nursing and interdisciplinary staff interactions. The purposes of this conference might be to better manage the client's discomfort and to establish a discharge plan. The conference participants would include direct nursing staff, family, and involved interdisciplinary team members, such as a clinical pharmacist, social worker, and discharge planner.

Another client might be an anxious, middle-aged adult experiencing a progressive degenerative disease, with serious complications requiring the use of assistive respiratory equipment, oxygen, suctioning, and postural drainage. Family care givers indicate that they feel tired, frustrated, and apprehensive about providing the needed care at home. The client has not improved noticeably during the first week of treatment. The purposes of the management conference might be to gather information about the client's current health problems and to make plans for long-term care. The conference participants might include direct-service staff, client, family, respiratory therapist, physical therapist, and discharge planner.

As these examples show, the client care manager uses the purpose of the staff meeting to guide the selection of conference participants (Palmer and Palmer, 1983, p. 30). Since they need to approve the overall plan, physicians are encouraged to attend such conferences. However, if they cannot, the client care manager collaborates with them to assure that they understand staff concerns and recommendations for improving the client's quality of care (Kerstetter, 1990, pp. 216–217). Or, the person leading the interdisciplinary team's efforts accepts responsibility for obtaining the medical approvals needed to carry out the team's plan (Herzog, 1985, p. 192).

Matching the purpose with needed skills is essential to increasing staff efficiency and success. The client care manager, who knows the roles and functions of various interdisciplinary staff members, can readily identify those who can contribute by and benefit from attending a management conference. It is important to include staff members who are authorized to make needed decisions about the client's care, rather than choosing substitutes or subordinates who lack the needed knowledge, skills, or authority. Subordinates benefit from participating in management conferences by learning about the importance of their observations and services. Their increased awareness helps them to carry out the client's plan of care. They also learn about the contributions made by various members of the interdisciplinary team. Discussion of the client's situation usually generates additional information that can be used immediately to improve the client's quality of care.

To promote efficiency, duplication of interdisciplinary staff knowledge, skills, and expertise is avoided. As an advocate and coordinator of the client's care, the nurse often expects and agrees to communicate staff concerns to attending physicians who are unable to attend these conferences. Sometimes, individual interdisciplinary team members discuss their specific concerns directly with attending physicians, depending upon their individual preferences and the complexity of the client's needs. These approaches promote the interdisciplinary collaboration and efficient exchange of information required to implement the client's overall treatment plan.

Before scheduling a management conference, the client care manager needs to consider whether there is a better method available to address the client's needs. Other agency resources might be used, such as telephone conferencing or computerization of interdepartmental communications. For example, if only one other discipline is involved, a telephone call might suffice to obtain the needed information. However, if multiple sources of input, discussion, and decisions are involved, a face-to-face conference might be most efficient and productive. If the participants are all nursing staff, the management conference might be scheduled to maximize involvement of members on two shifts to increase input and commitment to carrying out the desired approaches.

Once the planning is finished, a specific time is set that allows all participants to attend. To the extent possible, department routines are considered so that key staff members are not asked to leave their work area during periods of peak work activity. However, timeliness in addressing the client's needs has high priority. Generally, members of the interdisciplinary team are flexible in planning to participate in management conferences. Being invited to attend implies that their contributions are valued highly.

Each staff members accepts responsibility for using the available time wisely. Consequently, participants use their discretion when deciding to attend a client care conference. Duties and functions of various disciplines may overlap (Gunn et al, 1988, pp. 33–34). The client care manager considers suggestions by staff that other persons might be more appropriately selected as conference participants. Management conferences focus on the nature of the client's situation and on finding more effective approaches to priority

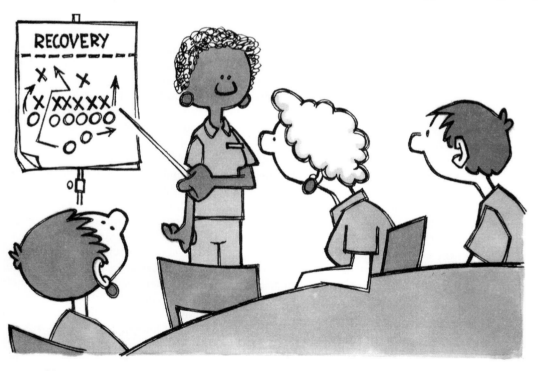

Management conferences focus on the nature of the client's situation and finding more effective approaches to priority needs.

needs. For the conference to be successful, client needs must be accurately matched with available staff knowledge and skills. Finding timely answers is critical; to confer after the client has been discharged from the unit or agency is unlikely to be of much practical use.

To the greatest extent possible, the participants are asked to meet within or near the clinical area. If the client is asked to attend the conference, the group often meets in the client's room. Sometimes, the staff confer briefly to organize their approach prior to reporting to the client's room. When staff and family meet, they frequently use the ward conference room, which is near the clinical area but subject to fewer distractions. It is important to note whether other activities are scheduled in the meeting area to avoid last-minute conflicts. When informing participants of the scheduled conference, let each of them know both the time and place. Also, let them know the purpose of the conference and the name of the client on whom it focuses. Try to notify participants far enough ahead, preferably 24 hours, so they can plan and prepare to attend. Let the participants know that the length of the conference will be 15 to 20 minutes, maximum, to help them plan for needed clinical "coverage."

Prior to the conference, the nurse needs to gather current information about the client as a person and about her or his health problems and needs. Such preparation includes meeting the client (preferably by prior participation in her or his care), and reviewing the clinical record and written plan of care. To increase self-confidence, the client care manager makes a few brief notes about her or his professional perceptions of the client's priority nursing diagnoses or collaborative problems.

CONDUCTING A MANAGEMENT CONFERENCE

Client care managers **conduct the meeting.** In contrast to many other types of meetings the participants already have been informed of the meeting's purpose, time, and place. Formal agendas are not used. However, it is important to start the conference at the scheduled time and place and to ensure that the participants are reasonably comfortable prior to beginning the discussion. Distractions such as noise, bright lights, extremes in temperature, or lack of chairs or space need to be addressed to avoid interrupting the conference later to attend to them. Such an approach conveys a genuine concern for the participants and an interest in their ability to contribute. Unless participants object, try to seat them in a circle or in such a way that they can face each other. Stress informality to the extent that it promotes open communication and encourages self-expression. All participants should introduce themselves if they have not been previously introduced. Familiarity with each other's disciplines helps participants to communicate with each other according to their roles and functions within the agency.

The client care manager appoints someone to take notes, especially to record priority concerns and proposed solutions. The conference leader refers to these notes to help summarize the discussion. The structure or sequencing of components of management conferences may vary. However, the components usually include background information about the client, discussion of the client's current needs, formulation of the care plan, and a summary. Generally, the conference is structured to address one or two top-priority client needs within the allotted time.

The leader begins by briefly reviewing the client's name, age, health problems, treatment plans, priority nursing diagnosis or collaborative problems, and any other information pertinent to the discussion. If helpful, the leader may note priority needs on an index card to use as a reference. Participants are invited to share concerns and identify their perceptions of

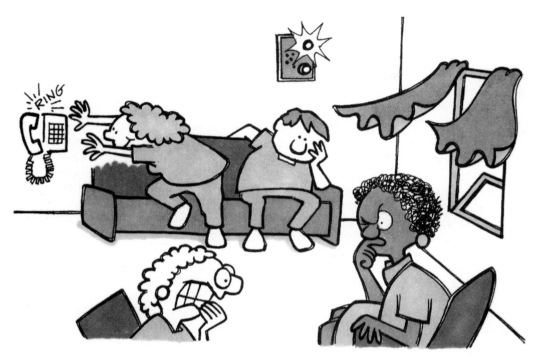

To maximize the effectiveness of a client conference, distractions should be kept to a minimum.

the client's priority needs. They are encouraged to discuss their feelings or any problems that they have experienced. Everyone is encouraged to contribute to the discussion.

The leader assumes responsibility for keeping the discussion client-centered. Accordingly, the leader minimizes digressions to other topics and avoids hidden agendas by returning the discussion to the client's situation and priority needs. When discussing the client's needs, participants are guided to avoid repetition, but they should take time for clarification. Participants are given sufficient time to describe their concerns but are guided to avoid lengthy explanations. The leader tries to prioritize the client's needs and address them one at a time.

The leader asks the staff, client, or family members to describe possible solutions and how the client's needs could best be met. Participants are asked to clarify comments that are unclear to others. They are encouraged to make a special effort to identify differences in perception of client needs and their proposed solutions by listening actively to each other. They are asked to describe what each believes should or could be done to address these needs.

To help the recorder, the leader summarizes what the client's priority needs are (one at a time), what revisions are to be made in the care plan, and who is to do what to carry it out to accomplish the desired outcomes.

The leader closes the conference on time, even if the discussion is still going. The discussion is closed early if completed ahead of schedule. This enables staff to return to their regular work as anticipated. The leader expresses appreciation for the participants' contributions and willingness to find workable solutions.

As soon as possible, the client care manager enters the revisions in the client's care plan on the appropriate agency form. In many agencies, these entries are documented directly in the client's clinical record or other communication tool used by staff providing the care. A summary of the conference results might also be recorded in the clinical record.

EVALUATING THE EFFECTIVENESS OF THE MANAGEMENT CONFERENCE

Client care managers **evaluate** the **effectiveness** of the meeting, which is influenced by its specific purpose. It is not unusual for conferences to produce additional benefits, such as staff development (or gaining insight into agency policies or procedures that are ineffective or inefficient) and identification of possible improvements in client care. Sometimes conclusions drawn from participating in several conferences stimulate "customer driven" organizational development. As staff gain experience working together, they are likely to become more efficient at responding to clients with similar needs and in using their conferencing skills. Several criteria can be used to judge the effectiveness of the management conference. Some can be used immediately after the conference, while others depend on the client's response to the revisions made in the care plan.

The conference should efficiently generate accurate information useful in planning and coordinating staff effort. The approaches established can reasonably be expected to benefit the client. If participants agree to the revisions, they are likely to follow up on the established care plan.

Figure 13-1 shows a brief conference evaluation form that might be used to help client care managers develop skills in conducting management conferences. Participants should be able to complete it in less than five minutes immediately after attending such a conference. Following effective management conferences, participants should expect to observe improvements in client care. They should also concur that the cost of the conference is worth the expenditure of agency resources, for example, the staff time consumed in completing the process. Ultimately, management conferences increase staff effectiveness and the quality of client care. With practice, skills used to conduct management conferences improve as well.

SUMMARY

Staff nurses are expected to coordinate staff efforts to meet client needs in a cost-effective manner. As client care managers, they can conduct management conferences to increase staff efficiency and effectiveness in providing cost-effective care. They need to develop and practice specific skills to use this management tool effectively.

The purpose of management conferences differs from that of conferences conducted for teaching purposes. The process of conducting management conferences involves four phases: identifying clients who could benefit, planning and preparation, implementation, and evaluation and follow-up. The client care manager needs to attend to various components in each phase to conduct a successful conference.

With experience, staff nurses learn to differentiate common individual variations in client responses from those that indicate serious risk of complication or inability to progress in achieving desired outcomes. The client care manager is in a strategic position to identify clients at special risk, those who are confronted by complex situations that are not adequately addressed by agency routines, or those who are not progressing within reasonable

EVALUATION OF CLIENT CARE CONFERENCE

1. Did the conference focus on the client?   Yes   No

2. List the main nursing needs of problems that were not discussed and should have been?

3. Did the participants develop a useful plan that you could follow? If not, give reasons.

4. Did you feel comfortable with the staff members contributions to the discussion? If not please explain.

5. Will the conference improve the client's care?   Yes   No

   In what ways?

About the Leader

1. Did the leader:

   A. Help the group identify client needs?   Yes   No
      What suggestions would you share to help the leader improve?

   B. (Guide discussion) or (control interaction)?   (Circle your response.)

   C. Summarize the care plan?   Yes   No

2. On a scale of 1 to 10 (10 being the highest), rate the conference.

Figure 13-1   Client care conference evaluation form.

time frames. Though any staff member can identify a need for a management conference, client care managers accept the responsibility and often take initiative for doing so when evaluation of client progress indicates need for more detailed consideration of the client's circumstances.

After identifying a client who could benefit from a management conference, the nurse begins to formulate the specific purpose for conducting one. After the conference's specific purpose is articulated, participants are selected. Selection criteria include knowledge and skills that match the nature of the client's anticipated needs and concerns. In addition, participants need authority to make the clinical decisions inherent in developing or revising care plans. To promote efficiency, duplication of staff expertise is avoided. Conferences are scheduled in or near the clinical area at times that are compatible with the participants' work flow. Participants are informed in advance of the subject, purpose, place, and time of the meeting.

Client care managers often lead management conferences. After completing introductions and assuring the comfort of the participants, a recorder is appointed. The discussion begins with a brief overview of the client's circumstances, priority needs, and concerns. Informality and open communication are encouraged. All participants are expected to contribute. The leader accepts responsibility for keeping the discussion focused on client needs and the plan of care. The leader also summarizes the discussion to reinforce the expectations of the staff who will implement the revisions in the client's care plan. Revisions are documented on the appropriate agency forms and communication tools to promote follow-through.

The success of the management conference relates directly to the purpose for which it was held. Though other benefits are often realized as well, results of the conference should improve the quality of care the client receives. Because of their involvement in developing specific approaches to the client's needs, participants expect the plan to benefit the client in a timely manner. Various methods of obtaining feedback from participants might be used to help the leader develop the skills used to conduct successful management conferences.

APPLICATION EXERCISES

a. Compare the purpose of a management conference with that of a change-of-shift report.
b. Identify one of your assigned clients who could benefit from a client care conference. Confirm the appropriateness of your selection with your instructor or supervisor.
c. Discuss how this type of conference differs from those that are regularly scheduled to monitor client progress toward treatment goals.
d. Plan and prepare a management conference so that needed participants can attend and contribute.
e. Evaluate the effectiveness of communication techniques you used during the management conference to promote implementation of the treatment plan.

Ceccio CM: Professional development for orthopaedic nurses through patient care conferences, *Orthop Nurs* 5(2):40–45. (May/June, 1986).

Coker EB, Schreiber R: The nurse's role in a team conference, *Nurs Manage* 21(3):46–48. (March, 1990).

Gunn R, Timms S, Terry J et al: A communication model in a day hospital, *J Gerontol Nurs* 14(8):30–36. (August, 1988).

Herzog KR: Documentation of hospice care plan development and team meetings, *QRB* 11(2):190–192. (June, 1985).

Jaeger TB: A head nurse's approach to multidisciplinary ethical conferences, *Nurs Manage* 19(1):60,62. (January, 1988).

Kerstetter NC: A stepwise approach to developing and maintaining an oncology multidisciplinary conference, *Cancer Nurs* 13(4):216–220. (August, 1990).

Palmer BC, Palmer KR: *The successful meeting master guide for business & professional people,* Englewood Cliffs, NJ, 1983, Prentice-Hall.

Reed C: Patient care conferences: 3 fast steps to better patient care plans, *Nurs 87* 17(3):66. (March, 1987).

Skurski V: *Interactive clinical conferences: nursing rounds and education imagery, J Nurs Educ* 24(4):166–168. (April, 1985).

PROFESSIONAL DEVELOPMENT

ADDRESSING ETHICAL AND LEGAL ISSUES

Completing this chapter should enable you to:

1. Describe fundamental ethical concepts.
2. Distinguish among ethics, spirituality, and law.
3. Describe the consequences of violating codes of conduct.
4. Describe appropriate responses to incompetent colleagues.
5. Describe legal ramifications of life-and-death issues that might stimulate conflict between co-workers.
6. Describe how health care financing methods might generate conflict.
7. Describe mechanisms used to protect subjects of nursing research.
8. List three emerging ethical issues affecting nursing practice.

KEY CONCEPTS

values
beliefs
cultural norms
ethics
ethical principles
essential professional values
  altruism
  equality
  esthetics
  freedom
  human dignity
  justice
  truth
common ethical concepts of nursing
  autonomy
  beneficence
  nonmaleficence
  justice

veracity
confidentiality
fidelity
moral conflicts
moral reasoning process
  moral issue
  moral dilemma
  moral uncertainty
  moral judgment
  ethical behavior
  ethical nursing practice
  moral distress
spirituality
law
code of nursing conduct
  ethical
  legal
quality of life

living will

durable power of attorney

providing aggressive treatment

   aggressive treatment

   extraordinary support measures

   resuscitative measures

withholding aggressive treatment

   death with dignity

   supportive measures

protecting the rights of human subjects

institutional research committees

using new knowledge

INCORPORATING ETHICAL DECISIONS IN NURSING PRACTICE

All nursing practice entails ethical decision making. Understanding common ethical concepts helps the nurse to practice nursing in accordance with ethical standards established by the profession. The purpose of this chapter is to discuss some of the common ethical issues confronting managers of client care.

Addressing ethical concerns requires application of knowledge of ethical concepts. These concepts frequently concern such topics as client autonomy, client participation in clinical decision making, justice in the context of the health care setting, and use of scarce available resources. Other common concerns relate to quality-of-life issues, "advance directives," "living wills," withholding aggressive treatment, and extraordinary means of prolonging life or promoting comfort. The health technology used to diagnose, treat, and substitute for human functions has also created a variety of ethical issues. In the future, the ethical issues inherent in nursing practice, which reflect social and technological changes, are likely to become increasingly complex.

As we make the transition from the industrial to the information era and the global economy continues to evolve, American culture is likely to become even more diverse. Increasing cultural diversity is reflected in prevailing societal values, norms, and mores (commonly accepted behaviors). Behaviors considered acceptable to members of one culture may be unacceptable to members of another. Furthermore, a persistent value held by Americans is the ideal of free choice. Consequently, each nurse needs to identify and clarify her or his own personal and professional values as a basic requirement for sound ethical reasoning.

The various nursing codes of conduct used to delineate ethical nursing practice are quite similar. According to Sawyer (1989, p. 148), who surveyed codes of nursing ethics, universal agreement exists in some areas. According to this study, there is universal nursing agreement that the nurse should

1. Accept responsibility for maintaining competence in nursing practice
2. Strive to maintain "good relations" with co-workers
3. Respect life
4. Respect the dignity of every client
5. Preserve confidentiality
6. Provide care in a nondiscriminatory manner

Differences in codes of ethics reflect the cultures of the nurses who adopted them (Sawyer, 1989, pp. 147–148). Accordingly, the ANA's Code for Nurses reflects the diversity of American culture and the expectation that the nurse will accept differences in lifestyles, standards of living, and the values of others. The ANA's Code for Nurses appears later in this chapter.

The principle of nondiscrimination prohibits stereotyping clients according to age, gender, race, ethnicity, economic background (including methods of financing care), or disability. How nondiscrimination affects nursing practice will be discussed in more detail later in this chapter. Nondiscrimination is an integral part of ANA's Standards of Practice.

Ethical skills are the foundation on which the entry-level staff nurse nurtures a sense of professional integrity. This is discussed in more detail in Chapter Fifteen.

COMPARING COMPONENTS OF CLIENT CARE MANAGEMENT AND ETHICAL NURSING PRACTICE

Though it was not often recognized until recently, the ethical components of the role of the nurse are integral to core nursing functions (Killeen, 1986, pp. 337–339). Some shared aspects of the nursing process and the ethical reasoning process have also been identified. The box below compares the phases of the nursing process with those of the ethical reasoning process.

Values and Beliefs

Nursing students usually receive instruction to help them identify and clarify their personal values. **Values** are difficult to define. They are characterized subjectively by the individual and reflect personal preferences, commitments, and patterns of using resources. The person considers certain beliefs, events, objects, people, places, or goals to have special meaning. An individual's values influence her or his choices, behaviors, and actions. They often serve as motivators.

Beliefs are the basic ingredients of values. **Beliefs** are basic assumptions or personal convictions that the individual perceives as truthful or factual or "takes for granted." Beliefs are not necessarily true or false. They frequently are handed down from generation to generation as cultural traditions (Jameton, 1990, p. 444). Cultural beliefs are commonly held by the others in the primary social groups (or subcultures) to which the individual belongs, such as families, work cultures, community interest groups, and church groups.

Cultural Norms

The individual's beliefs and values and those held by others in the same subcultures link the person to cultural norms. Predominant **cultural norms** prescribe expected behav-

---

Comparison of the Nursing and Ethical Reasoning Processes

Nursing process	Ethical reasoning process
1. Assessing	1. Recognizing the moral issues
2. Analyzing	2. Analyzing relevant facts, and identifying the moral dilemma
3. Planning	3. Formulating possible actions
	4. Selecting the action(s)
4. Implementing	5. Taking the morally right action
5. Evaluating	6. Evaluating the effectiveness of the moral action taken

ior of both clients and staff and provide guidelines for judging its acceptability. They strongly influence the person's actions and behaviors.

Cultural norms are rooted in values held by individuals. Figure 14-1 depicts the interconnectedness of individual values and cultural norms. When an individual accepts the beliefs and values of her or his work group or profession, the person is more likely to follow its codes of conduct without experiencing conflict. If the individual does not accept these predominant values or beliefs, potential for conflict exists.

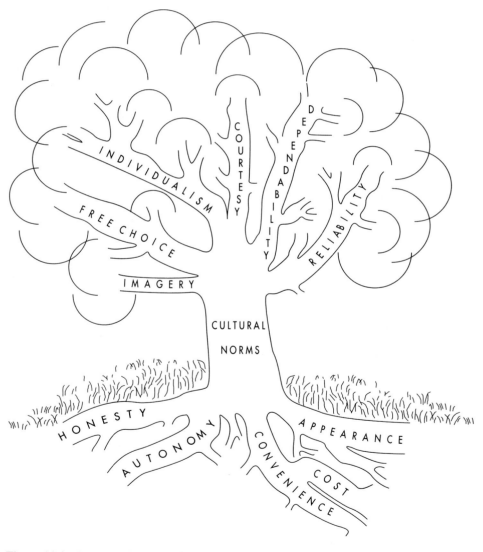

Figure 14-1   Interconnectedness of individual values and cultural norms.

Codes of acceptable conduct change in response to evolving cultural values and beliefs related to primary societal trends. For example, methods of child rearing are changing as increased numbers of women pursue careers. Explicit guidelines describing expected nursing conduct have been revised to correspond to evolving societal circumstances, economic constraints, and technological advances. The resulting situations are frequently inconsistent with ideal behaviors and significant differences in values and beliefs frequently give rise to moral conflicts.

Ethics

When conflicts occur, ethical principles or guidelines are used to distinguish right from wrong. **Ethics,** broadly defined, is the study of rightness of conduct, the processes used to judge moral behavior, and problems encountered when applying principles of morally correct behavior. As such, it incorporates cultural norms and mores. **Ethical principles** are used to judge right and wrong, good and bad, and to identify solutions to problems arising from conflicts (Fowler, 1989, p. 956). Ethics involves the study of values held by individuals and groups within social contexts. Nursing ethics reflect values held by members of the nursing profession within the social context of their practice. The ethical principles that guide the conduct of various disciplines differ according to the basic values espoused by members of the profession (Scanlon and Fleming, 1990, pp. 64–65). Accordingly, the nursing ethics incorporated in codes of conduct may differ from the ethics of other disciplines, including medicine.

As Curtin (1988, p. 7) so aptly stated, "Ethics, as applied to the profession of nursing, is concerned with the duties *voluntarily* assumed by nurses and with the consequences of nurses' decisions on the lives of patients and their families, on the lives of their colleagues, on the profession itself and on the health care delivery system as a whole." Nursing ethics involves the study of the principles and duties used to judge whether nursing motives and actions are right or wrong, good or bad in a specific client's situation and context of practice. As cultural plurality (diversity of values, norms, and mores) increases, the need to understand ethical principles will increase. Given current societal trends, the need to understand nursing ethics is likely to become more important.

The study of ethics requires a reasoning process that takes into account the values that guide behavior. **Essential professional values** commonly used to guide staff nurse behaviors include **atruisim, equality, esthetics, freedom, human dignity, justice,** and **truth** (American Association of Colleges of Nursing, 1986, pp. 5–7). These values guide the ethical behaviors expected of staff nurses. Translated into the nursing context, these values reflect **common ethical concepts of nursing.** They include

1. **Promoting autonomy** supporting the client's independence in making decisions affecting herself or himself
2. **Beneficence** doing good for the client
3. **Nonmaleficence** avoiding harm to the client
4. **Justice** using available resources fairly and reasonably
5. **Veracity** communicating truthfully and accurately
6. **Confidentiality** securing the client's privacy
7. **Fidelity** following through on one's word by carefully attending to details of the client's care (Gaul, 1989, p. 475)

Nurses study ethics to help them gain insight into how these concepts affect practice. Essential professional values influence the effectiveness of nurse-client relationships.

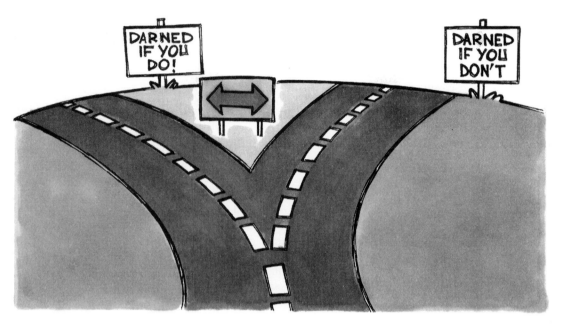

Nurses are frequently confronted with moral conflicts.

Ethical nursing practice is guided by professional values and corresponding "correct" behaviors. Attention to ethical concerns helps nurses resolve ethical conflicts through making morally correct decisions and taking corresponding moral actions.

Nurses are frequently confronted with **moral conflicts** between loyalties to clients and to employers; loyalties to employers and compliance with regulations of licensing bodies; responsibilities to clients and physicians, peers, or other interdisciplinary team members; and conflicting responsibilities to clients and their families.

To resolve moral conflicts, nurses follow a moral reasoning process to make moral judgments as the basis for ethical nursing actions. Nurses who do not use ethical reasoning skills are likely to respond to moral conflicts intuitively, on the basis of their personal values. Consequently, the nurse's behaviors are likely to serve her or his own needs instead of focusing on those of the client. This incorrect focus is even more likely when nurses work in settings that afford themselves and clients very little authority to participate in clinical decision-making processes.

THE MORAL REASONING PROCESS

Client care managers use moral reasoning to resolve moral conflicts. The specific steps in this process might vary, depending upon the nurse, the values involved, the client's circumstances, and constraints inherent in the situation. Basically, the **moral reasoning process** consists of the following phases:

1. Recognizing the moral issues
2. Analyzing relevant facts and identifying the moral dilemma

3. Formulating possible actions
4. Selecting the action that best resolves the moral conflict consistent with principles of ethical conduct
5. Taking morally right action
6. Evaluating the effectiveness of the moral action taken

Each phase of the moral reasoning process needs to be completed to successfully address the dilemma.

Recognizing Existing Moral Issues

A **moral issue** exists when questions of morals or values arise and seem to conflict, or when the compliance of one's actions with ethical principles is questioned. Common moral issues often pertain to such issues as quality of life, death, comfort, "to treat or not to treat," and the use of scarce resources in extraordinary measures of prolonging life.

To recognize a moral issue, the nurse needs to know which essential professional values are involved and how ethical principles can be used to sort out the key values of both the nurse and the client. This knowledge is in addition to that needed to perform nursing procedures, communicate and teach clients effectively, and manage client care.

Professional autonomy (nurse's freedom to make clinical nursing decisions) is gaining attention as nursing establishes itself as a profession. It is important that the nurse understand how professional autonomy enhances one's practice and how a lack of autonomy can limit the nurse's effectiveness in making clinical decisions. For example, nurses who have organizational authority to plan and evaluate care can make timely revisions as clients' needs change. On the other hand, nurses who are limited by the pattern of nursing service delivery, interdisciplinary team routines, or policies are less likely to exercise professional autonomy. As a result, clients may not receive as effective or efficient care nurses perceive to be possible. Consequently, these nurses may receive less satisfaction from the practice of their profession.

The staff nurse should also understand the various strategies that can be used to promote the client's autonomy. Limiting the client's participation in decisions affecting her or him can diminish the quality of care provided and affect the client's perceptions of the quality of care received. Strategies for maintaining client autonomy include protecting the rights of clients who depend on significant others to act on their behalf, due to age, illness, or disability. For example, the nurse may need to act as an advocate by providing information about client rights to families and significant others, communicating client concerns to the interdisciplinary team, and supporting clients in implementing advance directives (legally binding descriptions of the client's wishes regarding treatment).

In a similar manner, the nurse needs to understand how the ethical concepts of beneficence, nonmaleficence, justice, veracity, confidentiality, and fidelity are incorporated in nursing practice (Cassells and Redman, 1988, p. 465). These concepts are incorporated in standards of nursing practice, codes of conduct, and lists of clients' rights. The nurse should understand how these concepts guide nursing practice, influence staff perceptions of client's rights, and contribute to the design of strategies to protect them. For example, the concept of justice is incorporated in endeavors to provide quality care regardless of the source of payment. The concept of veracity is involved in informed consent. The principle of confidentiality protects clients experiencing socially isolating or stigmatizing conditions. In actual practice, clinical situations often involve more than one ethical concept.

To resolve such **moral dilemmas** (situations involving undesirable choices for personal behavior), the client care manager needs to decide which value or goal takes precedence. Prioritizing the conflicting values inherent in moral dilemmas requires the nurse to pay specific attention to who has responsibility for what in finding the solution, and to the extent to which the client and nurse have control over needed moral actions.

Research indicates that some nurses, for reasons not yet clearly identified, have difficulty separating their personal values from those that guide nursing practice. Personal values often change over time as individual circumstances evolve, whereas essential ethical guidelines persist over longer periods. Clarification of personal values is a prerequisite for recognizing moral issues in clinical practice. Not to differentiate personal and professional values leads to difficulty in perceiving moral issues. The client care manager who does not distinguish personal values from professional guidelines is less likely to recognize the need for ethical reasoning. Such a client care manager is also less likely to recognize the need to gather relevant facts.

Analyzing Relevant Facts to Identify the Moral Dilemma

Several research studies have indicated that many nurses experience difficulty when identifying ethical dilemmas in practice (Ketefian, 1989, pp. 518–519). In other words, **moral uncertainty** is common. Nurses are often unsure which essential values are at issue and which values or ethical principles are in conflict in a specific situation. To assure that the moral dilemma is accurately identified, the nurse needs to decipher the sources of conflict. These may include the client's values, organizational interest in controlling costs, and consumption of scarce resources such as staff time.

For example, consider the situation of a client who is a recent immigrant and has trouble communicating with staff due to language barriers and cultural differences. Suppose that the staff in this health care facility is consistently rewarded for discharging clients early. The nurse accepts responsibility for gathering information about the client's understanding of available health care options, their consequences, and the cost of each. Prior to formulating plans for addressing individual client needs, the nurse should be aware of staff perceptions of their obligations in preparing clients for discharge. If staff do not feel responsible for adequately preparing the client for discharge, the client may not receive information about treatment options, supervised practice of self-care activities, or needed referrals. These omissions are likely to jeopardize the client's well being or may even be life threatening. This situation involves the ethical concepts of client autonomy, beneficence, nonmaleficence, informed consent, justice, veracity, and fidelity. The nurse encourages the client to participate in selecting available options after receiving truthful and accurate information about them. The client needs information about anticipated outcomes of care and estimated times to reach them. If the client is to leave the hospital early, the nurse explains possible consequences; costs; need for special supplies, equipment, and skilled help associated with private home care services; hospital-based home care services, and other matters (autonomy, veracity). The nurse is mindful that reasonable plans are necessary to provide continuing services to avoid harming the client by early discharge, for example, risking complications due to lack of follow-up services (maleficence). In addition, the nurse advocates that sufficient organizational resources be used to implement the plan (justice). Finally, the nurse makes a specific effort to assure that the details of the client's plan are carried out to enable the client to adequately meet her or his specific health needs (fidelity, maleficence).

The nurse makes a **moral judgment** regarding the rightness or wrongness of the direction that the client's situation is taking. The judgment focuses on whether staff behaviors match standards of ethical conduct. The nurse evaluates the extent to which the client's rights are supported or violated and the extent to which staff behaviors adhere to standards identified in codes of conduct. For example, will the client be harmed by being unprepared for early discharge? By being uninformed of the treatment plan? By not comprehending what he or she needs to do to perform self-care procedures? If the answer to these questions is yes, the client's rights are being violated. The nurse begins prioritizing various activities needed to enable the client to participate in planning treatment, preparing for discharge, and performing self-care procedures.

Formulating Possible Actions

After the relevant facts are analyzed and the moral dilemma is identified, actions that could contribute to resolving it are considered. Specific actions that could change wrong actions into right actions are described. When first learning to formulate possible actions, the nurse should list the possibilities so that each can be readily recalled and considered. Each solution needs to be evaluated in terms of the extent that it meets the needs of the client, staff, and organization. The consequences of each possible solution are considered, including demands placed upon the client and support systems and use of agency resources and their costs.

For example, the attending physician might initially explain the treatment plan to the client in the presence of the staff nurse. To enable the client to fully comprehend the plan, staff on later shifts might need to explain the plan to the client's family (who, let us suppose, can only be available later in the day due to other commitments). This is done to increase comprehension of the plan and to evaluate its suitability given the client's needs, options, and financial resources. If language barriers exist, more time will be needed to communicate, reinforce, and follow through. The more complicated the plans, the more time it takes to establish them and the more agency resources (e.g., staff time) are consumed in following through. To not involve the client and staff (within organizational constraints) places the client at increased risk of harm. In addition, client rights are more likely to be violated if the client does not participate in making treatment plans.

If specific effort and time are not taken to formulate all possible actions, the best solution might go unrecognized. Consequently, the staff could become involved efficiently providing the wrong services. The client's needs might be treated as less important than agency efficiency or staff convenience.

Selecting the Action that Best Resolves the Moral Conflict

The nurse needs to select the action that best resolves the moral conflict consistent with codes of conduct. To select the best solution, the client's priority needs, values, and the consequences of these values need to be considered. Often the nurse uses advocacy skills to assure that the client's communication abilities, lack of comprehension of important information or decreased self-esteem or feelings of self-worth, do not result in hasty decisions that are not in her or his best interest. Particularly with clients experiencing difficulty comprehending information and explanations, staff working under tight time constraints can nonverbally communicate frustration and impatience to the client. It is important to provide the client with accurate information to enable the client to select the option that best meets her or his needs. The nurse also discusses possible consequences and demands on the client of the option selected. The client care manager should keep in mind that the client might not select the same solution the manager would select. The client needs support to select the solution that best addresses the person's health needs and also solves the moral dilemma under consideration.

The client care manager has an obligation to communicate accurately and truthfully. All relevant information should be presented. The client needs information about probable undesired or negative consequences of the options selected as well as positive consequences that are easy to hear. The client needs a realistic perspective to consider various factors that affect the potential success of the plan.

Taking the Morally Right Action

Once the best action is selected, it needs to be carried out. **Ethical behavior** is conduct consistent with the values inherent to the situation. **Ethical nursing practice** involves taking morally right actions within the context of the client's needs and values and nursing codes of conduct. Both the client and staff need to know what is expected of them—what they are to do and when. Frequently, solutions to moral dilemmas are not equally acceptable to both parties. The action might be best for the client but complicate demands upon the family or staff. Unforeseen responses may occur that might be more or less desirable than anticipated. The client care manager is obligated to follow through on the selected action.

Evaluating the Effectiveness of the Moral Action Taken

Then specific attention needs to be focused upon determining what happened after desired actions were taken. The client care manager, knowing what initial moral dilemma stimulated use of the moral reasoning process, is in a good position to judge whether the moral action taken resolved it. Did the actions help the client progress toward her or his goals? Does the client need further consideration and help to resolve the conflict? For example, in the situation described earlier, did taking more time to communicate effectively with the client help to clarify expectations and enhance the client's dignity and autonomy? Did the client's change in condition require that staff continue to take more time to explain and reinforce expectations related to the selected treatment options?

Reviewing the similarities between the phases of the moral reasoning process and those of the nursing process shows the relative ease with which ethical issues can be incorporated into nursing practice. Noting the similarities between the two processes should help to integrate moral reasoning into nursing practice (Murphy, 1989, p 74). Considerable attention has been paid to helping nursing students learn to use the nursing process. More effort is needed to help them integrate moral reasoning while using the nursing process to make clinical decisions. What is important is the nurse's sensitivity and recognition of moral dilemmas as they are evidenced by the client's expressed concerns and the staff's response to identified needs.

As mentioned earlier, health care settings exist that do not allow or promote ethical nursing practice. Nurses who know the moral values at issue and choose the right courses of action but are not allowed to take action to resolve them experience **moral distress**. Common constraints that cause moral distress include organizations that do not permit nursing autonomy in clinical decision making, policies that limit the nurse's authority, and lack of respect for nursing's ability to respond appropriately to moral issues (Fry, 1989, p. 490). As if the complexity of addressing moral dilemmas is not enough of a challenge to staff nurses, circumstances that cause moral distress complicate nursing practice and the ethical dilemmas confronting clients. Indeed, moral distress associated with such constraints can lead to tragic results. Wilkinson (1987/88, p. 27) reported, "Those nurses who are unable to cope with moral distress and who leave bedside nursing seem to be those who are most aware of, and sensitive to, moral issues, and who feel a strong sense of responsibility to patients for their own actions."

▇▇▇▇ DIFFERENTIATING BETWEEN ETHICS AND SPIRITUALITY

Staff nurses need to distinguish a client's spirituality from ethical issues. As discussed earlier, ethics is the study of the rightness or wrongness of behavior. It incorporates an understanding of beliefs and predominant cultural values that guide conduct. It considers variations in personal values, cultural norms and mores, and the context of the specific situations being studied.

Spirituality refers to a person's emotional investment, "attaching positive or negative importance to persons, places, objects, events, beliefs, and goals that seem to be relevant to the self" (Salladay and McDonnell, 1989, p. 544). A person's spirit relates to aspects of her or his mind or soul and is distinct from the body. Spirituality refers to the person's search for meaning from individual experiences. It is a basic human need that must be met to sustain a person's well-being. Often, spirituality refers to the human spirit's involvement with a greater power or divine spirit. One's spirituality reflects personal beliefs, values, and ethical choices made to realize goals and to make life worth living. Though religious practices rooted in spirituality may differ widely, the spiritual needs of valuing, seeking meaning, and setting personal goals are quite similar in all religions.

Both ethics and spirituality are concerned with values, with good and bad, right or wrong behavior. While ethics relates to a systematic approach to judging behavior, spirituality refers to the person's individual emotional investment in persons, objects, places, events, beliefs, and goals that make life meaningful. Ethics emphasizes cultural values, whereas spirituality focuses on those of the individual. Both ethical and spiritual considerations are usually involved in the moral reasoning inherent in nursing practice. The nurse attempts to adhere to ethical codes of conduct formulated by the profession and also to address the spiritual concerns of clients.

▇▇▇▇ DISTINGUISHING BETWEEN LAW AND ETHICS

As a study of conduct, ethics contributes to guidelines for desired behavior. The ethical behaviors expected of nurses, for example, are delineated in various codes of conduct. These codes describe various types of expected behaviors aimed at protecting client's interests, and, indirectly, those of nurses. They prescribe approaches to moral issues to avoid, reduce, or, resolve conflict. Ethical concepts change as cultures, values, and socially accepted patterns of behavior change.

Laws are rules for required behavior that define personal and professional relationships. Laws tell people what they may and may not do, alone, to, and, with others. Laws are generated by governments or by government sanction of customs. They change as social issues and concerns change. Various types of laws create different privileges, protections, and reponsibilities.

For example, constitutional law protects individual rights, such as freedom of speech, right to self-determination, and right to refuse treatment. Administrative laws define regulations for agencies, such as the authority of state boards of nursing to define and regulate nursing practice. Other administrative laws direct other agencies, such as those participating in Medicare and Medicaid health insurance programs. Criminal laws define actions such as murder, theft, or illegal possession of drugs. Nurses removing life support systems, consuming agency supplies for personal use, or abusing chemical substances violate criminal laws. Contract laws refer to legally binding agreements. Nurses may enter into contracts by agreeing to work schedules and job descriptions. Tort laws relate to compensating clients for harm or injury caused by malpractice.

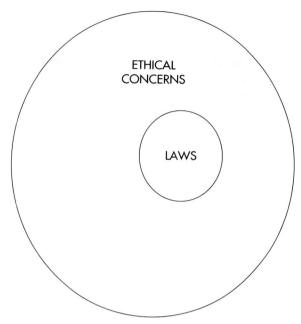

Figure 14-2   Law as a part of ethical concerns.

Laws reflect public policy. As such, they reflect society's view of what is good or bad, right or wrong behavior (Kjervik, 1990, p. 138). Good laws reflect desired ethical practices, including predominant cultural beliefs, values, and customs. Ethical guidelines are used by legislators to judge the rightness or wrongness of conduct and might be used in legal courts to determine the extent to which laws were violated. Ethics and law are not mutually exclusive. Figure 14-2 illustrates how law is conceptualized as being a part of ethical concerns.

As ethical issues emerge, professional organizations frequently prepare position papers on the issues to guide their members. Ethical guidelines are frequently used to inform policy makers and legislators of the expected behaviors of health care professionals (Fowler, 1988, p. 104). Laws change as legislators respond to social pressures to regulate behaviors that infringe on the rights, safety, or well-being of the public.

ADHERING TO NURSING CODES OF CONDUCT

Entry-level staff nurses are expected to adhere to both legal and ethical codes of conduct. A **code of nursing conduct** such as the ANA's Code for Nurses with Interpretive Statements is a description of standards of behavior required of nurses. See the box on p. 214 for a list of such standards. The consequences of violations of these codes depend upon which type of code of conduct was violated.

Legal codes of conduct are rooted in specific state nurse practice acts (which are often delineated in state statutes) and ANA Standards of Nursing Practice (established voluntarily by members of the American Nurses Association). To be licensed to practice nursing,

American Nurses Association Code for Nurses

1. The nurse provides services with respect for human dignity and the uniqueness of the client unrestricted by considerations of social or economic status, personal attributes, or the nature of the health problems.
2. The nurse safeguards the client's right to privacy by judiciously protecting information of a confidential nature.
3. The nurse acts to safeguard the client and the public when health care and safety are affected by the incompetent, unethical, or illegal practice of any person.
4. The nurse assumes responsibility and accountability for individual nursing judgments and actions.
5. The nurse maintains competence in nursing.
6. The nurse exercises informed judgment and uses individual competence and qualifications as criteria in seeking consultation, accepting responsibilities, and delegating nursing activities to others.
7. The nurse participates in activities that contribute to the ongoing development of the profession's body of knowledge.
8. The nurse participates in the profession's efforts to implement and improve standards of nursing.
9. The nurse participates in the profession's efforts to establish and maintain conditions of employment conducive to high-quality nursing care.
10. The nurse participates in the profession's effort to protect the public from misinformation and misrepresentation and to maintain the integrity of nursing.
11. The nurse collaborates with members of the health professions and other citizens in promoting community and national efforts to meet the health needs of the public.

From American Nurses Association: *Code for nurses with interpretive statements*, Washington, DC, 1985, The Association.

each nurse is required to meet requirements for licensure and registration. That is, each nurse must present evidence of capability to practice nursing safely. Initial licensure often involves meeting educational requirements that ensure that the individual has the knowledge and skills deemed critical for safe nursing practice. Registration requirements include information about the nurse's current name and address.

ANA Standards of Nursing Practice are often used in courts of law as *minimum standards* needed for safe practice. They provide guidelines that are often used to judge the reasonableness of actions taken by an individual nurse in a specific situation. They are frequently used to compare the practices of peers described by "expert witnesses" in court hearings. Additional institutional standards of care include those described in policy and procedure manuals and those delineated by quality assurance and improvement processes.

If convicted of violating the state nurse practice act, which is usually consistent with ANA Standards of Nursing Practice and other institutional standards, the nurse is legally responsible for the consequences. That is, the nurse is required to compensate injured parties for the damages or injuries resulting from these violations. Since these consequences can be very costly, most nurses obtain malpractice insurance to address these risks. In addition, depending upon the seriousness of the violation, the nurse's license could be suspended or revoked.

In contrast to legal requirements, **ethical** codes of conduct are developed by nursing organizations and describe expectations for *moral* conduct of a nurse. They are designed to protect the rights of all clients and to describe the moral obligations of nurses. They provide guidelines for making appropriate ethical decisions to provide quality care for clients with diverse spiritual, ethnic, racial, age, and gender characteristics, which often differ from those of the nurse. They also provide guidelines for nurses to avoid discriminating behaviors that could decrease the client's dignity or respect.

Violating ethical codes of conduct usually entails interference with the exercise of client rights. Violations of ethical codes of conduct could be described in courts of law as evidence of engaging in less than the minimally accepted standards of practice. However, not all violations of ethical codes of conduct result in legal disputes; sometimes they simply infringe on client's rights. Depending on the consequences of violations, legal disputes might follow.

To ensure that clients are informed of their rights as patients in acute care facilities or residents in long-term care facilities, federal regulations require that health care providers be familiar with these rights. In addition, federal regulations require that clients be informed of their rights upon admission to these facilities.

COMMON VIOLATIONS OF NURSING CODES OF CONDUCTS

Entry-level staff nurses are likely to encounter a variety of situations where violations of codes of nursing conduct could jeopardize client rights and safety. Several of these situations are described here to help client care managers promote safe care and protect client rights.

Identifying Life-and-Death Issues

In recent years, the media have sensitized the public to many of the technological advances in health care. Most adults express desire for "death with dignity" when good quality of life is not possible and the individual perceives the alternative as unacceptable. **Quality of life** is a subjective measure of acceptability of pain and suffering; it is difficult to define on more than an individual basis. Ethical codes of conduct require that the client's expressed desires for "death with dignity" be honored. Difficulties arise when the client has not legally established her or his wishes before the time when such life-and-death decisions need to be made.

Many American adults know that current medical technology can sometimes support physiological processes indefinitely on a mechanical level. Consistent with the Supreme Court ruling in *Nancy Cruzan vs. State of Missouri,* many individuals have completed living wills. A **living will** is a legal document that indicates individual directives for the care desired and indicates who is authorized to make medical decisions if the person becomes incapacitated. If these documents have been satisfactorily completed with appropriately witnessed signatures, they are legally binding in most states (Lammers, 1986, p. 629). Effective December 1, 1991, hospitals and nursing homes receiving Medicare and Medicaid funds were required to inform patients of their rights under state law to make living wills or other advance directives (Dolan, 1991, p. 7). Advance directives include designations of persons authorized to make decisions on the client's behalf, for example, durable power of attorney, should he or she be seriously injured, terminally ill, or in a persistent vegetative state. A person with adequately documented authority to act as **durable power of attorney** is legally empowered to carry out decisions and activities on behalf of the client. In most states (but not the District of Columbia), a person with durable power of attorney can perform all legal actions needed to fulfill the client's wishes as if he or she were the client (Lammers, 1986, pp. 629–630).

Client care managers are expected to adhere to these advance directives. In addition, they are expected to include designated individuals in decision-making processes involved in providing care in accordance with legitimate living wills and related directives. They need to clearly distinguish between measures that prolong life and those that hasten death. Measures prolonging life would be inconsistent with the goals of a client striving for "death with dignity." Measures that hasten death may be illegal. Nurses need to be prepared to defend their actions if their interventions are questioned. In addition, they need to explain such decisions and subsequent actions taken.

Distinguishing Treatment from Nontreatment Plans

Client care managers are expected to know the goals of each of their clients (Thompson, 1989, p. 344). That is, they need to clearly understand whether the measures taken are to restore health, treat symptoms of a disease, or provide supportive care for "death with dignity." Each type of goal implies different priorities. The nurse's activities and cares are adjusted accordingly. Generally, treatment includes measures taken to restore health or treat disease. Nontreatment plans emphasize measures designed to provide comfort or alleviate suffering. It is the purpose for which these measures are taken that is of paramount importance, not the type of measure. For example, a specific analgesic could be given to treat incisional pain postoperatively or to alleviate the discomfort of a terminally ill client. The nurse's evaluation of its effectiveness, including risks, benefits, and side effects, depends upon the purpose it was given.

In addition, client care managers need to distinguish between **providing** and **withholding aggressive treatment. Aggressive treatment** usually includes **extraordinary support measures** used to support physiological processes. One type of extraordinary life support measure includes any strategy used to maintain or restore a function of a person's vital organs. Another type includes **resuscitative measures** taken to reverse immediate, life-threatening situations, such as cardiopulmonary arrest. Resuscitative measures are performed to prevent death and are often considered heroic. Life support measures that are unnatural, such as mechanical respirators or enteral tube feedings, are usually considered to be extraordinary. Extraordinary life support measures are used to provide "aggressive treatment" and are designed to maintain and restore life and health.

When health care providers are requested to "withhold aggressive treatment," they are expected to eliminate all measures designed to maintain body function and restore health. This does not preclude the use of measures designed to promote comfort or alleviate suffering; such comfort measures do not deliberately prolong life or hasten death. Rather, the purpose of withholding aggressive treatment is to avoid prolonging life without dignity. A "nontreatment" program is designed to provide supportive care. **"Death with dignity,"** as perceived by the client, is a common goal of nontreatment programs. Such programs incorporate **supportive measures** that enable the client to achieve death with dignity.

Recognizing Ethical Issues Related to Health Insurance Benefits

As described in Chapter Two, health care agencies are heavily influenced by mechanisms commonly used to finance various treatment options. Consequently, clients frequently choose options that fit the design of their health insurance benefits. Clients assume that their insurance benefit programs determine the type of treatment they should receive. In fact, the purpose of insurance programs is to help pay for needed health care, not to determine what health care is needed. This fact has been somewhat obscured by the preadmission consultations required by many insurance programs.

Entry-level staff nurses as client care managers are expected to be accountable to the clients they serve. Codes of nursing conduct require client care managers to provide care without discrimination on the basis of economic status. That is, providing client care is nursing's primary function, for which nurses are ethically responsible and legally accountable. Financing health care, though important, is secondary. Accordingly, client care managers need to remain clearly focused upon providing care based on their assessments rather than emphasizing economic pressures originating inside or outside their practice settings (Cushing, 1989, pp. 471–472).

This approach is not to be taken to mean that the high cost of health care can be ignored. Rather, each client is entitled to cost-effective and efficient care, regardless of how it is financed. Client care managers, as advocates, are expected to help clients understand their needs and priorities and the various options available to meet them.

By requesting detailed documentation of the services provided, insurance companies have gained considerable influence over health care providers, sometimes to the detriment of their beneficiaries (Hines, 1988, p. 586). Insurance companies have sometimes attempted to reduce their costs by denying client benefits, refusing to reimburse clients or agencies for services provided that the insurance companies decided were inadequately or

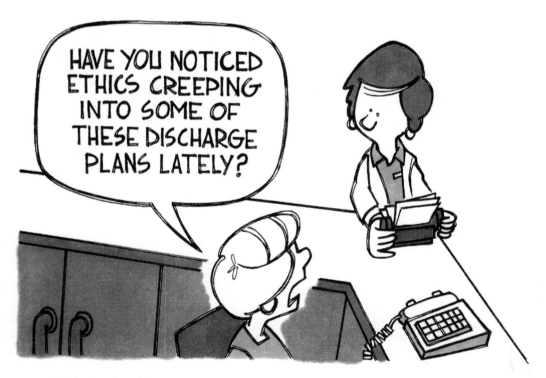

Each client is entitled to cost effective and efficient care regardless of how it is financed.

incorrectly documented. Client care managers, as advocates, assure that client progress and services provided are recorded accurately and reflect that standards of care were maintained (Murphy, 1987, pp. 537–538, 540). Nurses document client progress and care provided in order to evaluate them, however, not primarily to satisfy the demands of health insurance companies. To attempt the latter is not an appropriate use of scarce resources and consequently not in the client's best interest.

Responding to an Incompetent Colleague

Specific steps for resolving conflicts were detailed in Chapter Six. From time to time, every nurse encounters situations in which the safety of clients is endangered by the conduct of colleagues. To succeed as a member of a work group, everyone must work together cooperatively and with mutual respect. Consequently, when circumstances evolve in which a colleague's behavior is questioned, tension associated with intrapersonal and interpersonal conflict is likely. The unacceptable conduct of colleagues may also lead to intergroup conflicts. The differences causing the tension may relate to variations in perceptions of acceptability of personal behaviors, to lack of adherence to agency's standards of care, or to noncompliance with the specified interdisciplinary team's treatment plan. Coping with a colleague whose conduct and competence are under question always produces anxiety. Though entry-level nurses may lack self-confidence due to lack of experience, they are expected to evaluate the competence of their peers, especially if suspicious behaviors place client safety at risk. Codes of nursing conduct require the nurse to respond to colleagues whose behavior places the clients they care for at risk.

First, become familiar with the agency's policy for the management of unsafe practice. Usually, the nurse is expected to discuss her or his concerns with the colleague in question, noting whether it is the behavior or the outcomes of care that are problematic. Has the conduct resulted in harm to a client? Do client outcomes of care change under different workers? For example, is relief from narcotic analgesia reduced when the colleague is present, suggesting that the client might not have received the drug?

Are there policies or procedures that run contrary to the colleague's behavior? For example, is there a need to countersign for "wasted" controlled substances, or are alcoholic beverages prohibited before or during scheduled work hours? Obviously, the more endangered the client's safety and well-being, the greater the pressure on the nurse to respond to the colleague's conduct. In any event, the nurse needs to follow the agency's policy, if one exists.

Second, when the colleague is approached, follow the steps of conflict resolution. Your colleague may surprise you, either by agreeing with you or denying the problem. If you participate in a coverup of the colleague's behavior, you are ethically and legally accountable for the problem and its consequences.

Third, if you believe there is evidence of drug or alcohol abuse, submit a written report of your concerns and evidence to your supervisor. If your supervisor is unresponsive, report your concerns to your supervisor's supervisor, probably the director of nursing.

Fourth, you might want to seek guidance from unbiased sources, such as other client advocates, clergy, ombudsmen personnel, or the "employee directives committee." You may be protected from reprisal by state laws or administrative rules. Remember, your primary responsibility is your client's safety and well-being, for which you are ethically and legally accountable.

In sum, the presence of an incompetent colleague will engage you in conflict in behalf of client safety. You are expected to comply with agency policies related to unsafe, illegal, or unethical conduct. If you do not, you are also accountable for the consequences of the conduct in question. Use your communication skills to resolve conflict and ethical issues. In addition, report your concerns in writing to your supervisor.

PROTECTING THE RIGHTS OF HUMAN SUBJECTS

Beginning staff nurses may be expected to participate in research activities involving clients assigned to their care. Several important ethical concerns need to be adequately addressed, including **protecting the rights of human subjects,** protecting nurses as employees, and protecting the integrity of the specific research study. For example, staff nurses might be asked to witness client signatures on "informed consent" forms or to collect data consistent with the purposes of the study. If the staff nurse questions the adequacy of the protection afforded the human subjects, he or she needs to confer with his or her immediate supervisor to assure that the activities adhere to the agency's policies and procedures. Nurses assume responsibility for assuring that the research purposes and methodology preserve the dignity and rights of the individuals and social groups they are intended to serve. Wilson (1989) delineated guidelines for assuring ethical research practices using the acronym "SCIENTIFIC." See the box at the top of p. 220 for a description of these guidelines. If a research project satisfactorily addresses the criteria set forth in these guidelines, both the integrity and rights of the human subjects and nurses involved are likely to be protected.

While participating in research projects, nurses need to make a special effort to protect the rights of clients serving as human subjects. Clients must clearly comprehend when the nurse is providing care and when her or his activities are primarily of a research nature. The distinction is necessary to prevent clients from assuming that the nurse is acting in their best interests when, in fact, clients may be clearly taking risks while participating in specific research activities. For example, a nurse might administer prescribed experimental drugs treatments that pose potential risks to assigned clients.

Before implementation, all research projects that clients participate in as human subjects need to be approved by the organization's designated institutional board. Such groups are often known as the **institutional research committees** and are responsible for assuring that the purposes and procedures adequately protect the rights of the human subjects. The box at the bottom of p. 220 lists the rights of human subjects as participates in research, as delineated by the ANA.

Nurses need to know that clients as human subjects participate voluntarily after the risks and benefits of such involvement are truthfully disclosed to them. Clients can end their participation at any time without fear of punishment or reprisal. In addition, the nurse needs to know the specific plans to protect the subjects' anonymity and confidentiality and to assure that the researchers adhere to them.

Concurrently, while clients participate in research projects, staff nurses provide nursing care to them, in accordance with established standards of care. As mentioned earlier, accepted standards of nursing practice require the nurse to adhere to codes of nursing conduct to assure that ethical issues are adequately addressed. Protecting the rights of human subjects is undertaken in addition to providing established standards of care, not instead of it.

Evaluating research reports and **using new knowledge** are integral to sound nursing practice. Entry-level staff nurses are expected to review current literature and determine whether the findings have implications for their practice. Typically, staff nurses are re-

Guidelines for "Scientific" and Ethical Research Practices

Scientific objectivity. The investigator includes all data points, including those that are unsupportive; tries to be aware of personal values and biases; and doesn't preconceive a study's outcome or engage in any misconduct, fraud, or acts of bad faith in connection with the research.

Cooperation with duly authorized review groups, agencies, and institutional review boards. This means that you submit your proposed research to the appropriate committee in charge of reviewing provisions for the protection of subjects' rights and are willing to comply with their recommendations. Many journals require that study reports contain a statement that the research was approved from an ethical standpoint by the appropriate institutional committee.

Integrity in representing the research enterprise. This means that you do not withhold information about your study's possible risks, discomforts, or benefits, nor do you intentionally deceive study subjects on these matters.

Equitability in acknowledging the contributions of others. This means that you give credit where credit is due in publications, by listing coauthors, or in speeches and presentations, by acknowledging the work of others.

Nobility in the application of processes and procedures to protect the rights of human subjects. This means that you actively assume responsibility for protecting subjects from harm, deceit, coercion, and invasions of privacy, even when your own study may be inconvenienced.

Truthfulness about a study's purpose, procedure, methods, and findings. You do not attempt to disguise your research or conduct it "under cover."

Impeccability in use of any privileges that may be associated with the researcher's role. The investigator keeps data anonymous and confidential. The investigator is discreet about what is learned about people.

Forthrightness about a study's funding sources and sponsorship. You disclose all sources of financial support as well as any special relationship between a study and its sponsors in publications and presentations of research findings.

Illumination brought to the discipline's body of scientific knowledge through publications and presentations of research findings. Research should yield fruitful results.

Courage to publicly clarify any distortion that others make of your research findings.

From Wilson, HS: *Research in nursing,* ed 2, Redwood City, Calif, 1989, Addison-Wesley Publishing Company, pp. 67–69.

Rights of Human Subjects

1. Right to freedom from instrinsic risk of injury
2. Right to privacy and dignity
3. Right to anonymity

From American Nurses Association: *Human rights guidelines for nurses in clinical and other research* (Publication D-46 5M 2/85), Kansas City, Mo, 1985, American Nurses Association, pp. 6–7.

quired to comprehend the rationale underlying new policies, procedures, and techniques that incorporate research findings. Employers make resource persons available, often through committees and in-service programs, to help nurses maintain competencies based on evolving nursing knowledge.

BLENDING PRESENT AND FUTURE NURSING ETHICAL ISSUES

At the risk of overwhelming the beginning staff nurse with a wide variety of moral issues currently confronting client care managers, we believe that some future concerns merit a brief introduction. Anticipating potential moral dilemmas may help to prevent them or reduce their seriousness. Recognizing patterns of persistent moral issues focuses emphasis to help resolve them in a positive manner.

First, regardless of the contexts in which care is provided violations of client's rights will continue to be a common ethical concern of the public, and hopefully, of the nursing profession as well. If the public does not perceive that progress is being made in protecting human dignity, for whatever reasons, codes of conduct guiding ethical practice may be accorded less credence. Their value to the profession and their effectiveness in ensuring the common good are likely to be more frequently and seriously questioned.

Second, ethical issues related to controlling health care costs, to the constraining effects of costs on clinical decision making, and to the design of the technology that underlies health systems are likely to continue. Controlling cost at the expense of client well-being and satisfaction is likely to cause the public to question whether current laws regulating professional practice are adequate to protect the public. Is peer review of professional practice effectively addressing increasing complaints of unsafe, harmful, or insensitive care? Is the current system, which relies on nurses to practice ethically, working? If it is not, do solutions lie in changing ethical principles or laws?

Considerable evidence exists that, until recently, principles of ethical nursing practice have been neglected in educational programs (Cassells and Redman, 1989, p. 463; Fry, 1989, pp. 485–497; Gaul, 1989, pp. 476–477; Killeen, 1989, pp 334–340). The nursing profession is faced with many questions. Will including ethics in nursing curricula ensure ethical nursing practice? How can health care organizations contribute toward creating work environments that promote ethical nursing practice? What can individual nurses do to protect client rights?

Third, are ethical issues related to the individual nurse's commitment to health care goals? Are nurses, as members of the nursing profession and members of larger communities, demonstrating their commitment to health in their individual lifestyles and interactions with individual clients and community interest groups by promoting health and reducing the need for expensive illness care? If not, does their behavior reflect persistent personal values or preparation for professional nursing practice?

The interconnectedness of the global economy and its increasing complexity seem to indicate that economic constraints on the costs of care are likely to continue. As financing mechanisms continue to evolve, they may be allowed to usurp clinical decision-making authority in the guise of "managing care" for the purpose of reducing financial liabilities. Providers may be led to mistakenly believe that payers also voluntarily assume legal liabilities for the consequences of unsafe treatment decisions and ineffective services. Nurses need to continue to protect their legal authority, responsibility, and accountability for their professional practice and its consequences for clients served. Nursing interests need protection in political arenas as well as organizational settings. Protecting them requires responsible use of power and client advocacy.

Closely related to moral issues affecting ethical nursing practice are those that challenge the individual client's right to body integrity, which is nurtured by technology that has an increased capacity to substitute for bodily functions and parts. Increasing sophistication in successfully transplanting organs and inserting artificial body parts will require that individuals prepare advance directives to assure that their desires are addressed as their health conditions change. Moral dilemmas surrounding intergenerational donation of body parts are likely to become more common as advances in the life sciences continue. Questions concerning who can and should be authorized to permit donation of her or his body or any of its organs are likely to arise more frequently.

The staff nurse's involvement in nursing research is likely to expand as the management of data and information becomes easier and more efficient. Nurses need to develop creative methods of extracting the data used to evaluate nursing practice. Though data collected for clinical decision-making purposes are likely to differ from those gathered for research and evaluation purposes, nurses are likely to be asked to help collect data of both kinds. As client advocates, they will be required to ensure that the rights of clients as subjects of research studies are protected, in addition to clients' rights as recipients of nursing care. To maintain competencies, staff nurses will need to evaluate research reports as to the soundness of their findings and recommendations to determine whether following them is likely to improve the effectiveness of nursing care.

Special consideration is required to ensure that research designed to improve practice is distinguished from research designed to decrease costs. Another way to look at a research problem is to analyze whether its top priority is increasing economies in health care or designing more effective nursing strategies.

■■■■ SUMMARY

All nursing practice involves ethical decision making. Client care managers, as members of the discipline of nursing, need to incorporate ethics in their clinical decision making. Understanding common ethical concepts helps the nurse to practice in accordance with the ethical standards and codes of conduct established by the profession.

One's personal beliefs and values are rooted in cultural norms. These norms provide broad guidelines for judging whether one's conduct is right or wrong. Ethics is the study of rightness of conduct, the processes used to judge moral behavior, and the problems encountered when applying principles of morally correct behavior.

Ignoring moral conflicts does not cause them to cease to exist. Nurses need to develop sensitivity to moral issues and dilemmas. These moral conflicts usually involve misaligned personal and professional values that adversely affect clients and staff. Essential professional values include altruism, equality, esthetics, freedom, human dignity, justice, and truth. Translated into the nursing context, these concepts reflect commitment to promoting client participation in clinical decisions; doing good for the client; avoiding doing the client harm; using available resources fairly and reasonably; communicating truthfully and accurately; securing the client's privacy; and following through on treatment by carefully attending to details of the client's care. Once an existing moral issue is recognized, nurses use a moral reasoning process to seek appropriate solutions to resolve the conflict.

Ethical nursing practice involves taking morally correct actions within the context of the client's needs and values and nursing codes of conduct. Nurses suffer from moral distress when they know what moral values are at issue and choose the right courses of action but are not able to take action to resolve them. Excessive moral distress causes some nurses to leave bedside nursing.

Ethics differs from spirituality. Spirituality reflects personal beliefs, values, and ethical choices made to realize goals and make life meaningful. Religious practices are rooted in spirituality but ethics places more emphasis on cultural values.

Laws are rules for required behaviors that define personal and professional relationships. Laws reflect public policy. Good laws reflect desired ethical practices. Ethical guidelines are used to inform policy makers, legislators, health care professionals, and the public about desired behaviors.

The consequences of violating ethical and legal codes of conduct vary depending upon their effects on client safety and well-being. Client care managers are expected to adhere to directives described in living wills or provided by legally authorized persons. In addition, they are expected to distinguish between providing aggressive treatment and nontreatment, and among extraordinary life support measures, resuscitative measures, and supportive care measures.

Nurses focus on providing for client needs and documenting progress; they record client responses to treatment in a way that reflects that standards of care were maintained. Every client is entitled to efficient, cost-effective care. In a similar manner, nurses are expected to protect client safety by responding in an accountable manner to the conduct of incompetent colleagues. This response entails adhering to agency policies and following through with the steps of conflict resolution.

Nurses might be able to prevent future moral dilemmas and conflicts by learning about ethical nursing practice. By resolving current moral conflicts, health care organizations can develop mechanisms that more effectively address client needs and concerns. They can also participate in systematic studies designed to devise more effective nursing strategies using available technology.

◼︎ APPLICATION EXERCISES

 a. One of your peers believes that each individual has an inherent right to make as many choices as possible affecting one's lifestyle. Identify the nursing value reflected in this behavior. Discuss whether this value can be overemphasized to the detriment of other professional values. Give examples.

 b. One of your assigned clients repeatedly refuses to adhere to prescribed treatment. He has suffered several serious complications. Some staff have expressed frustration with the client's behavior, which they attribute to "not having to pay for it" since the client's care is funded by government programs. Identify which ethical nursing concepts are involved in this moral conflict.

 c. Describe how the moral reasoning process could be used to address the following moral issue. Your client has been ventilator dependent for two years and has expressed his wish to die on several occasions because his "life is no longer worth the effort." He has also asked several members of his immediate family to disconnect his respiratory equipment. Some nursing staff "don't think he really means it" and consequently, have ignored his request.

 d. Discuss practical ways that nurses might try to reduce moral distress.

e. Your client is a subject in a research project. However, he has suffered two serious setbacks since beginning his participation and now says he "wants out." The investigator is intent on retaining the client in the study for as long as possible, stating that the complications are not related to participation in the project. State whether you think the client's rights as a human subject are being violated. Give reasons for your answer.

REFERENCES

American Association of Colleges of Nursing: *Essentials of college and university education for professional nursing,* Washington, DC, 1986, American Association of Colleges of Nursing, pp. 5–7.

American Nurses Association: *Human rights guidelines for nurses in clinical and other research,* Publication No. D-46 5M 2/85, Kansas City, Mo, American Nurses Association.

Cassells JM, Redman BK: Preparing students to be moral agents in clinical nursing practice, *Nurs Clin North Am* 24(2):464–473. (June, 1989).

Curtin L: Ethics in nursing practice, *Nurs Manage* 19(5):7–9. (May, 1988).

Cushing M: Who's responsible for too early discharge? *Am J Nurs* 89(4):471–472. (April, 1989).

Dolan JF: Mounting interest in right to die issue, *AARP Bulletin: A Publication of the American Association of Retired Persons* 32(2):7, 1991.

Fowler MDM: Ethical Guidelines, *Heart Lung* 17(1):103–104. (January, 1988).

Fowler MD: Ethical decision making in clinical practice, *Nurs Clin North Am* 24(4):955–965. (December, 1989).

Fry ST: Teaching ethics in nursing curricula, *Nurs Clin North Am* 24(2):485–497. (June, 1989).

Gaul ALV: Ethics content in baccalaureate degree curricula: clarifying the issues, *Nurs Clin North Am* 24(2):475–483. (June, 1989).

Hines GL: DRGs: nursing documentation contributes to the bottom line, *Nurs Clin North Am* 23(3):579–586. (September, 1988).

Jameton A: Culture, morality, and ethics: twirling the spindle, *Critical Care Nurs Clin North Am* 2(3):443–451. (September, 1990).

Ketefian S: Moral reasoning and ethical practice in nursing: measurement issues, *Nurs Clin North Am* 24(2):509–521. (June, 1989).

Killeen ML: Nursing fundamentals texts: where's the ethics? *J Nurs Educ* 25(8):334–340. (October, 1986).

Kjervik DK: The connection between law and ethics *J Prof Nurs* 6(3):138, 185. (May-June, 1990).

Lammers P: Ethics euthanasia, suicide focus of ethics conference, *AORN J* 44(4):626–630. (October, 1986).

Murphy CP: Integration of diagnostic and ethical reasoning in clinical practice: teaching and evaluation, Chapter 14 in *Classification of nursing diagnoses: proceedings of the eighth conference,* edited by Carroll-Johnson RM. Philadelphia, Pa, 1989, J.B. Lippincott Company, pp. 73–76.

Murphy EK: Undocumented nursing care does not always indicate liability, *AORN J* 46(3):626–630. (September, 1987).

Salladay SA, McDonnell MM: Spiritual care, ethical choices, and patient advocacy, *Nurs Clin North Am* 24(2):543–549. (June, 1989).

Sawyer LM: Nursing code of ethics: an international comparison, *Int Nurs Rev* 36(5):145–148. (1989).

Scalon D, Flemming C: Confronting ethical issues: a nursing survey, *Nurs Manage* 21(5):63–65. (May, 1990).

Thompson TC: Rehabilitation: option or requirement? *Rehabil Nurs* 14(6):344. (November-December, 1989).

Wilkinson JM: Moral distress in nursing practice: experience and effect, *Nurs Forum* 23(1):16–29. (1987/88).

Wilson HS: *Research in nursing,* ed 2 Redwood City, Calif, 1989, Addison-Wesley Publishing Company, pp. 67–69.

chapter fifteen

NURTURING PROFESSIONAL INTEGRITY

OBJECTIVES

Completing this chapter should enable you to:

1. Discuss ethical issues related to accepting personal responsibility for self-management.
2. Describe a nurse's responsibility for lifelong learning.
3. Discuss common ethical issues associated with contributing to the nursing profession.
4. Describe adaptive attitudes used to cope and adjust to change.
5. Describe ethical issues related to meeting employee obligations.

KEY CONCEPTS

personal responsibility for self-management

advocate for the nursing profession

ethical obligations of an employee of a health care agency

loyalty

 he ethical concepts related to managing client care discussed in this chapter were selected to help the beginning staff nurse nurture a sense of professional integrity. These concepts concern personal and professional obligations.

ACCEPTING PERSONAL RESPONSIBILITY FOR SELF-MANAGEMENT

As a member of the discipline of nursing, client care managers are expected to accept **personal responsibility for self-management.** That is, they make a special effort to assure that their practice is characterized by the values accepted by nursing as a profession. Altruism—unselfish concern for the welfare of others—is one of those values. Being committed to altruism, client care managers accept obligations and need to rely on inner motivations to ensure that they practice nursing safely on their clients' behalf. Rather than waiting for others to request specific changes in their behavior, they are motivated by their inner desire to do what is right for clients.

Accepting altruism as a professional value carries the potential for serious personal risk. Placing the needs of others before one's own on a regular basis is very stressful.

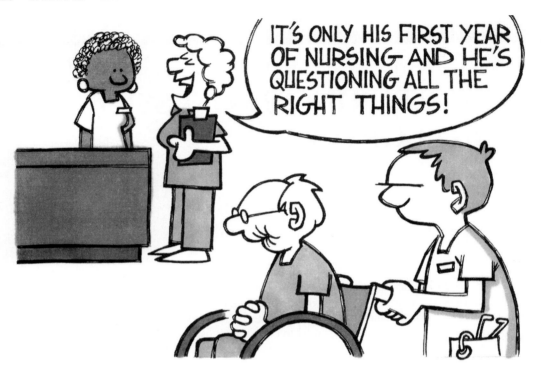

Client care managers make a special effort to ensure that their practice is characterized by the values accepted by nursing as a profession.

Indeed, one study found that "focusing on the needs of others, often to the exclusion of meeting personal needs, contributes to addiction" (Gelfand et al, 1990, p. 76). Nurses who have not incorporated these demands into their lifestyles may pay a high cost in terms of poor health and ethically questionable nursing practice. Nurses are responsible for the safety of clients. They are expected to recognize unsafe practice and monitor the practice of peers. They are also individually responsible for the quality of their own lives and nursing practice. Accordingly, each nurse is responsible for making the lifestyle changes needed to reduce the consequences of stress. Stress management can include a wide variety of relaxation techniques; physical exercise; and various diversional, recreational, and leisure activities. Effective stress management helps ensure that the demands of nursing practice do not destroy one's dignity and personal livelihood. Making the lifestyle changes required to effectively manage stress is challenging but critical to enjoying a successful career. Neglecting to manage stress increases the nurse's vulnerability to "burnout." "Burnout" is a term commonly used to describe behaviors that reflect lower levels of physiological, psychological, and emotional functioning. Nurses experiencing "burnout" might feel increasingly pessimistic and dissatisfied, chronically fatigued, frustrated, and irritable.

Successful staff nurses use several common strategies to maintain a sense of dignity. Perhaps the most obvious concerns appearance. The nurse needs an acceptable image as a mature adult. This image is enhanced by attire suitable for meeting the public and also adapted to the diversity of activities that nurses perform as part of their routine duties (such

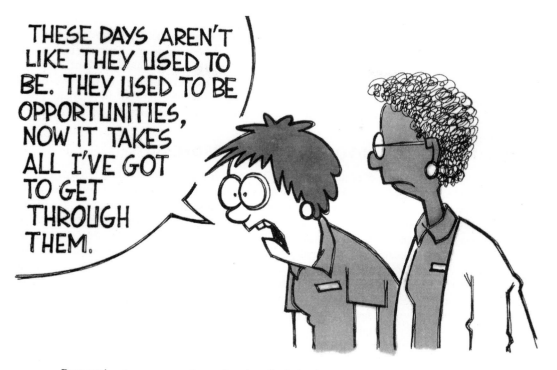

Burnout is a term commonly used to describe behaviors reflective of decreased physiologic, psychological, and emotional functioning.

as walking, reaching, bending, stooping, and stretching). The nurse's clothing needs to be comfortable, neat, and becoming.

A person's demeanor—tone of voice, facial expressions, and body movements—also contributes to her or his public image and needs regular attention. Focusing on others requires the nurse to separate home and work concerns. Clients expect to be the focus of the nurse's attention; they do not want to have to console or empathize with their nurse.

By attending to the public image projected by one's appearance and demeanor, the nurse can convey a positive attitude about nursing and display confidence when approaching others. Nursing students are amply aware of the widespread anxiety among clients and readily understand the need to display confidence in the clinical area. To do otherwise can increase client anxiety.

Nurses committed to the essential values of their profession take the initiative in identifying their individual strengths and limitations. Accordingly, they strive to develop their strengths as a means of creatively diminishing the influence of their limitations. It is virtually impossible to know and do everything! When effective nurses lack knowledge or skills needed to address client needs, they do not perceive the limitation as a personal inadequacy. Rather, they appropriately admit their limitations to others, so that needed resources can be obtained to assure that the quality of care received by clients is not adversely affected. They also accept constructive criticism. When strategies, procedures, or techniques exceed their capabilities, they seek help to develop needed knowledge and skills and help with giving care.

Another component of self-management relates to the nurse's responsibility to maintain nursing competencies. Staff nurses accept responsibility for lifelong learning by maintaining a positive attitude toward gaining insights from experience and participating in structured learning activities. Many strategies can be used to maintain current nursing knowledge and skills, including regularly reading professional journals, participating in systematic studies designed by others, and using research findings to improve nursing practice. Many nurses contribute to the evolving knowledge base of the nursing professional while implementing personal strategies for self-management.

SERVING AS AN ADVOCATE FOR THE PROFESSION

Many nurses serve as **advocates for the nursing profession.** They believe that they can and should contribute to nursing's evolving knowledge base. Accordingly, they belong to nursing organizations that advance their interests, and, indirectly, the interests of the various client populations they serve. They accept change as a challenge and understand that it is essential to the viability of nursing. They actively develop and maintain organized groups such as local nursing specialty groups to sustain the nursing profession as a valued component of society. Without continued support from special nursing interest groups, member socialization, advocacy, and development of meaningful relationships with other groups are not feasible. Nurses who do not belong to professional organizations (and some don't for a variety of reasons) limit their potential influence and contributions to society as members of their discipline. Their interests and concerns are more likely to be unrecognized, underrepresented, and unmet, since they lack strength through numbers. It behooves every nurse to join one or more nursing organizations and actively participate in special interest groups. Although organizational activities exact personal costs in terms of time, effort, and money, many nurses use this approach to actively address their obligations to the profession.

American society is politically pluralistic. That is, it incorporates many different, often conflicting views. These different views are often reflected in organized special interest groups. To ensure that the nursing profession's interests are expressed and responded to by policy makers, special organizations are necessary. In addition to the American Nurses Association, many other nursing specialty groups have been formed to represent diverse nursing interests and concerns. When elected officials are informed of their constitutents' concerns, they are in a better position to act on them. If they are not informed, concerns expressed by other vested interest groups are likely to take precedence. For example, the public, through the mass media, has expressed distress about the increasing costs of health care and consequent decrease in accessibility. Although the special interests of nursing might provide some solutions to these problems, nurses compete for the attention and resources of public policy makers and elected officials. To be successful, nursing interests need to be articulated in such a way as to promote the public good. Frequently, information-sharing by nursing groups enables legislators to fashion and approve legislation to address expressed concerns. In addition, nurses might participate on task forces to help governments initiate legislation to prevent or address emerging social problems—for example, advocating nutrition programs for preschool children or the elderly.

Nurses also contribute to public education through active involvement in local community activities. For example, by participating in recreational, volunteer, or religious groups, nurses frequently provide health education. They participate in programs designed to prevent diseases, promote health, and provide support for those with diagnosed diseases.

As discussed in Chapter Two, societal trends also affect nursing practice. Evolving technology has made it possible to handle more information and manage it such that those

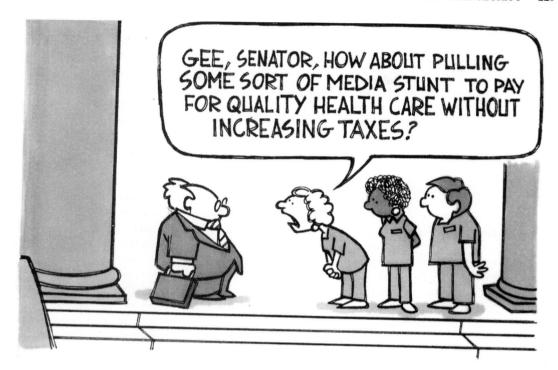

Nursing interests need to be conveyed in such a way as to promote the public good.

who are in decision-making positions have access to it. Several important ethical issues are emerging as a result of this trend.

MANAGING INFORMATION

Using Computer Literacy Skills to Influence Organizational Decision Making

Those who have the skills to use technology to acquire information are more likely to participate in organizational decision making than those who do not. To sustain autonomy in clinical decision making, it is very important that nurses develop computer literacy skills. Increased access to information about clients helps nurses use knowledge more efficiently to benefit clients. Processing detailed information more efficiently saves time to provide care. Much evidence, however, indicates that nurses have not carefully considered how best to use their time and skills to manage the data needed to enhance their nursing practice. Rather, nurses often spend considerable time and effort making detailed observations and entering data for other disciplines (Woolery, 1990, pp. 50–51). Using available technology is integral to nursing practice. The quality of client care will depend in the future upon the extent to which nurses efficiently manage data in accordance with established standards and nursing practice. These standards represent common nursing strategies and outcomes designed to guide the services provided to individual clients.

Using Available Technology Wisely

Nurses need to accept responsibility for maintaining nursing standards by using available technology wisely on their clients' behalf. Not to assert nursing interests when information systems are developed and purchased often results in decreasing the systems' availability to nursing staff. The design of information systems can influence what data is collected and who uses it. Taking initiative in expressing concerns about information systems and how they help or hinder client care can save nursing time and effort. Computerized information systems need to incorporate nursing's needs for accurate, current data to use in making clinical decisions in a timely manner. Nursing diagnoses of client needs must be incorporated into health care systems to guide planning, implementing, and evaluating the effectiveness of services provided.

Participating in Designing Information Management Systems

The nurse's effective use of technology and input into its design are rapidly growing, interrelated concerns (McConnell and Murphy, 1990, p. 333). An example of the influence of evolving technology is the design of the management information systems required to provide modern health care. Information management systems are evolving to address outcome criteria (individual client care goals) as well as gather the data needed to evaluate the quality of care provided. Such technology can be used to collect, store, and retrieve accurate, current information needed to formulate nursing diagnoses. Non-nursing activities, such as requesting and distributing equipment and supplies, compiling client charge lists, and staffing, can be done efficiently with available information technology. In the past, many nurses feared that information technology would consume scarce time and resources and detract from client care. These fears have proven to be unfounded.

Despite revolutionary technology, nurses will continue to coordinate client care. Careful consideration is needed to ensure that nursing skills and time are used efficiently so that the resources of support staff are used wisely. For example, rather than doing work themselves that can be safely and efficiently performed by support staff, client care managers can serve as resource persons helping other staff find ways to serve clients better. It is critical that nurses maintain autonomy if they are to be accountable for their own actions and those of staff working under their direction. Remember that nurses can maintain autonomy while delegating nursing tasks to others but not nursing responsibilities for client care. Each nurse shares the obligation of ensuring that available technology and equipment are used properly to adhere to established standards of nursing practice.

As the complexity of client care, organizational development, and nursing practice increases, the need for specialized nursing knowledge also increases. To assure the public of quality care, continuing efforts are being made to establish "practice guidelines" (standards of care established by the agency's nursing staff) to help nurses manage the client care process (Sharp, 1990, p. 22). Such guidelines are another way to resolve issues related to transforming scientific knowledge into clinical judgments, treatment effectiveness, and health care cost controls. Use of such practice guidelines may help to develop more efficient and economical health care systems that will improve nursing practice. Nursing practice strategies and organizational factors that contribute to or interfere with client care need continuous study. Each nurse shares responsibility for nursing research designed to improve nursing practice. Accordingly, each nursing research project should answer the following questions: How will the results of this study serve clients? How will it contribute to nursing knowledge?

Complexity also increases the demand for knowledge and skills. To maintain safe, effective, and efficient standards of care, nurses with advanced knowledge and skills are needed. The qualifications of such nurses are best determined by nurses practicing in similar specialized settings. Nurses with credentials for advanced practice beyond the competencies of beginning nurses are needed to provide specialized care. For the credentialing processes to be successful, nursing peer involvement is essential. Providing for this involvement is usually one of the functions of speciality nursing organizations. Though this is not often articulated, ethical nursing practice includes taking actions that support the profession in addition to those taken to provide quality care needed by clients. Ultimately, efforts directly made to enhance the profession indirectly benefit clients.

◼◼◼ MEETING PROFESSIONAL RESPONSIBILITIES AS AN EMPLOYEE

In addition to addressing responsibilities related to maintaining one's nursing competencies and actively supporting the profession, each nurse has several **ethical obligations as an employee of a health care agency.** At times in the past, nursing loyalty to the employer took precedence over client needs. Nurses continue to experience ethical conflicts when addressing client needs as their top priority. The client's ability to pay for services received is also of concern.

Identifying Moral Dilemmas Related to Health Care Financing

The code of nursing ethics requires the nurse to provide quality care without regard for the method of payment used. The current health care system and financing mechanisms are forcing many clients to accept, and nurses to provide, only the care that individual clients can afford. In an era when health care costs are spiraling upward, insurance mechanisms are designed to limit costs rather than satisfy client needs. If providing care according to parameters defined by insurers were acceptable, nurses would need to be prepared as insurance agents to assess and design insurance benefit programs, not as nurses who assess client conditions as the basis for care. Indeed, when current health care insurers try to control costs by interpreting benefits on a case-by-case basis, the situation comes to resemble that of the proverbial "tail wagging the dog." Nurses need to strive to be cost-effective, but not to the detriment of clients (Smeltzer, 1990, p. 5). Cost-effectiveness is a component of quality care.

Legal responsibility and accountability for the consequences of services provided continue to rest primarily with health care providers, not with health care insurers. Liability for the consequences of early discharge or selection of treatment options is likely to continue to rest with providers of care. Accordingly, nurses will serve clients well by expanding rather than limiting the accessibility and quality of health care. Nurses need to accurately assess client needs and plan to provide nursing services based on individual responses and anticipated client recovery patterns. For staff nurses, consideration of the methods of financing needed care is secondary to determining client needs and how they can be addressed by nursing staff. To align priorities in accordance with health care financing instead of client needs is unlikely to serve either the client's or the health care agency's interests.

Health care financing mechanisms often cause agency constraints that prevent client care managers from providing quality care. Nurses who understand what clients need but are prevented from providing quality care are likely to suffer moral distress. Complying with various administrative strategies to reduce expenses and increase revenue without acknowledging the consequences can require staff to neglect important details of quality client care. Common results are ineffective treatment, complications, or delayed client recovery. Rather than focusing on client needs, employees adjust by devising documentation strategies designed to obtain maximum reimbursement. Such operational strategies condition staff to ignore expressed client concerns or "cover up" inadequacies. Slowly, and often unnoticeably, the focus of staff efforts shifts from consumer satisfaction and quality client care to profit making. Such regressive shifts in organizational focus interfere with sustaining satisfying work cultures. Instead, employees devalue their work and find it difficult or impossible to remain committed to it. The staff encounter increasingly complicated moral dilemmas and legal difficulties (Hogue, 1990, pp. 317–318; Mallison, 1990, p. 25). Ethical solutions lie in administrative and nursing staff sensitivity to the specific moral dilemmas involved in current methods of discharge planning and their selection of available options.

Maintaining Loyalties

Loyal employees support the agency's philosophy, policies, and procedures. **Loyalty** to the employer involves commitment. It should not require submissive obedience or compromised values.

Loyalty does not include the obligation to provide unlimited overtime and effort without compensation. Taking into account the different circumstances causing the nurse to work overtime, the nurse has a moral obligation to determine what actions are in the best interest of clients, the self, and the employer. To continue to work extended hours without compensation or acknowledgment by the employer is likely to lead to even more overtime work. This moral dilemma is similar to many others that result from the expectation that the nurse will manage unreasonable conflicts, inconsistencies, and demands as an employee (e.g, lack of supplies, malfunctioning equipment, or inadequate staffing).

Promoting Client Interests while Communicating with Interdisciplinary Team Members

As the coordinator of client care, the nurse frequently becomes aware of interdisciplinary disagreements and role conflicts. Sometimes the nurse seeks to resolve these conflicts in an effort to serve the client's best interest. Some role conflicts relate to overlaps or gaps in the responsibilities involved in providing care over a 24-hour period on a daily basis. For example, nurses working during the evening and night shifts are often expected to "cover" for other disciplines in the interest of cost-effectiveness. Consequently, they are asked to provide physical, respiratory, pharmaceutical, or social services, in addition to fulfilling nursing responsibilities. Nurses need to articulate their concerns about these situations so that more effective approaches to quality client care can be devised. In addition, their need for adequate preparation to perform such services skillfully and safely must be made clear to the administration. The specific sources of each moral dilemma require analysis, and the options of ethical action to resolve the conflict must be identified.

Another type of moral dilemma presents itself when interdisciplinary communication patterns evolve into bureaucratic maneuvering for status instead of focusing on client care. High-quality care requires that health team members communicate effectively with each other in a spirit of collaboration. Among the universally accepted ethical behaviors are effective working relationships with co-workers (Sawyer, 1989, p. 145). Communication "games" do not serve clients or staff (Marsden, 1990, pp. 422–424). In fact, they typically increase stress, conflict, and potential for verbal abuse. Nurses have established a history of seeking autonomy in clinical decision making. Physicians have established professional boundaries that rely heavily on the expertise of other disciplines. What is important is that an environment be created and sustained in which team members focus on client needs as their top priority. Team members need to feel safe enough to communicate concerns and needs openly to each other. Such an atmosphere is likely to promote effective communication with clients as well. Open communication among team members serves to address client needs. Sensitivity to patterns of communication among health team members helps nurses identify those that detract from client care. A spirit of collaboration promotes quality client care by mobilizing costly human resources instead of allowing moral dilemmas to erode them.

Maintaining Confidentiality

Nurses have an obligation to maintain confidentiality about private and intimate client matters. As members of the larger society, nurses are affected by society's predominant anxieties and stereotypes. To practice ethically, the nurse needs to develop the sensitivity required to keep clinical information about individual clients private or secret from those not directly involved in providing their care. Indiscreet social interactions in nonclinical areas, or "shop talk," can be overheard or misinterpreted and result in considerable damage to clients, without the nurse's ever being aware of it (Glinsky, 1987, p. 24). Accordingly, "shop talk" is unethical because of its potential for violating client rights. Every nurse has a moral duty not to engage in "shop talk."

Nurses need to sort out the nature of the legal relationships of the client's family and significant others before sharing confidential information. Given the many variations in the composition of American families, this is no small achievement. To do otherwise poses serious risk of violating the client's rights, morally and legally.

Symptoms or diseases, such as AIDS, malignancies, or genetic disorders, frequently contribute to the social isolation or stigmatization of clients. These consequences present moral dilemmas and create the potential for violating client rights. Depending upon the severity of the negative stereotypes and the public's concern for the common good, laws are usually passed both to protect the individuals who are victims of the disease and to protect the public from contracting the dreaded diseases. For example, many states have laws concerning who is required to be "tested" for AIDS. In addition, many states have laws dictating how information about persons with the disease is to be handled to assure the privacy of individual clients (Grady, 1989, pp. 529–531). Associated with the issue of confidentiality are concerns for protecting the client's autonomy (beneficence, nonmalificence) and equal access to health care (justice). Nurses are obligated to provide services to clients in a nondiscriminatory manner. Expression of personal prejudices, evidenced by refusal to provide care or showing disrespect for the individual's characteristics or appearance, is prohibited.

Closely related to client rights to privacy are moral dilemmas associated with a person's right to bodily integrity. Nurses are involved in performing treatment programs in which tissue or organs are transplanted or artificial body parts are inserted. In addition to performing related nursing procedures correctly, nurses need to be sensitive not only to client responses but to how clients are selected for these procedures. What basic values are inherent in the ethical guidelines used? Is the client's autonomy protected, or do financial considerations predominate? Nurses need to be sensitive to which professional values and ethical principles are involved in protecting client rights and how they are prioritized in individual client circumstances.

Protecting One's Rights as a Provider of Health Care

Nurses obtain the privilege of practicing nursing after meeting specific licensure requirements. Nurses have rights related to the practice of their chosen profession, too. These rights are recognized and protected by position statements formulated by representative nursing organizations. Such position statements are written from time to time to inform the public and guide nurses in selecting moral actions inherent in ethical practice. For example, the ANA Committee on Ethics (1986) issued a "Statement Regarding Risk Versus Responsibility in Providing Nursing Care" to clarify parameters of nursing obligations and options in providing care involving risks to the nurse's life or well-being.

Nurses can morally justify refusal to participate in client care in some circumstances and need to be aware of the conditions required for doing so. The ANA statement delineated four basic requirements for determining the difference between doing good for another as a moral duty and doing so as a moral option. According to the ANA, the nurse is ethically required to provide care when:

1. The client is at significant risk of harm, loss, or damage if the nurse does not help.
2. The nurse's action or care directly prevents harm to the client.
3. The nurse's action will probably prevent harm, loss, or damage to the client.
4. The benefit the client will gain outweighs any harm the nurse might bring upon herself or himself and does not present more than minimal risk to the nurse (ANA Committee on Ethics, 1986).

To refuse to provide care for a client requires that the nurse understand the nature of the client's condition, the urgency of the need, and the likelihood that the nurse's help will make a significant difference. Obviously, ethical decisions require that the nurse make use of current and accurate information about client conditions, knowledge of the professional values involved, and understanding of the priorities in her or his personal values.

Another issue in maintaining confidentiality relates to the nurse's obligation to make reasonable efforts to use available technology to process information accurately and efficiently on the clients' behalf. To sabotage or undermine the use of the agency's technology for any reason, (e.g., fear, lack of information or skills) by omitting data or not using the system at all is ethically irresponsible when the quality of client care depends on it. Such behavior could jeopardize client well-being, result in lack of follow-through, or cause system inadequacies in meeting standards of quality care. As information technology develops, nurses need to be aware of their moral responsibility to use it for the purposes for which it was intended, which includes using the mechanisms for maintaining confidentiality.

Serving as a Role Model

As mentioned in Chapter Nine, nurses can lead and teach others about desired behaviors by modeling desired actions. Nurses' attitudes need to reflect their personal values and commitment to the values espoused by the profession in its ethical codes of behavior. This does not mean that individuals should expect others to mimic their behavior. Rather, functioning as a role model is a teaching strategy used to help co-workers learn about moral issues and acceptable methods of resolving them in the interests of all concerned. Instead of imitating the behaviors of role models, co-workers are encouraged to learn how to solve ethical issues to improve work performance and quality of client care. This approach reinforces respect for individual differences and the dignity of others. It also encourages employees to accept accountability for their actions.

The respect of others is earned, not given. Co-workers might indicate in several different ways that a nurse has earned their respect. One common indicator of respect is the nature of the communication patterns between co-workers, including demeanor and tone of voice. The right to privacy and to participate in clinical decision making are fundamental to meaningful relationships with peers, as they are to relationships with clients. Patterns of staff interactions can reflect positive attitudes toward clients. For example, staff nurses convey respect for peers and co-workers by using language that is commonly understood, incorporating accepted health care terminology and avoiding offensive expressions.

Another common indicator that co-workers respect a nurse is their responsiveness to supervision and instruction. Co-workers tend to actively seek guidance and direction from the nurse to help them complete their work assignments. They effectively communicate their concerns, acknowledge their limitations, and express the need to help or support when it arises. They do not delay such requests until the difficulties are unavoidable or overwhelming.

Another way to demonstrate respect for others might involve consulting with the agency's ethics committee to demonstrate the attitude that differing points of view are acceptable. The recommendations of such a committee can be incorporated in making appropriate clinical decisions for clients and staff when the situations encountered are difficult to manage using typical approaches. Nurses need to use an ethics committee to help them fulfill obligations of client advocacy, to clarify facts, and to improve communication (Murphy, 1989, p. 554). Respect for differences requires that they be acknowledged in the effort to find solutions, rather than suppressed or ignored. After the beginning staff nurse gains work experience and develops a special interest in addressing moral dilemmas, he or she might seek membership on such a committee.

Finally, co-workers who respect each other tend to use similar approaches to their work. Though they do not necessarily agree on many issues, their approaches to meeting diverse client needs become more similar than different. Respect for oneself and others creates work cultures designed to provide high-quality care and reinforces co-worker adherence to codes of ethical conduct.

Making Hard Choices

To be sure, nurses are required to make hard choices to maintain their personal livelihoods and nursing competencies, support the nursing profession, and remain loyal to their employers. Like many ethical issues in nursing practice, situations causing moral dilemmas are usually very complex. Solutions require careful attention to the identified differences and persistent commitment to resolving them. For example, making specific changes in one's lifestyle to effectively manage stress is usually very difficult, due to personal goals, time limitations, family needs, work schedules, commitment to various community groups, and recreational interests. However, these difficulties do not make the need to manage stress less critical. Similarly, societal trends (such as the increasing influence of the global economy) continue to influence nursing as a profession and require individual nurses to creatively support its evolution as a science and dynamic force in society. As economic constraints continue to influence the health care system (requiring more collaboration between various disciplines) the autonomy of all health care providers is likely to be affected, which will probably stimulate change in the role of nurses as employees.

As members of the nursing profession, beginning staff nurses are likely to be confronted with difficult choices. These decisions will significantly affect the quality of their lives, nursing practice, and employment. The best decisions for the involved individuals usually incorporate both personal and professional values. For example, a nurse's commitment to providing quality care may lead her or him to "bend the rules for the sake of the patient" (Hutchinson, 1990, p. 3). Doing so carries considerable risk to a nurse function-

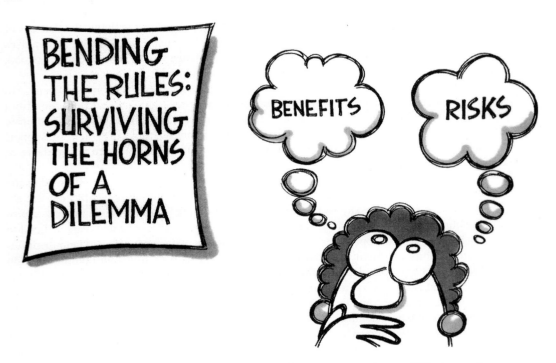

Beginning staff nurses are likely to be confronted with choices that are difficult to make.

ing as an autonomous professional and participant in a formal organizational system. The positive consequences of the actions taken are likely to be used to justify bending the rules even though there is no legal or organizational basis for doing so. Unfortunately, "responsible rule bending" may produce negative consequences and cause client injury or harm. Legal difficulties may arise if the situation is disclosed.

Employees who participate in "whistle-blowing" or criticize an agency's questionable practices accept both the positive and negative consequences of reporting situations that endanger client well-being (Fiesta, 1990, p. 38; Kiely and Kiely, 1987, p. 42). The positive consequences are the satisfactions and comforts of adherence with the nurses' professional code of ethics. The negative consequences concern the lack of organizational or legal support for doing so, which may ultimately result in being fired, career disruptions, license revocation, malpractice, and possible criminal charges. Whistle-blowing can imperil a career. Such risks, however, do not reduce the need to disclose unsafe practices. Hopefully, employers of nurses will become increasingly responsive to employee concerns about quality of care. Instead of firing concerned employees for disclosing questionable practices, administrative policies could provide alternatives to public disclosure, such as organizational communication systems and reporting procedures (Pinch, 1990, pp. 60–61).

Nurses need to remember that the ANA Code for Nurses is not law or public policy. Rather, it is "a policy document that constitutes the expression of principles that are geared to the enhancement of health care in general" (Blum, 1984, p. 150). Since it doesn't have legal status, ethical conduct consistent with established codes may not prevent an employer from dismissing an employee. By following nursing codes of conduct that support the public interest, staff nurses may benefit from societal support for needed legislation that currently does not exist (Fiesta, 1990, p. 38).

SUMMARY

Client care managers accept responsibility for self-management by participating in continued learning experiences to maintain nursing competencies. They are motivated to do what is right for the public and for their clients. They use several common strategies to maintain their health and sense of self-dignity, and they accept responsibility for managing their own individual strengths and limitations. They seek help to develop the needed knowledge and skills and help to provide care when the necessary strategies, procedures, or techniques exceed their capabilities.

Many nurses also participate in activities advocating the interests of the nursing professional. They join and become actively involved in nursing and special interest organizations. They participate in health education programs with community groups. In addition, nurses make a special effort to learn to use available technology, to maintain nursing standards, and to participate in research endeavors aimed at increasing nursing knowledge.

Client care managers also accept ethical obligations as employees of health care agencies. They support their agencies' philosophies and policies. They strive to maintain effective communication patterns with health team members to coordinate client care. They are expected to protect clients' rights as well as their own. They take the initiative to teach others about quality care and to demonstrate desired approaches. From time to time, client care managers must make hard choices regarding the ethical priorities of clients and their employers. They need to clearly distinguish behaviors advocated by ethical codes of conduct from those required by existing laws.

APPLICATION EXERCISES:

a. Interview three staff nurses about their self-management strategies. Ask them to discuss the methods they use to manage stress and set priorities. Compare your findings with peers. Identify predominant strategies and reasons for their popularity.

b. List ten different ways that nurses participate in lifelong learning. Rate them according to your personal preferences.

c. Your agency uses several different computer networks to store, retrieve, and access client information in an efficient and timely manner. One of your neighbors asks you about the recovery of a mutual friend, knowing that you have access to confidential information. List ethical alternative responses. Select the best option. Give reasons for your selection.

d. A colleague tells you that "things are getting worse instead of better since decentralization." You are new to the organization. When employed, you were informed of administrative plans for promoting professional autonomy and accountability. Describe how you would remain loyal to the organization and support your colleague's need for change.

e. While administering medications during the evening shift you overhear a client verbally abusing a nursing team member under your supervision. Describe criteria you would use to determine whether the nursing staff member can refuse to provide further care to the client.

REFERENCES

American Nurses Association Committee on Ethics: *Statement regarding risk versus responsibility in providing nursing care,* Kansas City, Mo, 1986, American Nurses Association.

Blum JD: The code of nurses and wrongful discharge, *Nurs Forum* 21(4):149–150. (1984).

Fiesta J: Whistleblowers: retaliation or protection?—Part II, *Nurs Manage* 21(7):38. (July, 1990).

Gelfand G, Long P, McGill D, Sheerin C: Prevention of chemically impaired nursing practice, *Nurs Manage* 21(7):76–78. (July, 1990).

Glinsky J: The perils of "shop talk," *Nurs Life* 7(6):24. (November/December, 1987).

Grady C: Ethical issues in providing nursing care to human immunodeficiency virus-infected populations, *Nurs Clin North Am* 24(2):523–534. (June, 1989).

Hogue EE: The liability of payors and providers in health care treatment decisions, *Pediatr Nurs* 16(3):317–318. (May-June, 1990).

Hutchinson SA: Responsible subversion: a study of rule-bending among nurses, *Scholar Inq Nurs Pract* 4(1):317. (Spring, 1990).

Kiely MA, Kiely DC: Whistleblowing: disclosure and its consequences for the professional nurse and management, *Nurs Manage* 18(5):41–45. (May, 1987).

Mallison MB: Controversies in care: a jury defines "Neglect" in nursing homes, *Am J Nurs* 90(9):25. (September, 1990).

Marsden C: Ethics of the "doctor-nurse game," *Heart Lung* 19(4):422–424. (July, 1990).

McConnell EA, Murphy EK: Nurses' use of technology: an international concern, *Int Nurs Rev* 37(5):331–334. (September-October, 1990).

Murphy P: The role of the nurse on hospital ethics committees, *Nurs Clin North Am* 24(2):551–556. (June, 1989b).

Pinch WJ: Nursing ethics: is "covering-up" ever "harmless"? *Nurs Manage* 21(9):60–62. (September, 1990).

Sawyer LM: Nursing code of ethics: an international comparison, *Int Nurs Rev* 36(5):145–148. (September-October, 1989).

Sharp N: National practice guidelines: what do they mean for nurses? *Nurs Manage* 21(11):22, 24. (November, 1990).

Smeltzer CH: The impact of prospective payment on the economics, ethics, and quality of nursing, *Nurs Admin Q* 14(3):1–10. (Spring, 1990).

Woolery LK: Professional standards and ethical dilemmas in nursing information systems, *J Nurs Adm* 20(10):50–53. (October, 1990).

MANAGING YOUR CAREER

Completing this chapter should enable you to:

1. Refine your personal nursing philosophy, interests, and talents.
2. Identify five-year goals.
3. Seek employment corresponding to your personal career goals.
4. Organize information about your qualifications and nursing credentials.
5. Determine the need for malpractice insurance.
6. Use available support systems to promote personal growth.
7. Establish licensure and maintain your registration as a registered nurse.
8. Write a letter notifying your employer of a desire to change or terminate employment.
9. Nurture an indefatigable sense of humor!

KEY CONCEPTS

nursing philosophy
  personal values
  beliefs
characteristics of nursing as a profession
  maintaining nursing competencies
  need for continued self-development
  personal life goals
five-year goals
nursing employment

qualifications and requirements
  credentials
malpractice insurance
support systems
licensure
registration
changing an employment status
humor

BLAZING A PERSONAL CAREER PATH

In addition to managing client care, successful staff nurses manage their careers to assure that they meet their personal goals. Neglecting personal goals contributes to personal frustration, which can diminish the quality of client care management. This epilogue is designed to help entry-level staff nurses gain perspective on their personal needs and begin to make choices and decisions conducive to a fulfilling career.

Many people believe a shortage of nurses persists. Accordingly, new graduates often have opportunities to select one of a variety of potential employers. They are challenged not so much by getting a job, but by identifying the best employer. To make the best choice, new graduates need to determine what employer characteristics and types of health

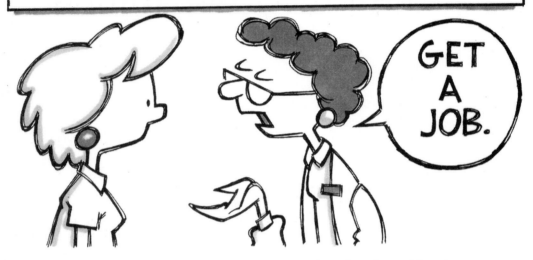

NURSE PREPARATION FOR THE NINETIES: ENTER A PROFESSION

New graduates often have opportunities to select one of a variety of potential employers.

care organizations best match their personal and career interests. By making an effort, entry-level staff nurses can match the desired characteristics of potential employers with their individual needs. Subsequently, new graduates can take the initiative to gain satisfaction from their employment and nursing practice.

The entry-level staff nurse realizes that (1) the employer will invest considerable resources to help the recent graduate succeed as an employee, and (2) in return, the employer expects the new graduate to remain employed long enough to obtain a reasonable return on such an investment. For example, many employers expect new graduates to remain employed for a year or longer to adjust to nursing practice and gain the experience required to develop confidence in their nursing knowledge and skills. Findings of at least one study indicate that new graduates had a higher probability of staying employed for one year than did experienced nurses (Prior et al, 1990, p. 27). To remain with one's first employer for less than a year may invite questions from subsequent employers as to the reasons for such a short term of employment. To avoid mismatches between individual goals and needs and the interests of the employer, each nurse needs to identify personal nursing beliefs and goals, as well as special interests and skills.

REFINING YOUR PERSONAL PHILOSOPHY, INTERESTS, AND TALENTS

With the evolution of an increasing variety of health care settings, recent graduates benefit from clarifying their personal **nursing philosophies** prior to seeking employment.

That is, each nurse needs to identify and clarify her or his **personal values, beliefs,** and assumptions about basic truths. Each nurse needs to know what he or she believes about human nature, societal needs, and what he or she believes nursing has to offer society, particularly as this relates to her or his personal goals, interests, and talents. A balanced appraisal of one's personal nursing philosophy also includes an assessment of what nursing is *not*. This entails considering one's biases, limitations, and vulnerabilities. For example, a nursing philosophy typically includes beliefs about people's basic needs and the extent to which the **characteristics of nursing as a profession** address them. If the nurse's personal belief is that people are inherently good and may be forced to change due to external circumstances, her or his nursing philosophy might include a commitment to altering external factors that interfere with satisfying basic human needs. On the other hand, if the nurse's personal belief is that people are neither inherently good or bad and that a person's features depends on the individual's inner resources and personality, her or his nursing philosophy is less likely to express as much commitment to altering external factors to satisfy basic human needs. Yet another nurse's personal belief might be that whether people are good or bad depends on both internal and external factors that need to be addressed. This person's nursing philosophy would more likely include a commitment to altering both external and internal factors that interfere with satisfying basic human needs. Thus, a nurse's basic beliefs affect her or his nursing philosophy and involvement in interest groups and professional organizations and activities consistent with it. One's personal nursing philosophy also reflects beliefs about each nurse's responsibility for contributing to the profession's knowledge base. Closely related to this responsibility is the moral obligation to **maintain nursing competencies** required to apply current nursing knowledge and skills to provide safe, high-quality client care.

One's nursing philosophy guides one's beliefs about the **need for continued self-development** and growth, which enable the nurse to practice effectively and efficiently. One's nursing philosophy also guides one's selection of an area of practice and settings that match one's values, beliefs, interests, and talents. Often, nursing students are asked to write brief descriptions of their individual nursing philosophies to help clarify beliefs about nursing, related values and assumptions, and **personal life goals.** Successfully completing such an assignment helps the student identify the characteristics of potential employers that match the individual's personal values, goals, and needs. The box on p. 242 lists characteristics of potential employers that staff nurses might consider when trying to identify those that best match their individual nursing philosophies, values, beliefs, nursing interests, and goals.

Critical Thinking

Developing a personal nursing philosophy entails critical thinking. The process of critical thinking requires an open mind and the ability to question basic "facts" (which may prove to be inaccurate), beliefs, and assumptions. The critical thinker accepts ideas, facts, and beliefs only after giving them careful thought, rather than casually accepting them as a matter of convenience. Critical thinking also involves elaborate problem solving, beginning with carefully identifying the problem or central issue, selecting the best available option, acting on it, and evaluating the outcomes.

The process of critical thinking is of great importance in providing and managing client care because the client care manager does more than perform care-giving activities. The effective client care manager constantly evaluates the outcomes of care and, using the processes involved in critical thinking, makes decisions regarding future care planning.

Characteristics of Potential Employers of Staff Nurses

Facility type

Episodic (acute) care/long-term (residential) care
Profit/non-profit
Private/public
Rural/urban community
Community-based/teaching/university

Agency image

Fast-paced/relaxed atmosphere
Organized/unorganized
Businesslike/friendly

Organizational culture

Reward innovation/maintain status quo
Opportunistic/ethical
High-tech/hands-on
Medical model/interdisciplinary health maintenance

Management style

Participatory/autocratic
Well-established/flexible/evolving
Short-term/long-term focus
Task-/People-oriented
Centralized/decentralized

Physical appearance

Meticulous/casually maintained
Old/new physical plant
High/low security
High/low safety concerns

Financial goals

Profit/avoiding loss
Private/publicly financed
Cost controls/creative spending
Survival/expansion plan

IDENTIFYING FIVE-YEAR GOALS

Each nurse has personal and career goals, whether he or she is aware of them or not. For example, Williams (1990, p. 104D) reported that nurses ranked pay, autonomy, professional status, and interaction with other nurses as very important contributors to "job satisfaction." If one clarifies personal and career goals, progress toward meeting them contributes to a sense of success and guides choices that increase the probability of reaching them.

Obviously, beginning staff nurses experience difficulty designing a lifelong career plan before they have experience practicing nursing in the area of their choice. However, each nurse enters the profession at a specific point in her or his life. For example, unmarried nurses who have no dependents and who hope to combine marriage, family, and career often have different personal goals from those who are married, rearing children of varying ages, and involved in various community groups. Personal needs for satisfactory child care, transportation, housing, and related community resources are likely to influence the nurse's selection of potential employers. Personal goals, such as finding a spouse or enabling children to obtain a particular type of education, influence where some nurses choose to live and practice.

To ensure that their personal goals are met, nurses need to assess both the requirements of potential employers and the extent to which the work environment and community characteristics match the nurse's goals, needs, and lifestyle, including recreational and

Matching Employers with Personal Career Goals

1. LOCATION: How do you plan to get to work? What are the anticipated transportation costs? Is the job conveniently close to grocery stores, restaurants, the school you plan to attend? How much security is needed to assure your safety?

2. VARIETY IN WORK ACTIVITIES: Are you looking for employment that will provide opportunity to perform a variety of tasks and develop new skills, or would you prefer to become an expert at a few specific skills? Will completing the work require well-developed organizational skills?

3. STRESS: Do you prefer a fast or slow pace? Do you enjoy change from day to day or a more steady, stable work environment? What are your preferences for shift and type or work schedule? Do you have work schedule requirements due to family or other commitments? How much advance scheduling is done? How many holidays and weekends will you be required to work?

4. AUTONOMY vs. AUTHORITY: Do you prefer to be self-directed or have procedures established in detail? Do you prefer to take the initiative in problem solving, identifying solutions and carrying them out, or prefer to hand over the responsibility for solving problems to others?

5. BENEFITS: How important is the amount of money you make? Would you prefer a full-time position with a predictable income or a part-time position with a fluctuating paycheck?

   Expendable Income: Get an idea of the income you will require, based upon a realistic budget. Allow extra money for expenses that crop up unexpectedly.

   Insurance Benefits: What kind of coverage do you and your family need? In addition to health and life insurance, are malpractice and disability benefits included? Can you participate in retirement and pension plans? How soon?

   Vacation and Sick Pay: What are the eligibility requirements?

   Support of Professional Growth: Will the employer reimburse some or all costs of continuing education or degree programs? Will further education help you climb this employer's career ladder?

6. OPPORTUNITIES FOR CHOICE OF CLINICAL AREA OF PRACTICE: Are clinical interests distinct specialties or are they integrated within the larger nursing practice group? How will the facility support your clinical interest? Are beginning staff nurses permitted direct entry into a specialty area of practice or is experience required?

7. RECOGNITION AND ADVANCEMENT: How does the facility reward individual excellence and dedication? Do you expect a monetary reward? What are the opportunities for advancement? Are you locked into an entry-level position or could you be promoted based on good work? Where do you want to be in five years? Will this employer help you get there? How?

8. HUMAN RELATIONSHIPS: How important to you are positive relationships among staff, management, and clients? How does this organization promote open communication and continuous problem solving? Does the culture encourage employees to make time-limited or lifelong commitments?

family activities. The box on p. 243 lists common employer characteristics that affect personal and career goals.

Individual nursing goals must also be considered. As so aptly stated by Manthey (1990, p. 17), "Once a nurse has become a member of the profession . . . career choices begin to appear almost immediately." Each staff nurse needs to carefully match beliefs about continuing education and personal growth with opportunities for meeting them, with or without the support and financial assistance of an employer. To be sure, personal and professional goals will not be realized unless they are identified, analyzed, and pursued with realistic plans that correspond to the availability of resources. Given the constant, rapid change in nursing and in life experiences, planning for **five-years goals** (rather than an entire lifetime) may be realistic. Such five-year plans might be compared to the building blocks of a personal career path. Formulating an initial five-year plan might be compared to taking the first step of one's career journey.

The beginning staff nurse needs to differentiate the career ladders often delineated by employers and those based on one's own nursing interests and talents. Many nursing career models exist. The Dalton/Thompson (Fig. E-1) model (Myers Schim, 1990, p. 96FF) is a good example. It provides an overview of the common stages of professional development of nurses and describes achievements during each phase and various choices made in pursuit of personal interests and goals. Usually, the employer's career ladder is only one of many available nursing career opportunities. Identification of goals for the next five years of one's career is paramount to determining how to achieve them. Personal growth depends

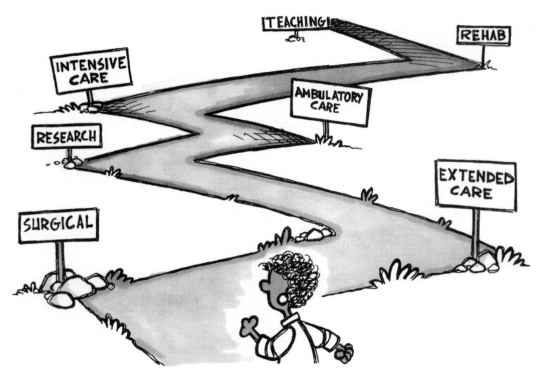

Nursing career path.

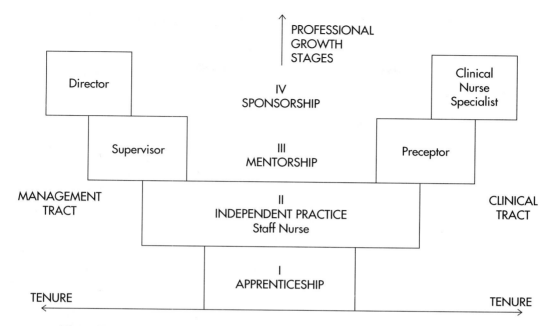

Figure E-1   The Dalton/Thompson Career Model. (From *Nursing Management*, May 1990.)

upon choices among nursing practice opportunities, personal development activities, and involvement in professional organizations that contribute to reaching individual career goals.

SEEKING EMPLOYMENT CORRESPONDING TO IDENTIFIED GOALS

After the beginning staff nurse clarifies her or his personal nursing philosophy and has identified both personal and career goals, she or he can seek **nursing employment** to match them. Prior to contacting a potential employer, the nurse needs to learn about the agency's characteristics. Since nursing students frequently begin seeking employment while completing required courses, they can use services available in the student affairs or placement offices. Such services can be used to help identify specific types of employers and employment opportunities in desired locations. In addition, employment opportunities are often posted on bulletin boards. Information about "career days" and other recruitment events is routinely posted as well. One might inquire about special programs and positions available to new graduates.

Once leads about employers of interest have been identified, the nurse can contact specific facilities and request information to compare potential employers. It is helpful to keep track of the names, addresses, and telephone numbers of those you contact to assist with follow-through on subsequent contacts. Keep copies of letters sent in the event that a potential employer contacts you about one of them.

Depending on the nature of the nursing employment desired, the nurse might compile a rèsumè or marketing letter or complete an application form. (A sample cover letter and rèsumè appear on pp. 246 and 247.) All correspondence *must* be neat and accurate. It needs to project a professional image and demonstrate attention to details.

1234 B Busy Lane
Somewhere, USA 58931
January 6, 1993

Director of Nursing
Grand Care Health Center
874 Quiet Street
Fun Spot, WI 53000

Dear Director of Nursing:

Attached is a copy of my rèsumè. You will note that I have begun to gain experience working with people and have completed requirements for my B.S. degree with a major in nursing. I am interested in obtaining a beginning staff nurse position on a general medical surgical unit at Grand Care Health Center because of the information I received about it from the Placement Office at Up-to-Date University.

I am very interested in gaining nursing experience in an innovative organization that enables nurses to provide high-quality care and grow professionally. I strongly believe that I could become a contributing member of your nursing staff.

Please contact me by telephone before 2:00 P.M. weekdays to schedule an interview. I look forward to hearing from you.

Sincerely,

Alyce R Nurse

Alyce R. Nurse, RN

Organize information about your credentials and related experiences to match the employer's *qualifications* and *requirements* for the desired position. Usually your **credentials** include a brief description of your educational background and previous employment, emphasizing pertinent accomplishments that contribute to the qualifications desired by the potential employer. Accurately communicate achievements and accomplishments that illustrate your qualifications for the desired position. Pertinent personal information on such topics as hobbies, special interests, awards, and organizational activities can also be included. Make sure to include your name, address, and telephone number.

It is as important that one's appearance communicate a positive professional image during employment interviews as it is while on duty. Prior to the interview, you need to learn about the agency and plan to ask at least two or three questions to help you determine whether to accept an employment offer. It is a good idea to follow up an interview with a brief letter thanking the agency staff for giving you an additional opportunity to express your interest in the position. If you make tentative plans to accept employment but later are

Alyce R. Nurse
1234B Busy Lane
Somewhere, USA 58931
(555) 987-6543

Position Objective:

To obtain an entry-level staff nurse position that would provide opportunities to gain experience and further develop my nursing interests, talents, and skills in general medical-surgical nursing.

Educational Background:

Graduated with honors from Middleton High School, in Elsewhere, Mass., in May 1987.

Received an associate degree in nursing, graduating cum laude, from Elsewhere Community College in Blue Skies, Mass., in December 1989.

Received a B.S. with a major in nursing from Up-to-Date University's College of Nursing located in Rolling Meadows, Wis., in January 1993.

While enrolled in nursing courses at Up-to-Date University's College of Nursing, I attended continuing education programs sponsored by the American Heart Association, American Cancer Society, and the University. Topics included "Managing a Heart-Healthy Lifestyle," "Detecting and Treating Breast Cancer," and "Using Nursing Diagnoses to Steer Nursing Practice."

Work Experience:

Employed part-time as a registered nurse at the Golden Gate Residential Center, in Rolling Meadows, Wis., since February 1990. I am typically assigned as a team leader, working with 1-2 LPNs and 3-4 NAs to provide care for 42 residents during the afternoon shift.

Employed part-time as waitress at Sizzling Pizza House in Blue Skies, Mass., from September 1988 until December 1989. I waited on customers from 5-10 P.M. 5-6 days per week.

Employed part-time as counter help at MacConald's Quick Burgers in Blue Skies, Mass., from September 1985 to May 1987. I took customer orders at the counter from 4:30 to 8:30 4-5 days each week.

Was a volunteer Candy Striper to deliver newspapers during the evenings at Blue Skies Memorial Hospital from September 1984 to August 1985.

Professional Organizations:

Currently, I am an active member of the National Association of Nursing Students. I served on the local chapter's Membership Committee from September 1991 until December 1992.

Served as student representative of my college class to the Student Government Association from September 1988 to September 1989.

References:

Available upon request.

unable to do so, common courtesy requires that you inform the agency of your changed plans at the earliest possible date. Such efforts typically distinguish applicants by showing consideration for the employer's needs. They also reflect professional integrity.

DETERMINING THE NEED FOR MALPRACTICE INSURANCE

Significant personal and financial risks are inherent in nursing as a career. Purchasing **malpractice insurance** is one strategy for managing these risks. Responding to legal accusations entails psychological and emotional costs as well as financial ones. Accordingly, strategies for preventing malpractice claims should be incorporated in every nurse's practice (Bernzweig, 1990, pp. 317–355; Luquire, 1988, pp. 61–62; Maher, 1989, pp. 34–41). Principle among these strategies are communicating effectively with clients and taking an active role in reducing their dissatisfaction as consumers. However, such efforts will not completely eliminate the potential for legal actions against you.

As discussed in Chapter Twelve, liability refers to legal accountability for client risks, danger, and injury caused by the nurse's negligent acts. Negligence entails actions or nonactions that the nurse could or should have taken to prevent harm or injury to the client. Malpractice involves nursing actions that are inconsistent with established standards and that are believed by peers to be unsafe or to place the recipient of such care at risk.

Every nurse decides whether to purchase and maintain personal malpractice insurance protection against the financial costs of legal accusations associated with nursing practice. The actual need for malpractice insurance is based on several factors. They include one's understanding of legal accountability or responsibility for one's actions and nonactions and perceptions of the associated risks to personal potential or actual assets. William O. Morris (Sandroff, 1983, p. 29) warns "With the current legal climate, it's downright foolish to practice in any profession today without professional malpractice insurance." Some nurses decide that the malpractice insurance protection provided by their employers is sufficient. Such insurance has limits. It might not cover financial costs of legal defense for actions taken outside of a job description; cover circumstances where the employer decides not to defend you; or cover actions taken that were presumed to be protected by "good samaritan acts" (state laws providing protection from liability associated with helping accident victims). Every nurse needs to know the actual protection afforded nurses providing emergency care as "good samaritans" in the state in which he or she practices (Northrop, 1990, pp. 50–51). In addition, consideration needs to be given to the liabilities involved in nursing activities performed as a volunteer.

Jane Greenlaw, a nurse and lawyer, offers a rational approach to using one's resources wisely: "I, myself, would not practice nursing without my own coverage" (Sandroff, 1983, p. 29). Several trends make such a decision appropriate. They include (1) the increasing public perception of nurses as professionals, who are therefore accountable for their own actions instead of being protected by their employers (Godkin, Wooten, and Godkin, 1987, p. 74); (2) the increasing complexity of skills nurses use when practicing in expanded roles (Bailey-Allen, 1990, p. 14); (3) patterns of documentation are changing to reflect actual care provided and client responses to treatment (Bailey-Allen, 1990, p. 15).

It is important to remember that purchasing malpractice insurance is only one way to manage the financial costs of legal disputes. It will not eliminate the need to practice nursing in accordance with established standards to prevent clients and their families, as well as employers or physicians, from making legal accusations. Employers or physicians may make legal accusations against nurses in an attempt to recover financial losses arising out of the process of settling legal disputes. Responding to a legal complaint made by others involved in the client's care typically requires considerable legal counsel and costs.

■■■■ USING AVAILABLE SUPPORT SYSTEMS TO HELP YOU GROW

Beginning staff nurses use many different strategies to grow professionally. To increase the likelihood of success, they need to use the **support systems** available at the agency and in their personal social circles. As mentioned in Chapter Fourteen, nurses participate in various structured learning programs while enrolled in nursing courses and in continuing education programs. In addition, they often actively seek learning opportunities to ensure that their nursing knowledge and skills remain current.

Frequently, nursing students participate in preceptorships during advanced nursing courses. Such one-to-one relationships with a more experienced nurse help the student practice nursing skills acquired in previous courses (Goldenberg, 1987/88, p. 11). Under close supervision, the student gains practical nursing experience. Preceptors provide regular feedback to guide learning. However, such experiences are usually limited by the time allotted for the course.

In addition to typical in-service orientation programs and financial support to participate in continuing education programs, many employers develop strategies that encourage nurse retention. These strategies are designed to help nurses develop their professional potential. Based on individual career goals, nurses are expected to use this agency support to the advantage of the individual and the benefit of the agency. For example, staff nurses typically share information gained during continuing education programs with other interested agency staff as a stipulation for receiving financial support. Another strategy used by an increasing number of nursing employers is a dynamic mentorship program. Mentorships are structured nurturing programs involving one-to-one relationships between inexperienced and experienced nurses. Preceptorships are typically part of a formal instructional program, whereas structured mentorships are frequently offered as part of an employer's in-service program.

Agencies that offer a structured mentorship program will be eager to inform nurses of its availability as a recruitment strategy. Employers have learned that mentorship enhances career development and retention of competent nurses (Caracuzzo and Kinsey, 1990, p. 45). Typically, the agency consumes resources to prepare mentors and implement mentorship programs to nurture beginning staff nurses during their initial employment and in-service programs. Such programs are designed to build supportive and meaningful relationships between new and more experienced nurses. By being a mentor, staff nurses gain satisfaction from teaching and feeling valued by peers (Law et al, 1989, p. 65). Mentors are generally viewed as respected role models who provide feedback to novices. Though mentorships are not for everybody, many nurses who worked with a mentor readily recalled positive learning experiences. Caracuzzo and Kinsey (1990, p. 45) reported, "protégés often report feeling replenished, refueled and inspired to make a significant contribution to their field or discipline." Accordingly, mentorships are gaining popularity among those nurses who strive to influence their profession.

Depending upon the nature of the community and its relationship with the health care agency, many other resources may be available. These resources often involve opportunities to work with groups of people with interests similar to those of nurses. Common interest groups include local chapters of the American Heart Association, American Cancer

Society, and groups involved in caring for disaster victims, controlling communicable diseases, or assisting the homeless. Nurses frequently are invited to participate in efforts to solve the many complex problems affecting the health of a neighborhood or community. They are asked to share their knowledge of desired health practices and teach techniques for adopting them. Ultimately, such experiences help the nurse to further develop personal talents, self-confidence, knowledge, and skills.

ESTABLISHING LICENSURE AND MAINTAINING REGISTRATION

While completing the curriculum requirements for graduation from a nursing program, nursing students receive assistance in compiling the credentials needed to obtain **licensure** as registered nurses. Each applicant accepts responsibility for becoming licensed and maintaining **registration** when practicing nursing for compensation. State nurse practice acts, while broadly defining the legal scope of practice, also establish requirements for obtaining and maintaining a nursing license. Though these requirements vary from state to state, the agency authorized to regulate nursing practice also carries out the activities involved in licensing nurses. These activities include implementing plans for administering licensure examinations by screening applicants and carrying out the testing program; compiling educational records; and maintaining records of candidates who satisfactorily complete the licensure examination.

When nurses wish to practice in another state, they need to contact the agency regulating nursing practice in that state. Such agencies provide information about the requirements and process involved in becoming licensed as well as maintaining registration as an RN in that state.

Employers verify the licensure and registration status of nurses upon initial employment and at regular intervals thereafter. If any questions arise about the veracity of a nurse's license and registration status, they can usually be readily answered by the state agency regulating nursing practice.

NOTIFYING EMPLOYERS ABOUT CHANGING OR TERMINATING EMPLOYMENT

Most new graduates focus attention on various strategies that might be used to seek employment. However, to establish a reputable work record, they also need to know how to notify an employer of a desire to change positions or terminate employment. Whenever feasible, the employee is asked to adhere to the agency's established personnel policy when **changing an employment status.**

The box at right lists several guidelines for writing a letter regarding changing positions or terminating a relationship with an employer. The letter needs to be addressed to the person responsible for managing such personnel changes within the agency. One must also notify one's immediate supervisor. Giving sufficient advance notice allows time for the employer to change work schedules and plan for adequate staffing. If appropriate, the notification letter should include reasons the employee is requesting the change. These reasons should be given in such a way that they reflect positively upon the employee. Reasons might include career advancement, evolving family needs, or relocation.

When composing the letter, the nurse needs to be mindful that it may be used by the employer to provide future reference information. The letter is likely to become part of the individual's personnel file with the employer. The content of the letter should clearly state

Guidelines for Changing Positions or Terminating Employment

1. Adhere to the employer's agency personnel policy when specifying the date the resignation or change is effective.
2. State your reasons, if appropriate.
3. When composing the body of the letter, remember that the letter is likely to become part of your personnel file with this employer and may be used to provide reference information.
4. State the name of the position you are leaving.
5. Project a positive image and desired qualities of clarity and neatness, both in person and on paper.
6. Use quality paper for the written notification.

the position that the nurse is leaving. When possible, the nurse should include a brief, accurate, positive statement about the employment relationship.

It is important for the nurse to project a positive image as a valued employee who consistently demonstrates desired qualities of neatness and attention to detail. Such attention includes accurate spelling and proper grammar and punctuation. It is also important that

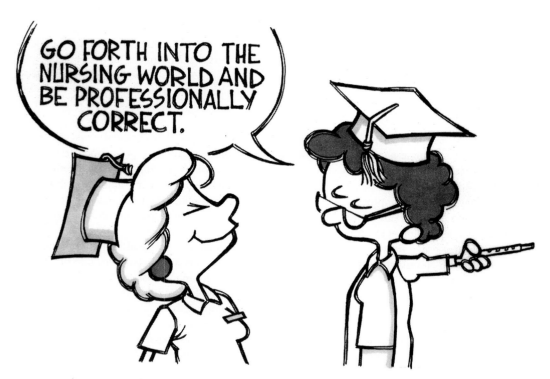

It is important for the nurse to project a positive image.

the letter be written on quality paper—not on notebook paper or dinner napkins! The letter's overall appearance reflects the character of the employee.

Perhaps the real issue in notifying an employer of a desire to change or terminate a relationship rests with the employee's attitude toward managing her or his career. Obtaining and maintaining the credentials required to practice nursing as an RN involves a large investment of time, effort, and money. Careful attention to preserving and increasing the value of this investment reflects an appreciation of sound career managment principles.

USING HUMOR AS AN INTEGRAL NURSING MANAGEMENT STRATEGY

Client care management is often very stressful. Though its importance is frequently unrecognized, **humor** can be used as a deliberate strategy to elicit favorable responses from others in the work environment. As Lee (1990, p. 86) so aptly stated, "The positive physiological and psychological benefits of laughter cannot be overestimated." She emphasized that humor as a management tool needs to positive instead of negative. Positive humor stimulates laughter as a favorable response from an individual or group. Negative humor deliberately attempts to elicit a destructive reaction from an individual or group, leading the individuals involved to engage in "put-downs" or self-deprecation. Insensitive, inappropriate joking can diminish effective working relationships. Positive humor promotes effective working relationships.

The aim of humor is to increase laughter, get in touch with one's feelings, and increase the acceptance of others. When positive humor is used, staff morale increases, as does the work group's cohesiveness. Clearly, since positive humor reflects a healthy attitude it can be nurtured and rewarded. It is not used so much to reduce stress as to maintain vitality. There is truth to the belief common among direct nursing staff that if you don't laugh, you don't survive! Accordingly, it behooves every nurse, beginning and experienced, to "nurse" an enjoyable sense of humor.

SUMMARY

Successful staff nurses manage their careers to ensure that personal goals are met. To do so, each nurse needs to clarify her or his personal and nursing philosophy. Each beginning staff nurse is encouraged to identify five-year plans as steps toward meeting career goals. Completing these requirements helps to establish a career foundation and prepare the nurse to seek employment. Successful staff nurses match their goals with the characteristics of potential employers. In addition, they organize and communicate their credentials in such a manner as to reflect a positive image.

Each nurse decides whether to purchase and maintain personal malpractice insurance protection against the financial costs of legal accusations associated with nursing practice. This is only one of several methods of managing the financial costs of legal disputes.

Effective staff nurses use support systems available through their employing agencies and social circles to help them grow. One common method is participation in dynamic mentoring programs. In addition, they accept responsibility for obtaining licensure and maintaining registration while practicing nursing. This responsibility continues throughout the nurse's career. Employers verify that every employed nurse is licensed and registered.

Humor is a skill worth nurturing; it helps to increase staff morale and develop coping skills used to manage the diverse stresses inherent in a nursing career. One's nursing liveli-hood depends on it!

■ APPLICATION EXERCISES

a. Write a description of your nursing philosophy. Compare it with the beliefs and goals you aspired to when you applied for admission to a nursing program.

b. Daydream about your career. List your five-year goals. Rank their importance to you.

c. Write a résumé for a position as a staff nurse in a long-term care agency. Include your nursing career goals, qualifications, credentials, and personal interests. Match them with the characteristics of your assigned agency as a potential employer.

d. Debate the pros and cons of malpractice insurance. Identify other methods of man-aging the risks inherent in practicing nursing.

e. Laugh a lot!

REFERENCES

Bailey-Allen AM: Changing liability of the nurse over the past decade, *Orthop Nurs* 9(2):13–15. (1990).

Bernzweig EP: Part seven: principles of mal-practice claims prevention, in *The nurse's liability for malpractice: a programmed course,* ed 5, St. Louis, 1990, C.V. Mosby, pp. 317–355.

Caracuzzo Kinsey D: Mentorship and influ-ence in nursing, *Nurs Manage* 21(5):45–46. (May, 1990).

Godkin L, Wooten B, Godkin J: The jury de-cides: are registered nurses legally liable for their job-related actions? *Nurs Manage* 18(5):73–74, 76, 79. (May, 1987).

Goldenberg D: PRECEPTORSHIP: a one-to-one relationship with a triple "p" rating (preceptor, preceptee, patient), *Nurs Forum* 23(1):10–15. (1987/88).

Law MS, Smith MO, Igoe SN, Caplin MS: Nurses helping nurses, *Imprint* 36(2):65, 67–68, 71–72. (April/May, 1989).

Lee BS: "Humor relations" for nurse man-agers, *Nurs Manage* 21(5):86, 88, 90, 92. (May, 1990).

Luquire R: 6 common causes of nursing lia-bility, *Nurs* 88 (11):61–62. (November, 1988).

Maher VF: Your legal guide to safe nursing practice, *Nurs* 89(11):34–42. (November, 1989).

Manthey M: 1990 nursing: a profession of choice, *Nurs Manage* 21(9):17–18. (September, 1990).

Myers Schim S: Nursing career management: the Dalton/Thompson model, *Nurs Manage* 21(5):96BB–96DD. (May, 1990).

Northrop CE: How good samaritan laws do and don't protect you, *Nurs* 90(2):50–51. (February, 1990).

Prior MM, Cottingham EM, Kolski BJ, Shogan JO: Nurse turnover as a function of employment, experience and unit, *Nurs Manage* 21(7):27–28. (July, 1990).

Sandroff R: Why you really ought to have your *own* malpractice policy, *RN* 46(3):29–33. (June, 1983).

Williams C: Job satisfaction: comparing cc and med/surg nurses, *Nurs Manage* 21(7):104A–104H. (July, 1990).

INDEX